Complex Knee Ligament Injuries

Fabrizio Margheritini
João Espregueira-Mendes
Alberto Gobbi
Editors

Complex Knee Ligament Injuries

From Diagnosis to Management

INTERNATIONAL SOCIETY OF ARTHROSCOPY, KNEE SURGERY & ORTHOPAEDIC SPORTS MEDICINE · 1995 ·

Springer

Editors
Fabrizio Margheritini
Orthopaedics and Traumatology
University of Rome "Foro Italico"
Rome
Italy

João Espregueira-Mendes
Clínica do Dragão
Espregueira-Mendes Sports Centre - FIFA
Medical Centre of Excellence
Porto
Portugal

Alberto Gobbi
O.A.S.I. Bioresearch Foundation NPO
Milan
Italy

ISBN 978-3-662-58244-2 ISBN 978-3-662-58245-9 (eBook)
https://doi.org/10.1007/978-3-662-58245-9

This Springer imprint is published by the registered company Springer-Verlag GmbH, DE part of Springer Nature
The registered company address is: Heidelberger Platz 3, 14197 Berlin, Germany

Acknowledgments

We are very proud to introduce this new book on the management of complex knee injuries, which still represent a clinical challenge for the orthopaedic surgeon. Complex knee injuries are not frequent but have a high socioeconomic impact and often imply knee residual functional deficits. The impact is especially high in professional athletes has it may imply an early end of the sportive career. Thus, managing correctly these injuries is crucial to decrease the risk of these residual deficits and prevent the early development of knee osteoarthritis. Thus, to correctly treat these complex knee injuries—which should follow treatment algorithms and be individualized to the patients and injury characteristics—the orthopaedic surgeon must understand the correct knee normal anatomy and pathomechanics, know the available diagnosis options, identify associated injuries and accurately measure any deficits to perform an informed decision of which is the most suitable treatment. Many recent innovations have emerged for the treatment of knee injuries that will equip the orthopaedic surgeon with a different and effective arsenal of management options to provide the patients with the best possible treatment.

Finally, we want to thank all who have contributed in this great team work: the contributors first, who made this book so powerful by sharing their skills and knowledges; the Springer staff, who helped us in preparing the book in the best way possible; and Dr. Gaetano Lo Bue, MD, who was behind the work of the editors in a restless way, and a special thanks to ISAKOS who made possible to bring this project to life.

We hope that the readers will enjoy the content of this book, as we did while preparing.

Rome, Italy — Fabrizio Margheritini
Porto, Portugal — João Espregueira-Mendes
Milan, Italy — Alberto Gobbi

Contents

Part I

Management

Knee Dislocations: Classification and Treatment Algorithm

1

Dinshaw N. Pardiwala, Sanjay Soni, and Alhad Raut

1.1 Introduction

Knee dislocations are defined as clinical or radiological loss of tibiofemoral congruity. Since many knee dislocations reduce spontaneously and are associated with multiple ligament tears, multi-ligament injuries are now synonymous with knee dislocations. Although knee dislocations account for less than 0.02% of all orthopedic injuries in the general population [1] and less than 0.5% of all joint dislocations [2], these are complex injuries associated with serious short-term complications like neurovascular injuries and long-term consequences such as persistent residual instability and degenerative joint disease. Over the years the treatment of knee dislocations has evolved from nonoperative treatment to surgical repair and reconstruction, which has now been shown to yield better results. The heterogeneity, relatively rarity, and serious nature of these injuries have prevented consensus of treatment. Controversies still exist on the timing of surgery, need for ligament repair, augmentation, or reconstruction, single-stage or two-stage surgery, use of autografts or allografts for reconstruction, and postoperative rehabilitation protocols. Over the past ten years, our service has treated and prospectively analyzed 93 knee dislocations, and this experience forms the basis for the treatment algorithm proposed in this chapter.

D. N. Pardiwala (✉) · S. Soni · A. Raut
Centre for Sports Medicine, Kokilaben Dhirubhai Ambani Hospital, Mumbai, India

1.2 Classification

Knee dislocations can be classified based on either the direction of tibial displacement relative to the femur (Kennedy position classification system) or the ligaments disrupted in the process (Schenk anatomic classification system).

The Kennedy system classifies knee dislocations into anterior, posterior, lateral, medial, and rotatory [3] (Table 1.1). Rotatory dislocations were later subclassified into anteromedial, anterolateral, posteromedial, and posterolateral. Although this classification system is well established, is useful in determining the reduction maneuver needed, and correlates to potential associated injuries, it has limitations. Often knee dislocations are spontaneously reduced prior to medical evaluation and, hence, unclassifiable by the position system. Secondly, this system only suggests likely ligamentous involvement, and the many possible combinations of cruciate and collateral ligament disruptions are not defined.

Hence, Schenck classified knee dislocations in terms of ligaments involved (Table 1.2), and this is best done during the time of presentation or during examination under anesthesia [4]. This anatomic classification system describes the ligaments torn and is useful in deciding treatment. The higher the number, the more severe the injury. Thus a classification of KD3LCN denotes a bicruciate injury with torn LCL and posterolateral corner, and an injury of the popliteal artery, and neural injury (most commonly, peroneal

F. Margheritini et al. (eds.), *Complex Knee Ligament Injuries*,
https://doi.org/10.1007/978-3-662-58245-9_1

Table 1.1 Kennedy "position" classification system for knee dislocations

Anterior	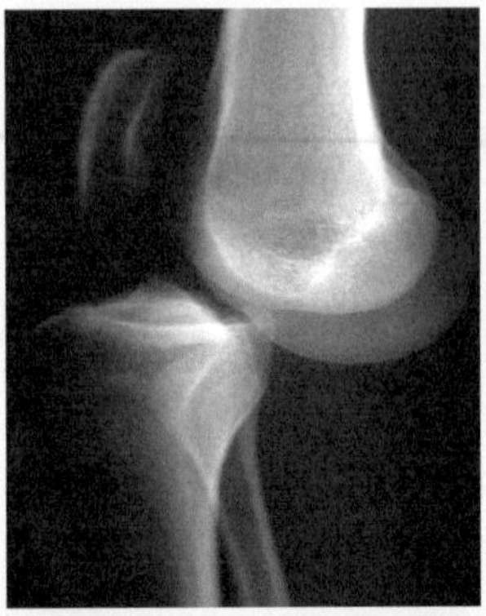	• Most frequent, 40% • Mechanism: hyper extension • No medial or lateral ligament damage • Sometimes intact PCL • Vascular damage common
Posterior	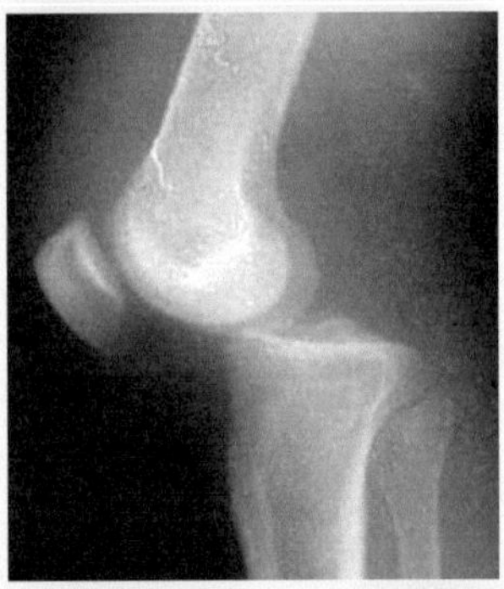	• Common type, 30% • Mechanism: direct posterior drawer • Sometimes ACL intact • Vascular damage at times
Medial/lateral	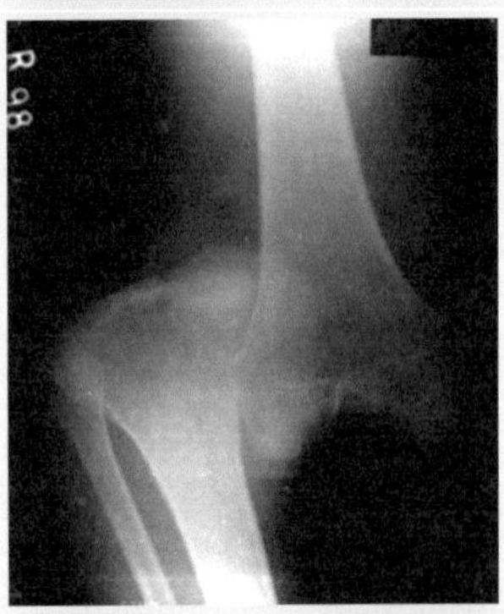	• Rare occurrence if pure • Most of the time posteromedial or posterolateral • ACL + PCL always torn • Vascular damage if posterior • Nerve damage common
Rotatory	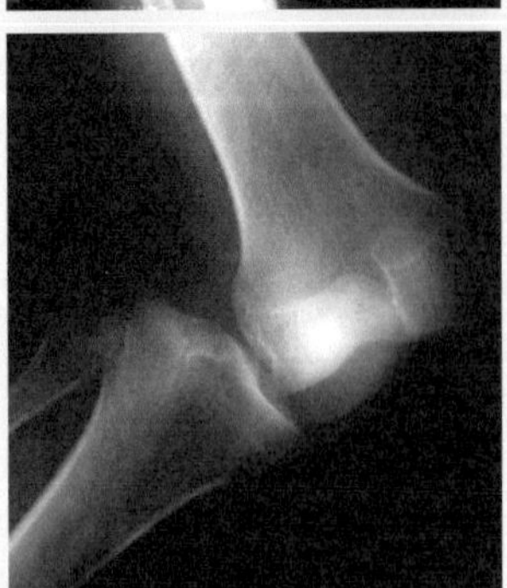	• Rare occurrence • Associated with high-velocity trauma • Complex associated lesions • May be irreducible due to soft tissue interposition

Table 1.2 Schenck anatomic classification system for knee dislocations

Type	Description
KD1	Knee dislocation with either cruciate intact
KD2	Bicruciate injury with collaterals intact
KD3	Bicruciate injury with one collateral ligament injury
	• KD3M—Bicruciate injury with medial-sided ligament injury
	• KD3L—Bicruciate injury with posterolateral ligament injury
KD4	Bicruciate injury with both collateral ligament injury
KD5	Periarticular fracture dislocation

Associated injuries: *C* arterial injury, *N* neural injury

nerve). This classification system allows for accurate discussion of injuries and allows for comparison of like injuries in the wide spectrum of knee dislocations. This classification, however, does not include extensor apparatus injuries that are sometimes seen with knee dislocations.

1.3 Treatment Algorithm and Its Rationale

1.3.1 Acute Knee Dislocations

Patients may present with a dislocated knee (Fig. 1.1a) or a spontaneously reduced knee following a dislocation. All severe knee injuries sustained in motor vehicular accidents, contact sports, combat sports, and high-speed sports such as gymnastics and skating should be viewed with suspicion as these may be spontaneously reduced knee dislocations and can be associated with neurovascular complications. Any high-energy injury or polytrauma should be first managed with standard advanced trauma life support protocols to rule out and manage other injuries like brain concussion and head injury. Grossly deformed limbs should be gently repositioned. Often this itself reduces the joint. No attempt at formal reduction of the joint at the accident site or on the sports field should be attempted prior to confirming the radiographic status of the knee unless the deformity is severely compromising the skin and soft tissues. Limb perfusion and neurological status of the knee should be evaluated.

In the acute setting, after limb perfusion is confirmed, an immediate radiograph should be performed (Fig. 1.1b) to understand the type of dislocation and whether there is any associated fracture. The dislocation should then be reduced under anesthesia on an emergency basis. Usually, traction followed by gentle extension is all that is required to achieve reduction; however, this would be dictated by the type and direction of dislocation. Following reduction, a detailed examination under anesthesia of knee ligament stability should be performed. The Lachman's test (ACL), posterior sag and posterior drawer test (PCL), valgus stress test (MCL), varus stress test (LCL), and dial test (PLC) usually suffice in the acute testing. The other tests, which involve a greater degree of manipulation of the knee, are not warranted. If the knee is not grossly unstable and there is no indication for emergency intervention, the knee is immobilized in full extension a long knee brace. If the knee is extremely unstable or dislocates after reduction, then temporary external fixation may be required. At times, the knee may require immobilization in 20° of flexion to avoid posterior subluxation of the tibia due to an incompetent posterior capsule [5].

After reduction in the emergency room, it is advisable to get anteroposterior and lateral radiographs to confirm joint reduction, identify avulsion fractures around the knee, and assess the need for associated fracture surgery. In the presence of fractures, further evaluation with a CT scan may be useful. An MRI is mandatory in knee dislocations to determine the extent of soft tissue injury and characterize the injury to the ligaments and muscles-tendons [6]. This significantly aids in surgical planning and should be done early in the treatment process. Stress radiography may be considered in select cases to document the extent of ligamentous laxity. Regular monitoring of the distal pulsations and ABI (ankle brachial index) (measured as ankle

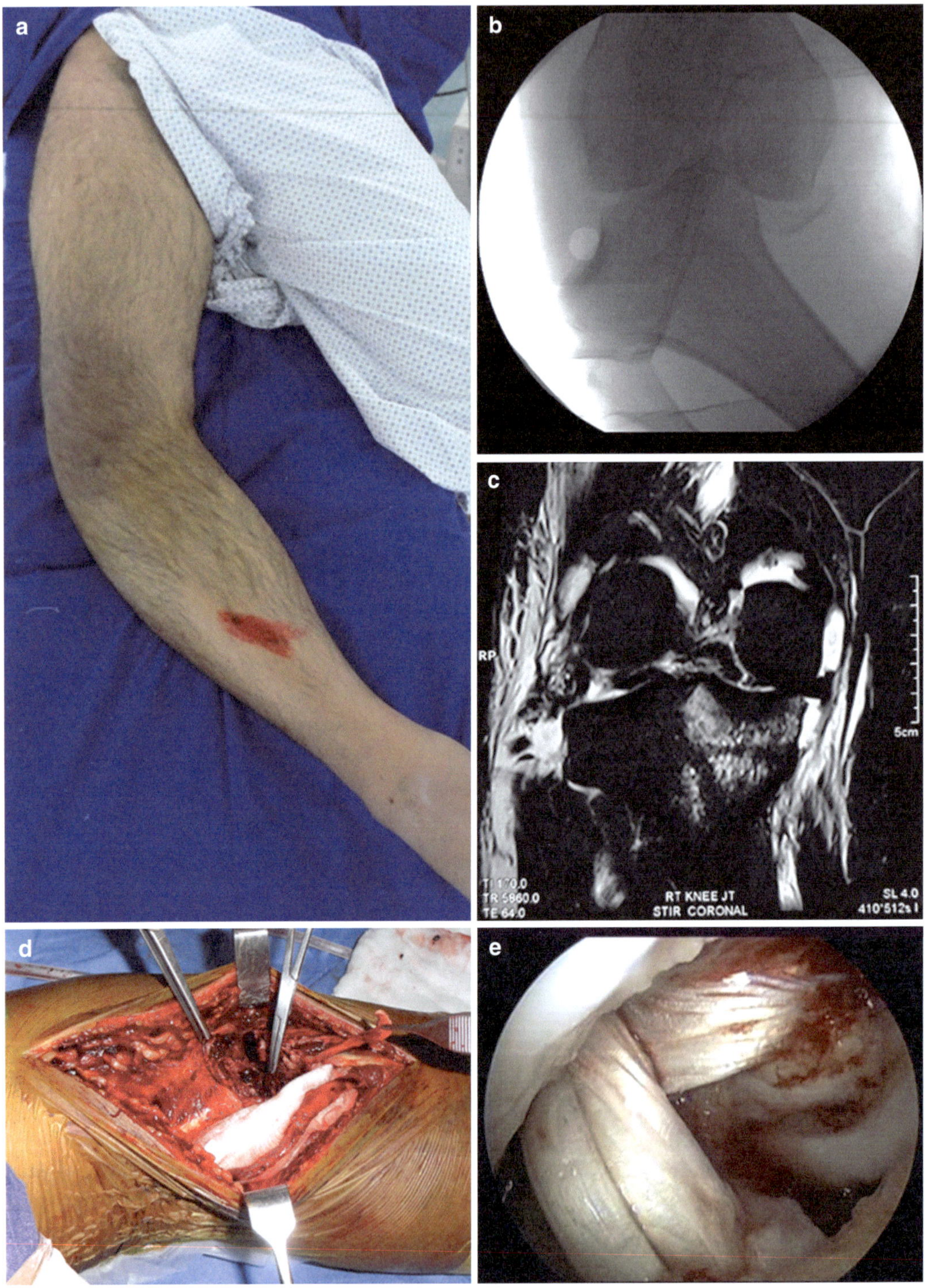

Fig. 1.1 Acute knee dislocation following a motorcycle accident. KD3LN-type injury. (**a**) Clinical presentation; (**b**) immediate radiograph prior to closed reduction under anesthesia; (**c**) MRI defines tears of the PLC, ACL, and PCL with an intact MCL; (**d**) the patient underwent a two-stage surgical procedure—stage 1 included early open PLC repair with peroneal nerve neurolysis followed by stage 2 arthroscopic bicruciate reconstruction (**e**)

Table 1.3 The surgical algorithm for knee dislocations that present in the acute phase. Although specific indications warrant emergency surgical treatment, most patients require elective single-stage or staged ligament surgery

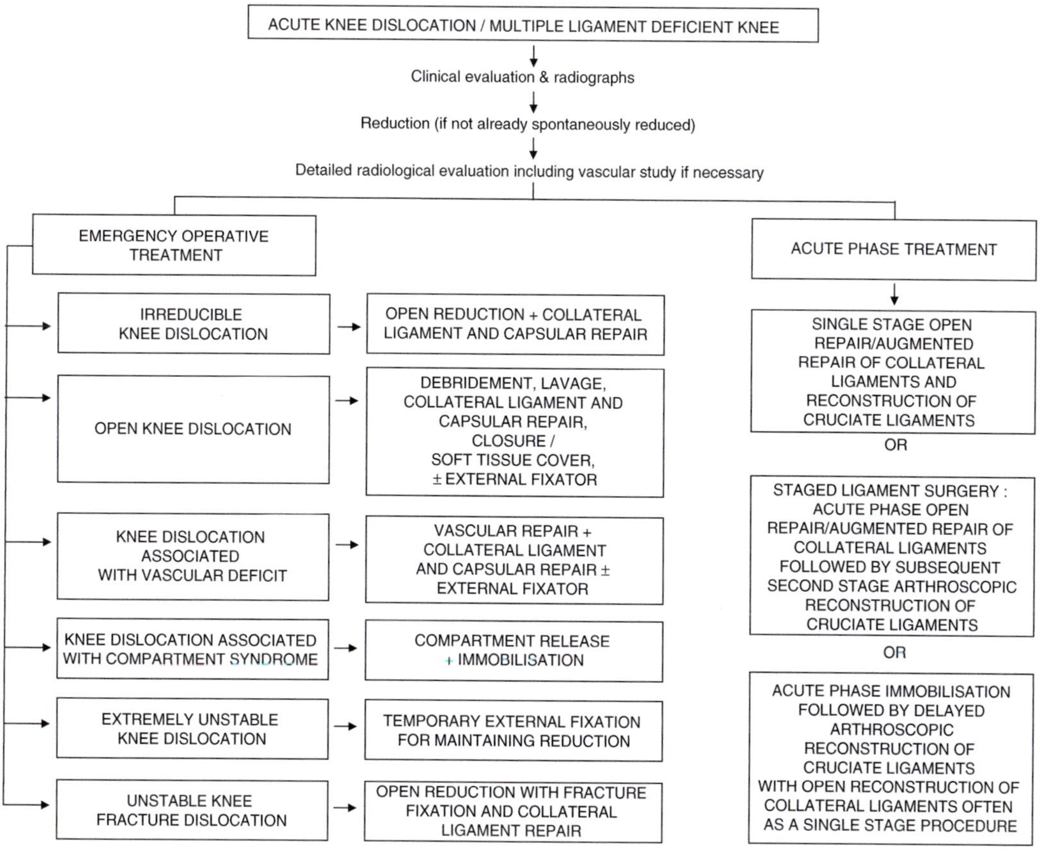

systolic blood pressure/arm systolic blood pressure) should be done in acute setting for at least 72 h. Any fall of the ABI below 0.9 is an indication for angiography. Many centers advocate routine vascular studies for any multiple ligament injured knee. The treatment algorithm for knee dislocations that present in the acute phase is elaborated in Table 1.3.

1.3.1.1 Emergency Surgical Intervention in the Acute Dislocated Knee

The indications for emergency surgical intervention in the acute phase [7] are as follows.

1. Irreducible knee dislocation—Soft tissue or bony incarceration is the usual cause for irreducibility following a knee dislocation. A posterolateral knee dislocation with MCL invagination causing medial femoral condyle buttonholing is well described (Fig. 1.2). There is a skin dimple on the anteromedial aspect at the level of the joint. This becomes prominent when the knee is extended as the MCL is sucked into the joint. We have also encountered popliteus muscle interposition causing irreducibility in a patient with a KD3LN type of injury (Fig. 1.3) and a displaced tibial eminence fracture causing irreducibility in a KD5 type of injury. All irreducible knee dislocations warrant urgent open reduction. Extra-articular repair of torn collaterals and the extensor apparatus should be completed at this first stage. Bony avulsion repair of cruciates may be performed at this stage; however, we do not recommend ACL/PCL reconstruction in the emergency setting.

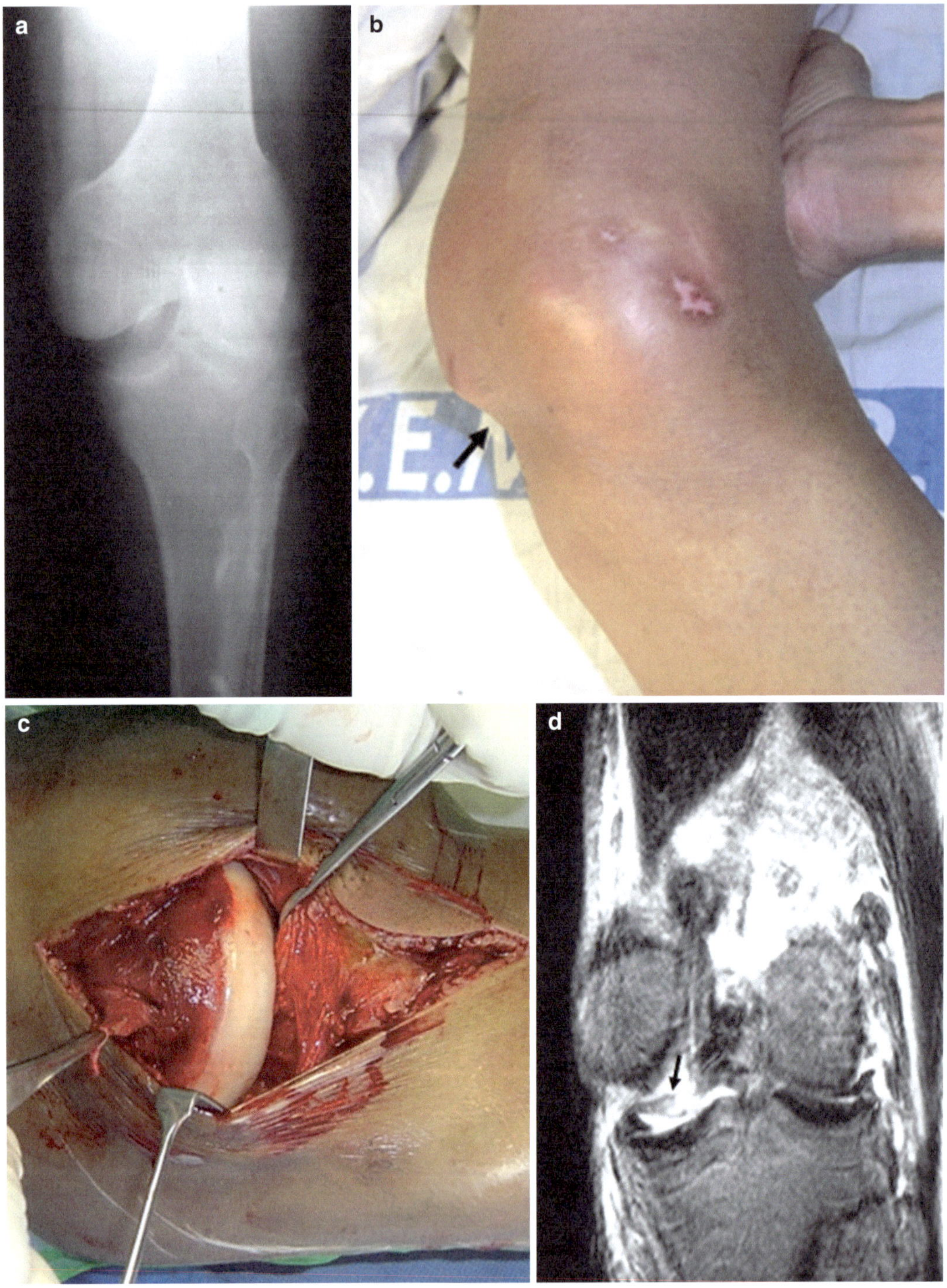

Fig. 1.2 Irreducible posterolateral knee dislocation (**a**) with classical transverse furrow (**b**). It is a complex joint dislocation in which the medial femoral condyle buttonholes through the medial capsule (**c**) and the MCL invaginate into the knee joint (**d**), preventing closed reduction

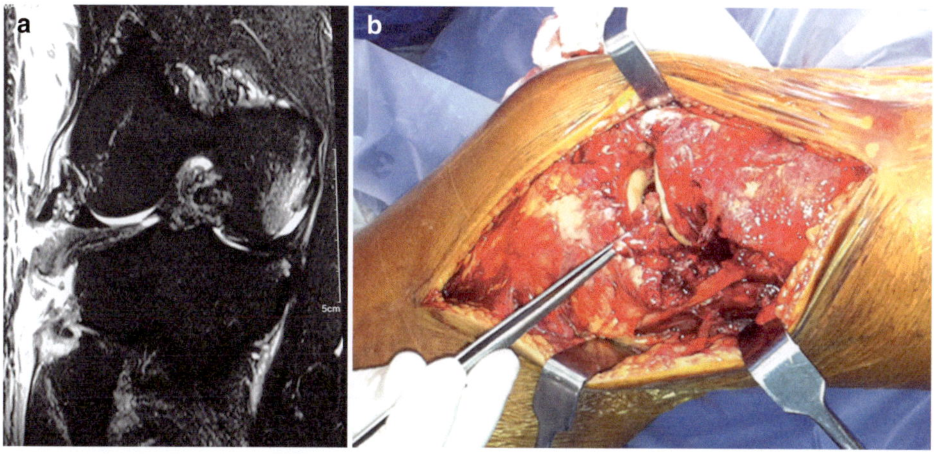

Fig. 1.3 Irreducible KD3LN knee dislocation with popliteus interposition preventing closed reduction. (**a**) MRI reveals injury to the posterolateral ligament complex with submeniscal popliteus interposition within the lateral tibiofemoral joint (**b**) intraoperative image—extensive PLC tear with the popliteus invaginated into the knee joint

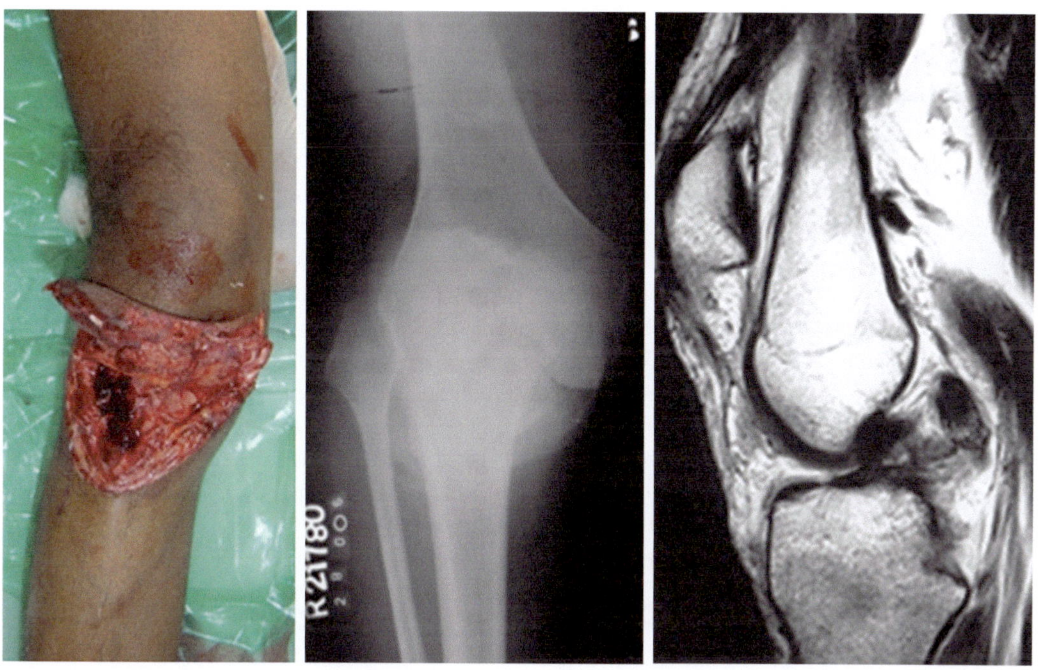

Fig. 1.4 Open anterior knee dislocation (KD4) following a jump from height. This young male underwent emergency reduction, lavage with debridement, patellar tendon repair, skin closure under drains, external fixator immobilization, and antibiotic cover in the first stage. He underwent second-stage multiple ligament reconstruction once his wounds had healed and knee range was normal

2. Open knee dislocations (Fig. 1.4)—These warrant emergency lavage, closure or soft tissue cover under drains, and immobilization, with antibiotic cover similar to open fractures. Extra-articular repair may be attempted if the wound is clean after debridement. If an external fixator is applied, then a margin of 10 cm above and below the joint line is to be kept so as not to interfere with future tunnel placement for ligaments [8]. The external fixator is

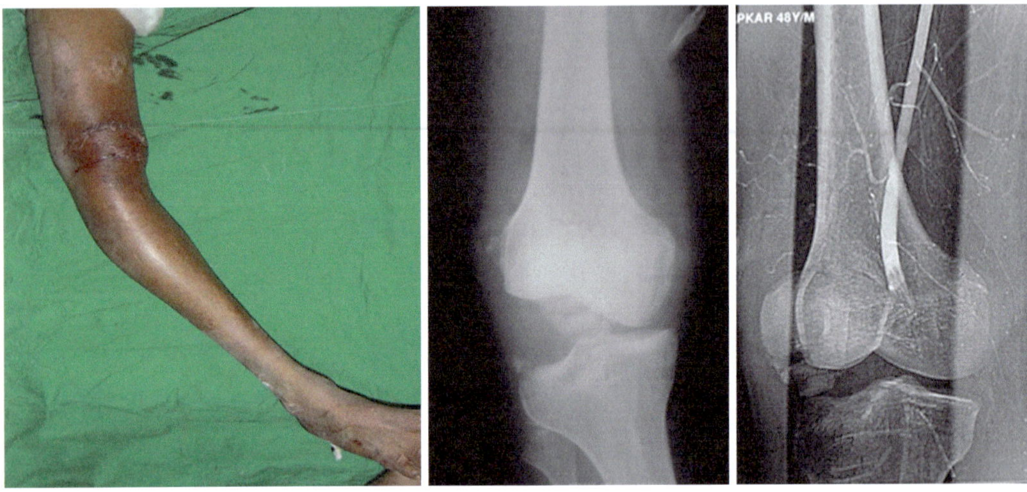

Fig. 1.5 High-velocity knee dislocation with popliteal artery injury (KD4C) with extensor apparatus disruption. The patient underwent emergency vascular repair, extensor apparatus repair, and collateral ligament repair in the first stage, followed by arthroscopic bicruciate reconstruction in the second stage

kept till acceptable soft tissue healing or till vascular reconstruction healing is achieved, without jeopardizing the time duration within which ligament repair, if required, is to be done.

3. Vascular injuries (Fig. 1.5)—If distal pulsations are not palpable and are not present on bedside Doppler examination despite reduction, the patient is shifted to the operating room, and intraoperative angiography is done. Arterial repair or bypass grafting with four compartment fasciotomy is performed. A temporary joint spanning fixator may be required.
4. An extremely unstable knee may warrant a temporary joint spanning external fixator for knee immobilization till soft tissue healing is achieved.
5. Unstable fracture dislocations may warrant immediate reduction and fracture fixation to prevent vascular and soft tissue complications.
6. Compartment syndrome warrants immediate release of all four leg compartments.

1.3.1.2 Approach in Knee Dislocations Associated with Vascular Injuries

A systematic review has found that 18% of knee dislocations have an associated vascular injury [9] with reported incidence being as high as 64% [5]. 80% of these patients underwent a vascular repair, and 12% of the patients underwent an amputation. Most of the amputations were a consequence of failed repair or an infection. Patients with maximum incidence of vascular injury were KD3L (32%) and posterior dislocations (25%). Patients with an open injury and increased BMI have been found to have increased incidence of vascular injury [10]. In general, sports dislocations have a lower rate of vascular injury as compared to high-velocity injuries [11].

Early detection and treatment of vascular damage are critical as amputation rates following early intervention (within 8 hours) are 11% and a delay beyond 8 hours results in 86% amputation rates [12]. Even so, residual amputation rates after surgery are 10% [13]. The most common arterial injury involves the popliteal artery. This is due to the fact that the popliteal artery is tethered proximally at the adductor hiatus and distally at the soleus arch.

A patient with definite signs of ischemia (absent distal pulsations of the dorsalis pedis or posterior tibial artery) needs to be shifted to the operating room immediately where an intraoperative angiography is done and treated accordingly. Arterial repair for short-segment injuries and interpositional grafts (usually contralateral saphenous vein graft) for long-segment injuries are often needed.

Patients with either asymmetric pulsations or ABI < 0.9 need further workup with either a CT or MR angiography. There has been a long-standing debate between the proponents of routine angiography and selective angiography with the former claiming that small intimal tears leading to delayed thrombosis may be missed, leading to disastrous complications. However studies have shown that selective angiography is the standard of practice [14]. Angiography is an invasive procedure with its associated risk. Recent advances have enabled CT angiography to be highly sensitive and specific (up to 100% sensitive and specific) [6] while being less invasive and involve lesser radiation [15]. MR angiography is our investigation of choice since it is equally accurate [16] without the risks of radiation and can be performed in the same sitting, as all patients would be evaluated with an MRI. Patients with palpable dorsalis pedis and posterior tibial pulse with ABI of 0.9 or greater were found to have a sensitivity of 100% to rule out vascular injury. However even these patients need to monitored for at least 48 h to rule out delayed thrombosis and vascular insult.

1.3.1.3 Approach in Knee Dislocations Associated with Peroneal Nerve Injury

The common peroneal nerve is the most commonly injured nerve in knee dislocations. The incidence, in general, is 14–25%, with as high as 41% cases reported after posterolateral complex (PLC) injuries [17]. Approximately 8% of peroneal nerve injuries have been attributed to sports-specific knee fractures and dislocation with skiing (50%) and football (27%) being the most common sports [18]. Further, out of these patients, 25% patients needed a neurolysis, and the rest needed nerve grafting. Patients who needed nerve grafts less than 6 cm fared better than those who needed longer grafts [18].

Approximately 30% of cases have a complete neurological palsy, and the rest have a partial peroneal nerve palsy [19]. Only 38.4% of patients with a complete palsy and 87.3% of patients with incomplete palsy have been found to have functional recovery (MRC grade > or = 3) [20].

Treatment options for complete nerve palsy include ankle-foot orthotic support, neurolysis, tendon transfer, nerve transfer, and combined nerve/tendon transfer. The treatment for partial nerve palsy includes nonoperative, neurolysis, nerve transfer, and combined nerve/tendon transfer [21].

1.3.1.4 Elective Surgical Intervention in the Acute and Subacute Phase After Knee Dislocations

In patients with an acute knee dislocation that has been reduced and observed or patients who present after 72 h of injury with a spontaneously reduced knee, the pain has usually subsided, and concerns over vascular injury have abated. Patient evaluation then is concentrated over the ligaments injured, the soft tissue condition, and to rule out neurological injury. A detailed radiological evaluation including radiographs, MRI, and if necessary a CT scan is indicated.

The principles of treatment of multi-ligament injury include identification and treatment of all torn ligaments often with surgical repair or reconstruction followed by a supervised rehabilitation program. An early single-stage surgery with repair of collaterals and reconstruction of cruciates may be appropriate for a high-grade injury in a young patient capable of extensive and prolonged supervised rehabilitation (Fig. 1.6). In all others, it may be prudent to consider staged treatment—either initial nonoperative treatment followed by subsequent reconstruction of all residual ligament deficiencies or acute stage open repair of collaterals and extensor apparatus followed by second-stage arthroscopic bicruciate reconstruction (Fig. 1.1). The complex anatomy of the knee with wide variation in severity and extent of injury, coupled with various treatment protocols and multiple outcome scores reported in literature, has resulted in controversies in treatment in knee dislocations.

Operative Versus Nonoperative

Systematic reviews have conclusively demonstrated that operative treatment results in better functional outcome as compared to nonoperative treatment (IKDC excellent/good results 58% vs. 20%) and a higher return to

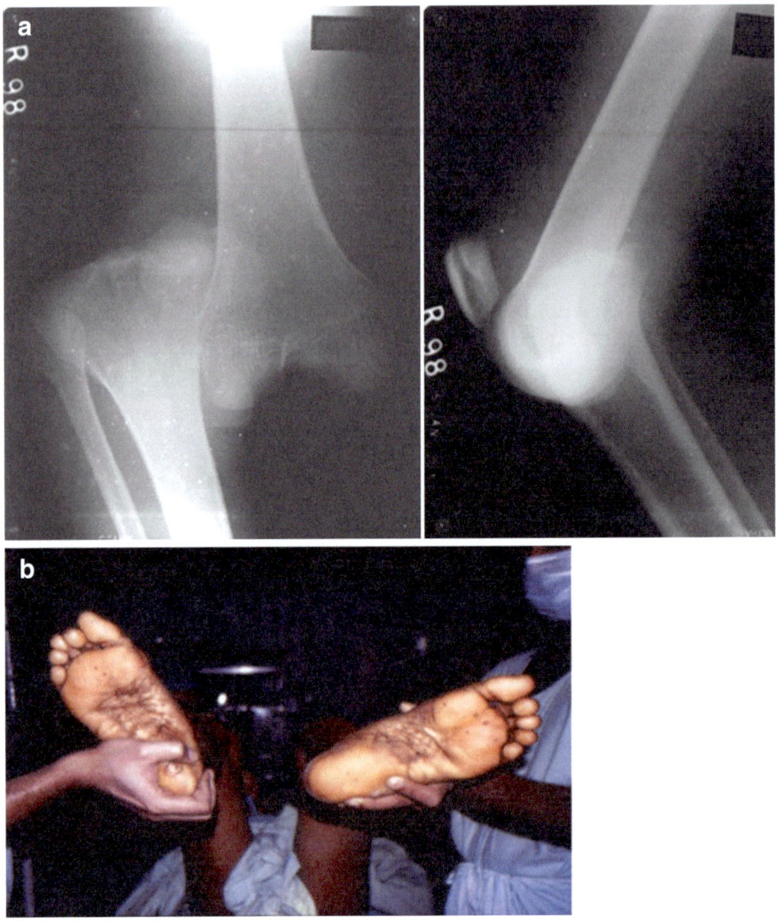

Fig. 1.6 Acute single-stage surgery for a lateral knee dislocation (KD4N). This was a closed injury with no vascular deficit. In January 2001 the senior author performed an open reconstruction of both cruciates, augmented repair of MCL, VMO repair with PLC repair, and peroneal nerve decompression. His menisci and articular cartilage were normal. He returned to competitive kabaddi (a traditional Indian combat sport) 18 months following his injury with a stable knee and full range of movements. His 17-year follow-up reveals no secondary degenerative joint disease despite competing in sports for 8 years following his injury (**a**) Preoperative radiographs—true lateral knee dislocation (**b**) The dial test reveals significant posterolateral rotatory instability following closed reduction (**c**) Clinical outcome 1 year after surgery (**d**) Radiological outcome 17 years following surgery

c

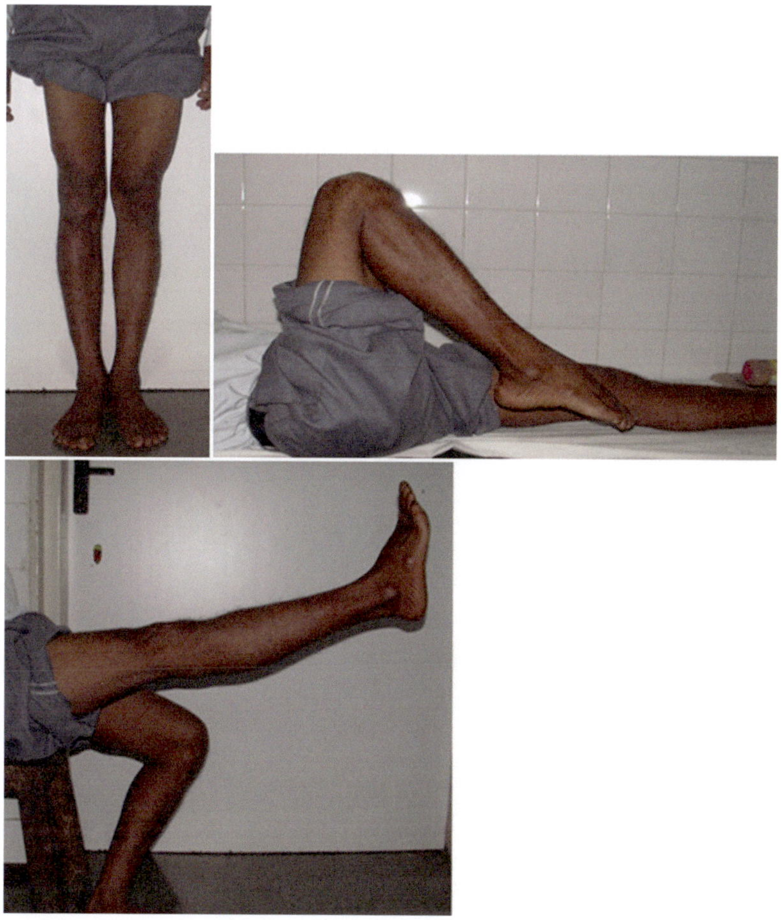

Fig. 1.6 (continued)

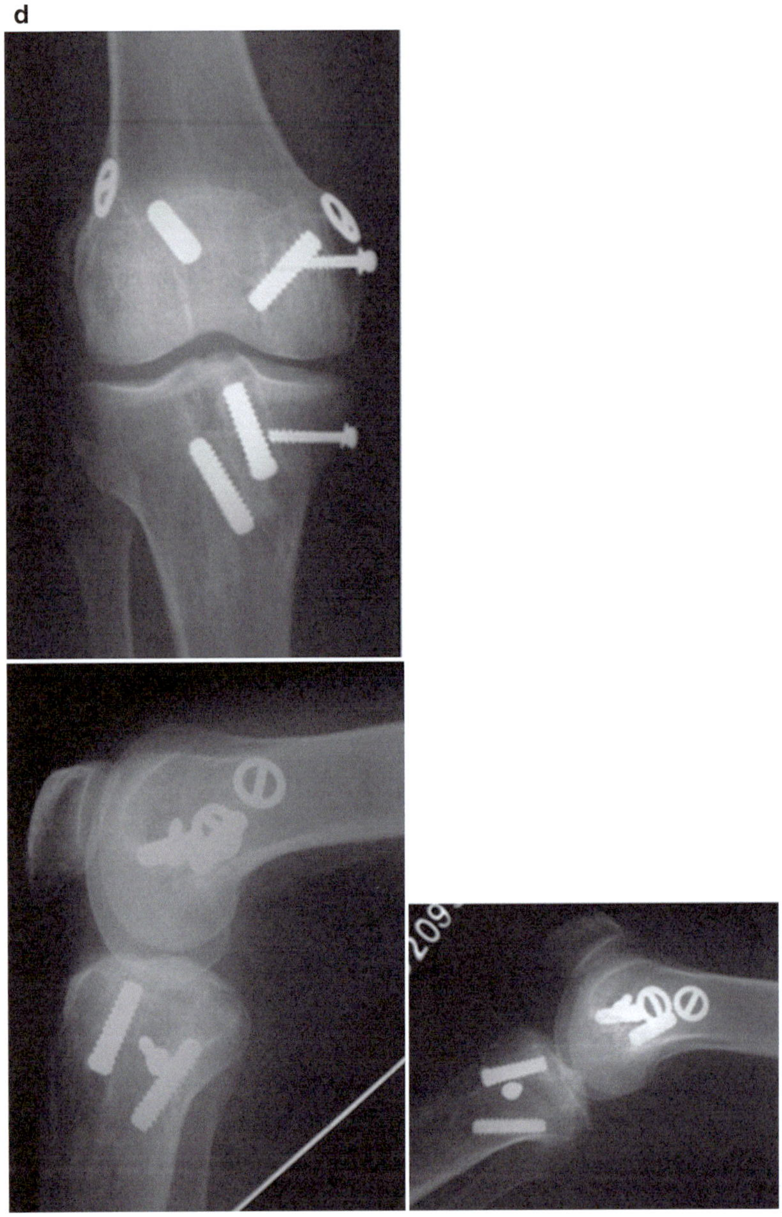

Fig. 1.6 (continued)

sports (29% vs. 10%). However the mean range of motion (126° vs. 123°) and flexion loss (4° vs. 3°) do not seem to be significantly different in both the groups [22]. A meta-analysis also supported the concept of operative treatment over nonoperative treatment as it yielded better outcome scores and range of motion [23].

Early Versus Late Surgery

Sports persons undergoing surgery within 3 weeks of injury have been shown to have higher return to sports as compared to those who undergo surgery in the chronic stage (>3 weeks usually, at a mean of 51 weeks). However the functional outcome scores and outcome measures were reported to be similar in both the groups [22].

Repair Versus Reconstruction

In a study comparing ligament repair with ligament reconstruction especially for the posterolateral corner (PLC), it was found that PLC repair had a higher failure rate than reconstruction (37% vs. 9%). Return to sports was higher with reconstruction than repair of the PLC (51% vs. 23%) [24]. Another study has demonstrated that while the functional outcome scores may be similar in ligament repair and reconstruction groups, patients who undergo repair have a greater flexion loss, posterior sag, and lower return to pre-injury activity level [25]. However a systematic review found no difference between outcomes of repair and reconstruction of ACL and PCL for these injuries [22]. Shelbourne's technique of en masse repair of lateral side structures in multi-ligament injuries has reported a 81% return to sports rate at a mean follow-up of 55 months with excellent functional outcomes [11]. When multiple graft options including allografts are available, it may be preferable to choose reconstruction over repair; however, when graft options are limited especially in acute KD4 situations, it may be prudent to primarily repair the collateral ligaments and preserve autograft options for same stage or subsequent cruciate reconstruction.

Early Simultaneous Repair Versus Staged Repair and Reconstruction

While early intervention has been shown to give better results, there has been debate whether all the ligaments should be repaired and reconstructed or whether the procedure should be staged. Patients who undergo early simultaneous repair and reconstruction of three or more ligaments are at higher risk of knee stiffness after surgery. A systematic review of 12 articles and 150 patients has reported that staged repair gives better clinical outcomes (79.1%) than simultaneous ligament surgery in acute cases (58.4%) and chronic cases (45.5%). Similarly there was no difference in outcomes of KD3M and KD3L knees [26]. In a study on staged reconstruction of multi-ligament injuries in general population consisting of sports persons, 70% of patients had an IKDC score of more than or equal to B [27].

Staged surgery includes collateral ligament repair and/or reconstruction in the acute stage (<3 weeks) followed by supervised rehabilitation for 3–6 weeks. Once knee range of motion is achieved beyond 100°, the second-stage ACL and PCL reconstruction is performed. The advantages of staged surgery include shorter operative time, decreased chances of infection, and decreased chances of arthrofibrosis [28, 29].

1.3.2 Knee Chronic Dislocations and Multiple Ligament Instability

Patients may present in the chronic phase (> 6 weeks) with a reduced knee dislocation and multi-ligament instability or rarely with a chronic unreduced knee dislocation. The treatment algorithm for chronic phase presentations is elaborated in Table 1.4.

In the chronic (but reduced) multiple ligament-deficient knee, assessment of single-stance limb alignment in both the coronal and sagittal plane is important. For patients in whom limb alignment is normal, a single-stage or staged multiple ligament reconstruction is indicated. This often involves an arthroscopic bicruciate reconstruction with medial-sided and/or posterolateral corner reconstruction.

Table 1.4 The surgical algorithm for chronic knee dislocations and multiple ligament injured knee

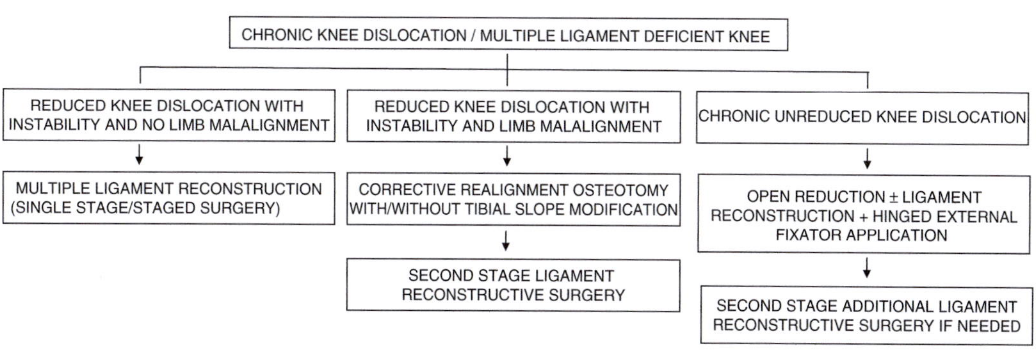

Patients with limb malalignment (commonly varus malalignment in a PCL-PLC-deficient knee) should undergo corrective osteotomy (usually with slope modification) in the first stage prior to any subsequent ligament reconstruction. Increasing tibial slope reduces tibial sag in a PCL-deficient knee, whereas decreasing tibial slope has a protective effect on the ACL-deficient knee [30]. Often limb alignment with slope correction itself is sufficient to afford functional knee stability in low-demand individuals. In patients with residual instability following corrective osteotomy, a second-stage ligament or multiple ligament reconstructive surgery may be warranted.

Chronic unreduced knee dislocations are rare and are often missed injuries in a polytrauma patient. These cases are extremely challenging since achieving stability and range of motion warrants complex management techniques including open reduction, hinged external fixator application, with or without staged ligament reconstruction, and prolonged rehabilitation [31]. In the past 20 years, the senior author has treated 26 chronic unreduced knee dislocations, and each has required an individualized approach. To reduce the chronically dislocated knee, complete circumferential capsular release and scar tissue excision are required. To prevent extensive arthrofibrosis, early mobilization is mandatory, and this is possible only with a hinged external fixator that helps maintain the reduction and reestablish stable anatomic range of motion. Moreover, if ligament reconstruction is planned at the same stage, a hinged external fixator is critical to prevent increased stress on the grafts (Fig. 1.7).

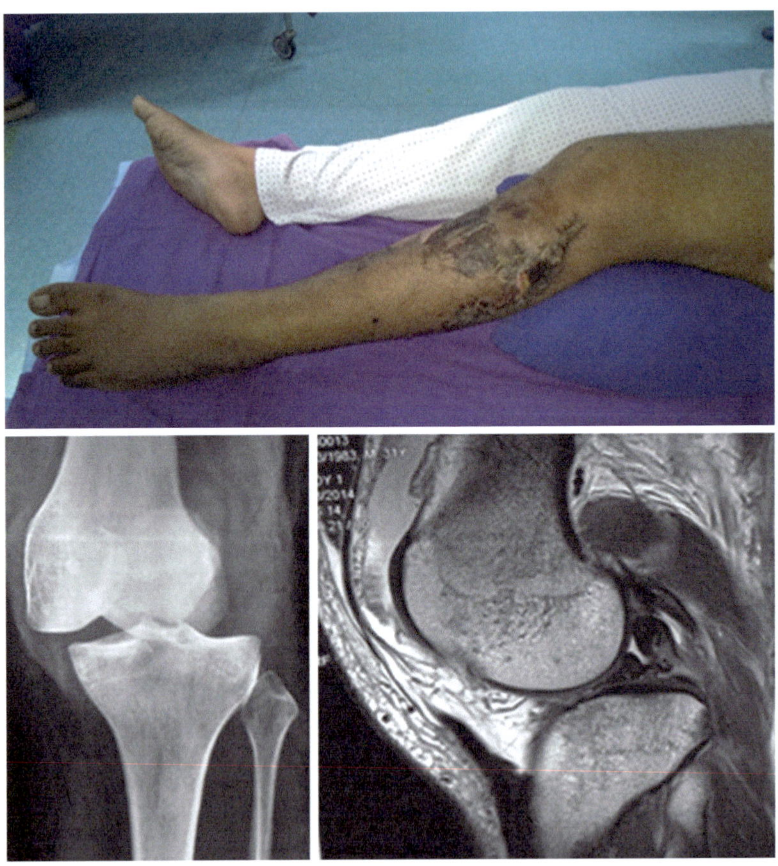

Fig. 1.7 A 3-month-old unreduced posterolateral knee dislocation following a high-velocity motorcycle accident with polytrauma. The injury occurred at a remote high-altitude location and resulted in a missed knee dislocation. He required open reduction, hinged external fixator application, and staged multiple ligament reconstruction with allografts. He returned to rally racing 18 months following index surgery

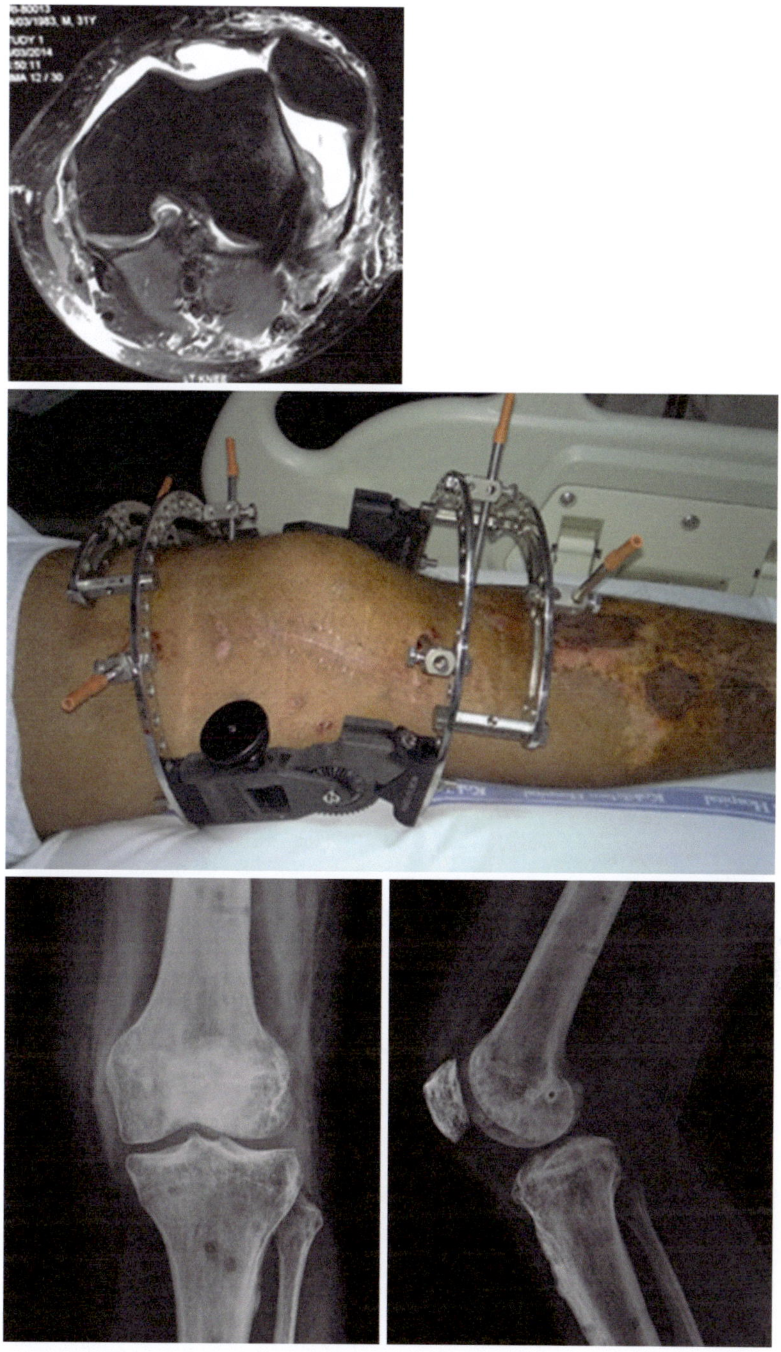

Fig. 1.7 (continued)

References

1. Rihn JA, Groff YJ, Harner CD, Cha PS. The acutely dislocated knee: evaluation and management. J Am Acad Orthop Surg. 2004;12(5):334–46.
2. Richter M, Lobenhoffer P, Tscherne H. Knee dislocation. Long-term results after operative treatment. Der Chirurg. 1999;70(11):1294–301.
3. Kennedy JC. Complete dislocation of the knee joint. J Bone Joint Surg Am. 1963;45:889–904.
4. Schenck RC. Classification of knee dislocations. In: Fanelli GC, editor. The multiple ligament injured knee. New York, NY: Springer; 2004.
5. Seroyer ST, Musahl V, Harner CD. Management of the acute knee dislocation: the Pittsburgh experience. Injury. 2008;39(7):710–8.
6. Fanelli GC, Stannard JP, Stuart MJ, MacDonald PB, Marx RG, Whelan DB, et al. Management of complex knee ligament injuries. J Bone Joint Surg Am. 2010;92(12):2235–46.
7. Pardiwala DN, Rao NN, Anand K, Raut A. Knee dislocations in sports injuries. Indian J Orthop. 2017;51:552–62.
8. Howells NR, Brunton LR, Robinson J, Porteus AJ, Eldridge JD, Murray JR. Acute knee dislocation: an evidence based approach to the management of the multiligament injured knee. Injury. 2011;42(11):1198–204.
9. Medina O, Arom GA, Yeranosian MG, Petrigliano FA, McAllister DR. Vascular and nerve injury after knee dislocation: a systematic review. Clin Orthop. 2014;472(9):2621–9.
10. Weinberg DS, Scarcella NR, Napora JK, Vallier HA. Can vascular injury be appropriately assessed with physical examination after knee dislocation? Clin Orthop. 2016;474(6):1453–8.
11. Shelbourne KD, Klootwyk TE. Low-velocity knee dislocation with sports injuries. Treatment principles. Clin Sports Med. 2000;19(3):443–56.
12. Green NE, Allen BL. Vascular injuries associated with dislocation of the knee. J Bone Joint Surg Am. 1977;59(2):236–9.
13. Boisrenoult P, Lustig S, Bonneviale P, Leray E, Versier G, Neyret P, et al. Vascular lesions associated with bicruciate and knee dislocation ligamentous injury. Orthop Traumatol Surg Res OTSR. 2009;95(8):621–6.
14. Nicandri GT, Chamberlain AM, Wahl CJ. Practical management of knee dislocations: a selective angiography protocol to detect limb-threatening vascular injuries. Clin J Sport Med. 2009;19(2):125–9.
15. Redmond JM, Levy BA, Dajani KA, Cass JR, Cole PA. Detecting vascular injury in lower-extremity orthopedic trauma: the role of CT angiography. Orthopedics. 2008;31(8):761–7.
16. Potter HG, Weinstein M, Allen AA, Wickiewicz TL, Helfet DL. Magnetic resonance imaging of the multiple-ligament injured knee. J Orthop Trauma. 2002;16(5):330–9.
17. Niall DM, Nutton RW, Keating JF. Palsy of the common peroneal nerve after traumatic dislocation of the knee. J Bone Joint Surg Br. 2005;87(5):664–7.
18. Cho D, Saetia K, Lee S, Kline DG, Kim DH. Peroneal nerve injury associated with sports-related knee injury. Neurosurg Focus. 2011;31(5):E11.
19. Bonnevialle P, Dubrana F, Galau B, Lustig S, Barbier O, Neyret P, et al. Common peroneal nerve palsy complicating knee dislocation and bicruciate ligaments tears. Orthop Traumatol Surg Res OTSR. 2010;96(1):64–9.
20. Woodmass JM, Romatowski NPJ, Esposito JG, Mohtadi NGH, Longino PD. A systematic review of peroneal nerve palsy and recovery following traumatic knee dislocation. Knee Surg Sports Traumatol Arthrosc. 2015;23(10):2992–3002.
21. Krych AJ, Giuseffi SA, Kuzma SA, Stuart MJ, Levy BA. Is peroneal nerve injury associated with worse function after knee dislocation? Clin Orthop. 2014;472(9):2630–6.
22. Levy BA, Dajani KA, Whelan DB, Stannard JP, Fanelli GC, Stuart MJ, et al. Decision making in the multiligament-injured knee: an evidence-based systematic review. Arthrosc J Arthrosc Relat Surg. 2009;25(4):430–8.
23. Dedmond BT, Almekinders LC. Operative versus nonoperative treatment of knee dislocations: a meta-analysis. Am J Knee Surg. 2001;14(1):33–8.
24. Stannard JP, Brown SL, Farris RC, McGwin GJ, Volgas DA. The posterolateral corner of the knee: repair versus reconstruction. Am J Sports Med. 2005;33(6):881–8.
25. Mariani PP, Santoriello P, Iannone S, Condello V, Adriani E. Comparison of surgical treatments for knee dislocation. Am J Knee Surg. 1999;12(4):214–21.
26. Jiang W, Yao J, He Y, Sun W, Huang Y, Kong D. The timing of surgical treatment of knee dislocations: a systematic review. Knee Surg Sports Traumatol Arthrosc. 2015;23(10):3108–13.
27. Suh JT, Ahn JM, Lee JM, Kim NR. Staged surgical management of multiple ligament injury of the knee. Arthrosc Orthop Sports Med. 2014;1(2):111–9.
28. Ohkoshi Y, Nagasaki S, Shibata N, Yamamoto K, Hashimoto T, Yamane S. Two-stage reconstruction with autografts for knee dislocations. Clin Orthop. 2002;(398):169–75.
29. Subbiah M, Pandey V, Rao SK, Rao S. Staged arthroscopic reconstructive surgery for multiple ligament injuries of the knee. J Orthop Surg Hong Kong. 2011;19(3):297–302.
30. Giffin JR, Vogrin TM, Zantop T, Woo SL, Harner CD. Effects of increasing tibial slope on the biomechanics of the knee. Am J Sports Med. 2004;32(2):376–82.
31. Simonian PT, Wickiewicz TL, Hotchkiss RN, Warren RF. Chronic knee dislocation: reduction, reconstruction, and application of a skeletally fixed knee hinge. Am J Sports Med. 1998;26(4):591–6.

Management in the Emergency Room

2

Michael E. Hantes and Konstantinos Banios

2.1 Introduction

Knee dislocation, or multi-ligamentous injury of the knee, is recognized to be a rare injury, quoted to represent between 0.02% and 0.2% of all orthopedic trauma [1, 2].

However, this figure probably does not represent the whole truth, because of a (common) missed diagnosis after a spontaneous reduction of the dislocation [3].

Dislocation entails the complete disruption of the tibio-femoral articulation (Fig. 2.1), which most commonly presents as an anatomically reduced but highly unstable knee, requiring rupture of a minimum two major stabilizing ligaments.

Knee dislocations are potentially limb-threatening injuries, with a high risk of vascular compromise, varied widely, ranging from 3.3% to 64% [4].

Radiographic evidence of dislocation is not always available, and the clinician has to be aware of other signs of a dislocation that may have spontaneously reduced like an hematoma of the popliteal fossa (Fig. 2.2). Approximately 50% of knee dislocations are spontaneously reduced prior to the examination of a clinician.

Most knee dislocations are the result of high-energy mechanisms [5]. However, nowadays as obesity becomes a worldwide medical issue, even low-velocity injuries such as ground level falls may lead to knee dislocation. Therefore, evaluating physicians should maintain a high suspicion for a knee dislocation in any obese patient who presents with knee pain following a seemingly innocuous injury. Careful history and physical examination in a systematic approach will aid in identifying patients at risk for this injury.

The three most common mechanisms of these injuries include:

(a) High-energy trauma due to motor vehicle collision (almost 50%).
(b) Sport injuries (33%).
(c) Simple falls (12%).

A patient with a dislocated knee should be approached very carefully in the emergency department in order to recognize, deal with this severe injury, and avoid misdiagnosis or other complications.

2.2 History and Physical Examination

The mechanism of injury is an important factor in guiding evaluation of a knee injury in the emergency department (ED) and in predicting the

M. E. Hantes (✉) · K. Banios
Department of Orthopedics, Faculty of Medicine, University of Thessaly, Larisa, Greece
e-mail: hantesmi@otenet.gr

F. Margheritini et al. (eds.), *Complex Knee Ligament Injuries*,
https://doi.org/10.1007/978-3-662-58245-9_2

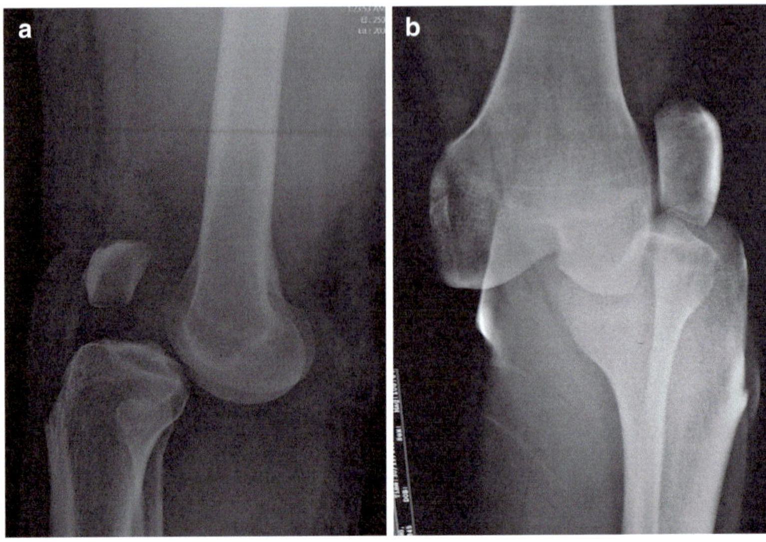

Fig. 2.1 Anteroposterior (**a**) and lateral (**b**) X-rays of a dislocated knee

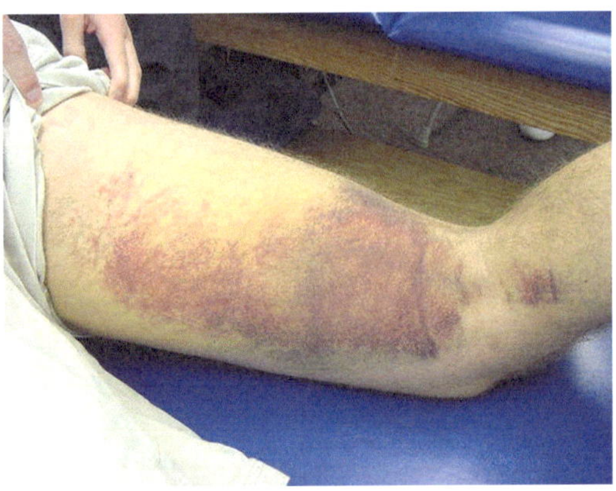

Fig. 2.2 Extensive hematoma of the popliteal fossa and posterior thigh after a knee dislocation

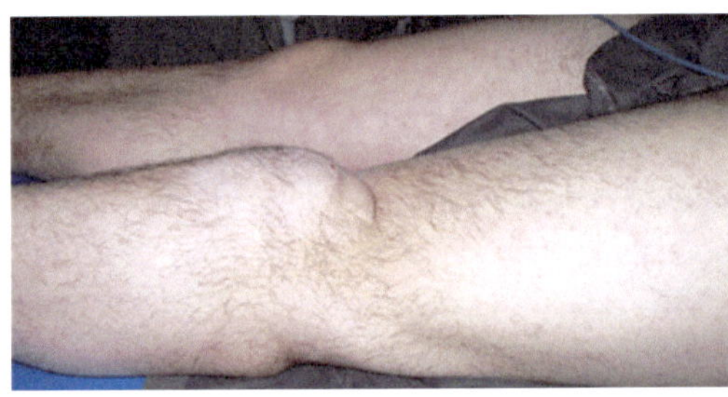

Fig. 2.3 Gross deformity of the knee due to knee dislocation and anteriorly dislocated tibia

ultimate diagnosis. Consider the direction of the force applied to the knee and the position of the knee at the time the force was applied. Inquire about the ability to bear weight immediately after the injury, the development of restrictions of range of motion, the location of pain, loss of sensation, any new swelling and the period of time over which it occurred, and whether a "pop" was felt or heard by the injured patient.

As knee dislocations are usually associated with other injuries, the clinician must initially follow the ATLS principles. So it is crucial not to concentrate only to the injured knee but inspect the whole body for any concomitant injury. Hemodynamic instability may result from internal injury or fractures and is the most important consideration for the orthopedic surgeon.

As the patient is stabilized, it is important to inspect the affected limb so as to recognize any skin injury (15–30% of knee dislocations are open) [6, 7]. Moreover, the presence of any obvious deformity can reveal the direction of the dislocated tibia (Fig. 2.3). Compare the affected knee with the contralateral one for reference and symmetry.

- Palpate bony structures of the knee and note any tenderness.
- Patellar tap test can reveal joint effusion.
- Note the range of motion (passive and active).
- Assess distal pulses and capillary refill distal to the injured knee.
- Check for any sensory and motor dysfunction of the affected limb.

2.3 Vascular Examination

The incidence of popliteal artery injury is 3.3%–64% [4].

Popliteal artery is fixed proximally onto the medial femoral epicondyle at the fibrous insertion of adductor magnus and distally tethered by the tendinous arch of soleus; movement of the artery is restricted leading to traction injury.

Because vascular injury is potentially limb threatening, early identification of vascular injury is critical. A delay in the diagnosis increases the time of warm ischemia and the risk for irreversible injury, resulting in the possible need for an above the knee amputation.

Up to 20% of patients with vascular compromise will eventually require amputation, increasing to more than 80% with an ischemic time of over 8 h; therefore, early recognition and management of a compromised limb is vital [8].

A recent review of available literature did not demonstrate any association between direction of dislocation and vascular insult [9].

A clinician who suspects a knee dislocation has to examine the leg for two essential things in order to assess vascular integrity of the leg. First, palpate dorsalis pedis and posterior tibial pulses bilaterally and assess for any asymmetry. In the absence of any asymmetry, further assessment is not necessary [10, 11].

Second, the *ankle-brachial index (ABI)*, which is the ratio of the systolic blood pressure measured at the ankle to that measured at the brachial artery, should be calculated. To perform this, a clinician needs a manual blood pressure cuff and a Doppler probe. With the patient in the supine position, a blood pressure cuff is placed on the affected ankle above the malleoli. The ultrasound transducer is used to locate the dorsalis pedis or posterior tibial artery signal. The blood pressure cuff is inflated while listening to the Doppler signal. Once the signal has disappeared, the pressure in the cuff is slowly released until the Doppler signal can be heard again. The pressure at which the Doppler signal in the dorsalis pedis or posterior tibial artery returns is the systolic blood pressure value for the ankle. For the brachium, the blood pressure cuff is placed on the arm, and the brachial pulse is located in the antecubital fossa using the ultrasound transducer. The cuff is inflated until the Doppler signal from the brachial artery disappears. The cuff is then gently relieved of pressure until the signal in the brachial artery returns. The pressure at which the Doppler signal returns is the systolic blood pressure in the brachium. To calculate the ABI, the systolic blood pressure measured at the ankle is divided by that measured at the brachial artery. A ratio of less than 0.9 is considered abnormal and necessitates further investigation with arteriography. On the contrary, if the ABI is greater than 0.9, it has been shown that the risk of major arterial lesion approaches 0% [12].

For further investigation, CT angiogram (CTA) is mostly preferred (Fig. 2.4), as it provides a higher sensitivity and specificity and almost one fourth less radiation than conventional one [13].

MR arthrography also shows potential in this setting through its convenience of including venous contrast while conducting a conventional MRI to evaluate ligamentous injury [14].

An algorithm employed at the University of Washington Medical Center for the diagnosis of vascular injury following multiple-ligament knee injuries is presented in Fig. 2.5.

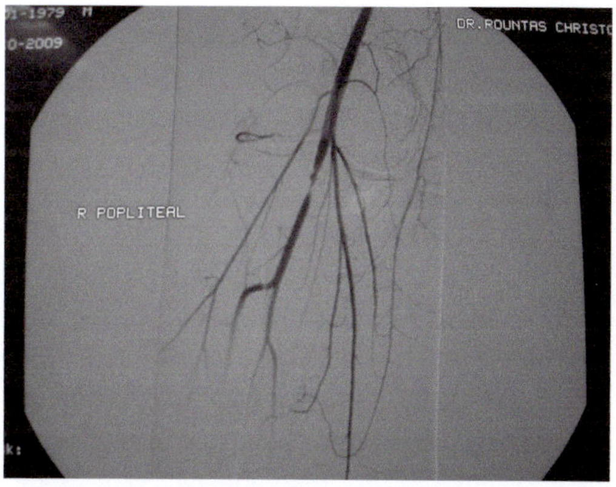

Fig. 2.4 CT angiogram image of a patient with popliteal artery occlusion after a knee dislocation

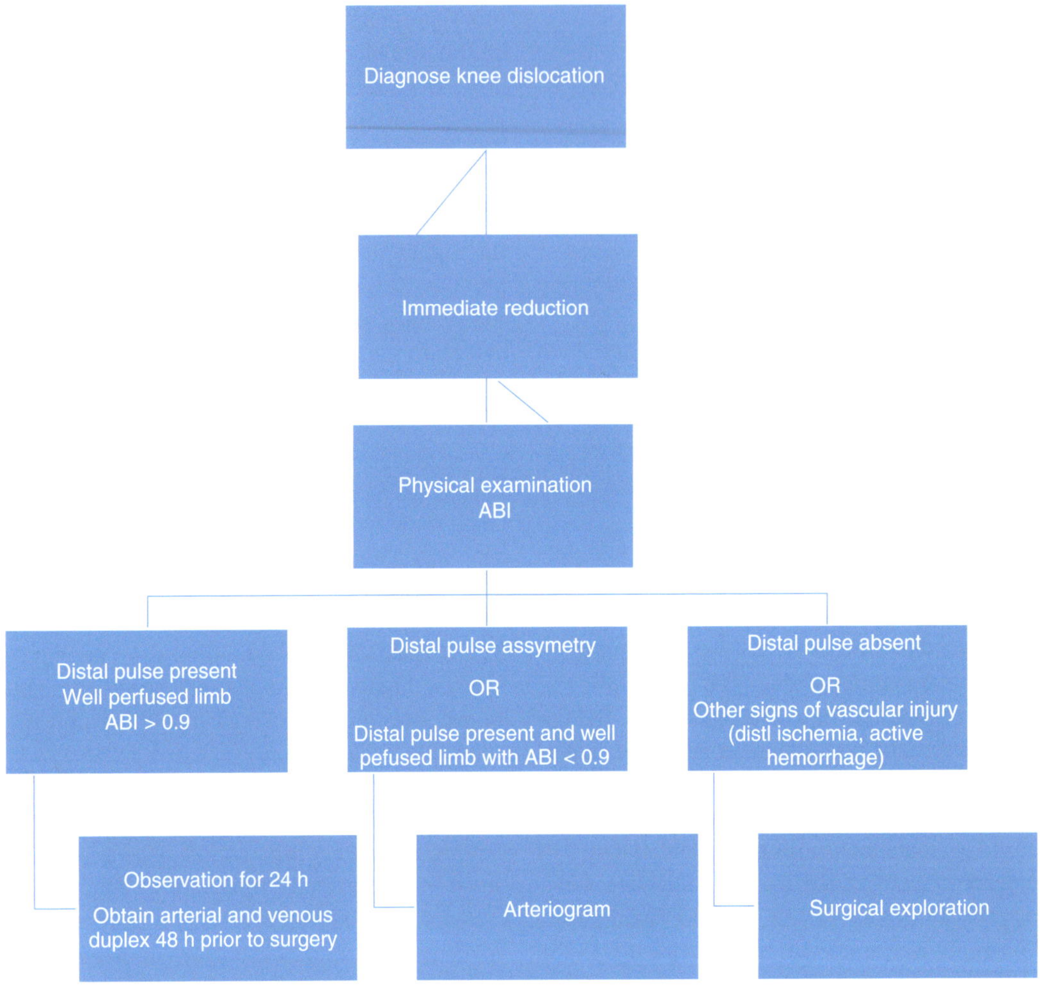

Fig. 2.5 Algorithm employed at the University of Washington Medical Center for the diagnosis of vascular injury following multiple ligament knee injuries

2.3.1 Neurologic Examination

The physical examination should include a detailed neurologic examination including sensation in the tibial, deep peroneal, and superficial peroneal distributions to light touch, pinprick. Motor examination including the flexor and extensor hallucis longus, tibialis anterior, and gastrocnemius as well.

The incidence of nerve injury associated with knee dislocation ranges from 4.5% to 40.0%. Most commonly, the common peroneal is the injured nerve. The nerve is at risk for injury as well, similar to the artery, due to its anatomic constraints both proximally and distally. The fibular neck tethers the nerve proximally, and the fibrous arches of the intermuscular septum form the distal tether.

Common causes of nerve injuries are fractures (e.g., lateral tibial condyle, fibula head) and tractions of the nerve due to varus stress or hyperextension.

Unfortunately, recovery of patients with a neurologic deficit is unpredictable. The outcome depends on the location, the severity, the time of injury, and the age of the patient. Peripheral peroneal nerve injuries in young patients are associated with a better prognosis.

2.4 Plain X-Rays

Frontal and lateral plain films are performed as a standard in the emergency department. These should be performed before (evaluation for concomitant fractures such as Segond or other fractures and direction of displacement) and after reduction to confirm proper joint articulation and congruency. CT after performing reduction is recommended if a fracture is revealed at X-rays.

MRI is helpful preoperatively for the diagnosis of ligamentous, meniscal, and articular damage, but it is not necessary in the emergency department. However, it is mandatory after initial management to reveal the whole spectrum of injuries.

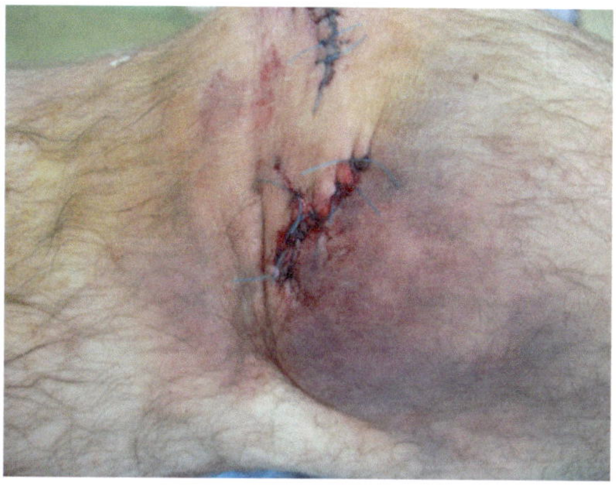

Fig. 2.6 The *dimple sign*: skin dimple between the medial femoral condyle and the medial tibial plateau. This patient had an open unrecognized knee dislocation and managed with wound closure initially

2.4.1 Reduction of the Dislocation

After X-ray confirmation of a knee dislocation, a reduction of the dislocation should be performed. The reduction of the knee should be attempted with the patient under sedation either in the emergency department or at the operating room, for a successful reduction is essential to make a maneuver that reverses the deforming force. Often, gentle in-line traction attempting to bring the knee into extension is enough to reduce a dislocated knee. No manual pressure should be used to aid in any direction, especially in the popliteal fossa, to avoid iatrogenic neurovascular injury.

After reduction is done, the knee should be splinted in 20° of flexion so as to provide stability of bony and neurovascular structures, relaxation of soft tissues, and pain relief to the patient. Moreover the splint must prevent posterior subluxation of the tibia to minimize traction of vessels. Opening a window to splint is crucial to allow vascular evaluation of the foot. Successful reduction is confirmed with knee X-rays.

If the reduction is unsuccessful, the patient should be taken urgently to the operating room for a reduction under general anesthesia (in many cases, the irreducible knee has pinched or threatened skin, particularly on the medial aspect of the knee). If closed reduction performed under anesthesia is unsuccessful, the surgeon should proceed to an open reduction of the knee. One of the reasons for an irreducible knee dislocation is the so-called dimple sign.

The *dimple sign*: When the knee is gently brought into extension, a worsening skin dimple between the medial femoral condyle and the medial tibial plateau can be a sign that closed reduction will be unsuccessful. The skin dimple is a sign that the medial femoral condyle has buttonholed through the medial joint capsule, and the MCL has become entrapped and is being pulled into the joint with the gentle traction (Fig. 2.6). Multiple case reports cite this as a sign for an irreducible knee dislocation and recommend open reduction in the operating room [15]. Unfortunately, it may not be visualized in many cases due to diffuse swelling of the knee. A midline surgical incision with a medial parapatellar arthrotomy is useful to address the acute dislocation and later ligament reconstruction.

A recent review of the literature identified that KD-III is the predominant injury pattern in irreducible dislocations, which refer to ruptures of ACL, PCL, and MCL or LCL (79.5%) [16]. The interposed tissue is likely to be MCL or medial retinaculum, but all surrounding structures cannot be neglected.

Once the knee is reduced, repeat neurologic and vascular examination are done immediately. With any vascular compromise or asymmetry in ABIs whereby the affected leg is less than 0.9, surgical exploration is warranted.

Compartment syndrome development is another potential complication of a knee dislocation. High suspicion of compartment syndrome and close monitoring of the leg, through clinical examination or through invasive measurements of the intra-compartmental pressure (ICP), should be performed. In case of compartment syndrome development, immediate fasciotomy of all four compartments is necessary, and it should be performed without any delay. Moreover, care must be taken not to elevate the injured limb above heart level in order to avoid perfusion depression.

2.5 Examination of Knee Stability

Examination of ligamentous integrity is usually limited secondary to patient discomfort, and some of the most specific diagnostic tests require patient cooperation, which is difficult under these circumstances. However, the physician could attempt a gentle examination, and probably intra-articular injection of lidocaine after aspiration of any hemarthrosis can aid in patient's comfort.

Clues to ligament injury in a spontaneously reduced knee dislocation are any asymmetry in the joint space, minor subluxations in any direction, and Segond fractures.

The Lachman test and the anterior drawer test (ACL rupture), varus/valgus stressing (MCL/LCL compromise), and posterior sag (PCL disruption) are the most reliable maneuvers in the acute setting.

The pivot shift, dial test, reverse pivot shift, and weight-bearing examinations are impractical at the bedside but can aid in the diagnosis while under anesthesia.

2.6 Emergent Surgery

Absolute surgical indications in patients with a knee dislocation include (a) vascular injury, (b) irreducible dislocations, (c) gross instability on examination with failure to maintain joint reduction, (d) open injuries, and (e) inability to tolerate mobilization in a brace, whether due to pain or noncompliance [17–19]. Associated fractures, avulsion-type injuries, and ligamentous hypermobility often benefit from surgical repair, although this can be done in a later stage.

The determination of instability is made with a thorough ligamentous examination and an examination under anesthesia with fluoroscopic stress views in the operating room. If a patient has gross instability and reduction cannot be maintained, then there is a risk of repetitive trauma to the posterior vascular structures (popliteal artery) making them more vulnerable for thrombosis, and this is an indication to apply an external fixator to maintain stability.

As for the vascular injury, the rationale for external stabilization is:

(a) To stabilize the vascular repair in case of a vascular injury which requires surgical intervention.
(b) To protect from further vascular trauma when a vascular surgery is not necessary.

In case of an open dislocation, it is obvious that as an open trauma the surgeon has to do a thorough irrigation and debridement of foreign material and nonviable tissues. Furthermore placing an external fixator prevents from further trauma to the soft tissues and also makes mobilization of the patient possible.

Another indication for placing external fixator is patient's inability to tolerate mobilization in a brace either due to pain (probably the brace does not hold the limb in a stable fashion) or due to incompliance especially in obese patients.

As external fixator is applied, it is mandatory to perform X-rays in order to confirm the correct articulation of the joint and the correct positioning of the pins.

The advantages of using spanning external fixation include skin assessment, compartment pressure observation, and monitoring the neurovascular status of the affected limb.

The main indications for initial application of external fixation are:

1. Arterial injury requiring repair.
2. Compartment syndrome.

3. Open dislocation.
4. Irreducible dislocation.
5. Polytrauma patients during damage control.
6. Obese patients with insufficient stability after brace.

References

1. Howells NR, Brunton LR, Robinson J, Porteus AJ, Eldridge JD, Murray JR. Acuteknee dislocation: an evidence based approach to the management of the multiligament injured knee. Injury. 2011;42:1198–204. https://doi.org/10.1016/j.injury.2010.11.018.
2. Lachman JR, Rehman S, Pipitone PS. Traumatic knee dislocations: evaluation, management, and surgical treatment. Orthop Clin North Am. 2015;46:479–93.
3. Peskun CJ, Whelan DB, Fanelli GC, et al. Diagnosis and management of knee dislocations. Physician Sports Med. 2010;38(4):101–11.
4. Natsuhara KM, Yeranosian MG, Cohen JR, Wang JC, McAllister DR, Petrigliano FA. What is the frequency of vascular injury after knee dislocation? Clin Orthop Relat Res. 2014;472:2615–20.
5. Harner CD, Waltrip RL, Bennett CH, et al. Surgical management of knee dislocations. J Bone Joint Surg. 2004;86-A:262–73.
6. King JJ, Cerynik DL, Blair JA. Surgical outcomes after traumatic open knee dislocations. Knee Surg Sports Traumatol Arthrosc. 2009;17(9):1027–32.
7. Wright DG, Covey DC, Born CT, et al. Open dislocation of the knee. J Orthop Trauma. 1995;9(2):135–40.
8. Patterson BM, Agel J, Swiontkowski MF, Mackenzie EJ, Bosse MJ. Knee dislocations with vascular injury: outcomes in the lower extremity assessment project (LEAP) study. J Trauma. 2007;63:855–8.
9. Wascher DC. High velocity knee dislocation with vascular injury: treatment principles. Clin Sports Med. 2000;19:457–77.
10. Klineberg EO, Crites BM, Flinn WR, et al. The role of arteriography in assessing popliteal artery injury in knee dislocations. J Trauma. 2004;56(4):786–90.
11. Hollis JD, Daley BJ. 10-year review of knee dislocations; is angiography always necessary. J Trauma. 2005;59(3):672–5.
12. Mills WJ, Barei DP, McNair P. The value of the ankle-brachial index for diagnosingarterial injury after knee dislocation: a prospective study. J Trauma. 2004;56(6):1261–5.
13. Redmond JM, Levy BA, Dajani KA, et al. Detecting vascular injury in lower-extremity orthopedic trauma: the role of CT angiography. Orthopedics. 2008;31:761–7.
14. Johnson ME, Foster L, DeLee JC. Neurologic and vascular injuries associated with knee ligament injuries. Am J Sports Med. 2008;36:2448–62.
15. Wand JS. A physical sign denoting irreducibility of a dislocated knee. J Bone Joint Surg Br. 1989;71-B:862.
16. Xu B, Xu H, Jun T, Guo R. Initial assessment and implications for surgery: the missed diagnosis of irreducible knee dislocation. J Knee Surg. 2018;31(3):254–63. https://doi.org/10.1055/s-0037-1602135. Epub 2017 May 1
17. Levy BA, Fanelli GC, Whelan DB, et al. Knee dislocation study group. Controversies in the treatment of knee dislocations and multiligament reconstruction. J Am Acad Orthop Surg. 2009;17(4):197–206.
18. Levy BA, Krych AJ, Shah JP, Morgan JA, Stuart MJ. Staged protocol for initial management of the dislocated knee. Knee Surg Sports Traumatol Arthrosc. 2010;18(12):1630–7. https://doi.org/10.1007/s00167-010-1209-y. Epub 2010 Jul 16
19. Nicandri GT, Dunbar RP, Wahl CJ. Are evidence-based protocols which identify vascular injury associated with knee dislocation underutilized? Knee Surg Sports Traumat Arthrosc. 2010;18:1005–12.

An Advanced Device for Multiplanar Instability Assessment in MRI

3

Renato Andrade, Hugo Duarte, Rogério Pereira, Claudia Arias, Ricardo Bastos, Sérgio Rodrigues-Gomes, Joaquim Miguel Oliveira, Rui L. Reis, and João Espregueira-Mendes

R. Andrade
Faculty of Sports, University of Porto, Porto, Portugal

Clínica do Dragão, Espregueira-Mendes Sports Centre - FIFA Medical Centre of Excellence, Porto, Portugal

Dom Henrique Research Centre, Porto, Portugal

H. Duarte
Faculty of Medicine, University of Porto, Porto, Portugal

R. Pereira
Faculty of Sports, University of Porto, Porto, Portugal

Clínica do Dragão, Espregueira-Mendes Sports Centre - FIFA Medical Centre of Excellence, Porto, Portugal

Dom Henrique Research Centre, Porto, Portugal

University Fernando Pessoa, Porto, Portugal

C. Arias
Hospital Edgardo Rebagliati Martins, Lima, Peru

International Clinic San Borja, Lima, Peru

R. Bastos
Clínica do Dragão, Espregueira-Mendes Sports Centre - FIFA Medical Centre of Excellence, Porto, Portugal

Dom Henrique Research Centre, Porto, Portugal

Fluminense Federal University, Rio de Janeiro, Brazil

3B's Research Group–Biomaterials, Biodegradables and Biomimetics, University of Minho, Minho, Portugal

Headquarters of the European Institute of Excellence on Tissue Engineering and Regenerative Medicine, Barco/Guimarães, Portugal

S. Rodrigues-Gomes
Clínica do Dragão, Espregueira-Mendes Sports Centre - FIFA Medical Centre of Excellence, Porto, Portugal

Dom Henrique Research Centre, Porto, Portugal

J. Miguel Oliveira · R. L. Reis
3B's Research Group–Biomaterials, Biodegradables and Biomimetics, University of Minho, Minho, Portugal

Headquarters of the European Institute of Excellence on Tissue Engineering and Regenerative Medicine, Barco/Guimarães, Portugal

ICVS/3B's–PT Government Associate Laboratory, Braga/Guimarães, Portugal

J. Espregueira-Mendes (✉)
Clínica do Dragão, Espregueira-Mendes Sports Centre - FIFA Medical Centre of Excellence, Porto, Portugal

Dom Henrique Research Centre, Porto, Portugal

Headquarters of the European Institute of Excellence on Tissue Engineering and Regenerative Medicine, Barco/Guimarães, Portugal

School of Medicine, University of Minho, Braga, Portugal
e-mail: espregueira@dhresearchcentre.com

F. Margheritini et al. (eds.), *Complex Knee Ligament Injuries*,
https://doi.org/10.1007/978-3-662-58245-9_3

3.1 Introduction

Multiligament knee injuries are uncommon [1]. Duc to the severity of the lesion and the difficulty to reestablish the complex ligamentous anatomy and native stability, multiligament injuries represent a great challenge for orthopaedic surgeons. Many anatomical and morphological factors may contribute for knee stability independently of the ligamentary structures and should be considered during diagnosis and treatment [2–4]. These lesions are associated to high-energy (motorcycle accidents) or low-energy (cutting and pivoting mannuevers) traumas which young patients are considered at high risk since this population is very active in sports [5, 6]. The consequences of these injuries can result in knee ligamentary malalignment, association with meniscus injuries, cartilage defects and joint instability, which has a strong correlation with early onset of osteoarthritis [7, 8]. Therefore, an accurate and comprehensive diagnosis plays a key role in treatment algorithm [9, 10]. In this chapter, we discuss the use of Porto-knee testing device (PKTD) in both diagnosis of knee ligament lesions and instability assessment.

3.2 Diagnosis of Multiligament Knee Injuries

The clinical history and the physical examination play a key role in determining the existence of the injury; however, they are insufficient to determine the extension of the lesion [11]. Radiographs are used to rule out fractures and to confirm the reduction of the knee joint [12]. Magnetic resonance imaging (MRI) is still the method recommended to determine the extent of lesion and carefully plan the treatment [13]. Nonetheless, despite its high sensitivity (78–100%) and specificity (68–100%) for anterior cruciate ligament (ACL) injuries [14–17], when multiligament are considered, these predictive decrease significantly [18–20]. Instrumented manual devices (such as the KT-1000/2000) may be used to assess the knee sagittal laxity, but are unable to provide accurate objective quantification of tibiofemoral sagittal and rotational laxity [21, 22]. Moreover, due to their material composite, it is not possible to use them in association with MRI. In this sense, the concomitant use of both instrumented laxity and MRI examination may provide the greatest diagnostic value [23]. Therefore, new approaches are needed to overcome these difficulties.

3.3 Porto-Knee Testing Device (PKTD)

The PKTD is an innovative diagnostic tool (Fig. 3.1), made of polyurethane composite material and designed to be compatible imaging devices, such as MRI and computed tomography. It evaluates knee instability as it is capable of measuring the tibiofemoral sagittal and rotational laxity. It offers the possibility to adjust the knee

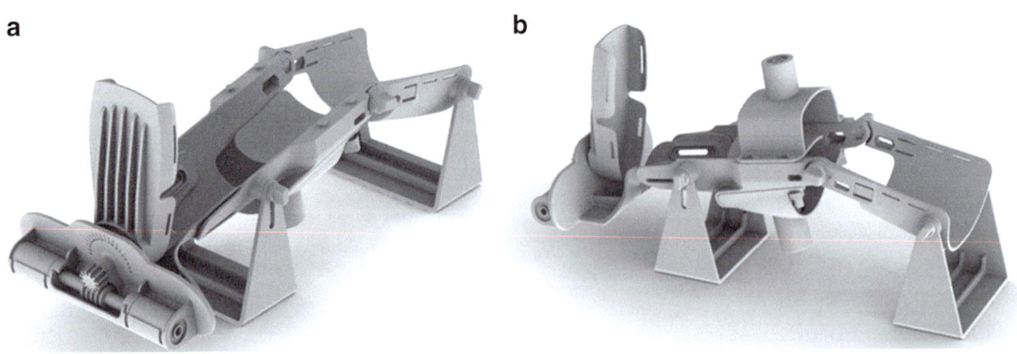

Fig. 3.1 Photograph of Porto-knee testing device. (**a**) PKTD setup for ACL assessment; (**b**) PKTD setup for PCL assessment

at different degrees of knee flexion and to combine the anteroposterior (AP) or posteroanterior (PA) translation with tibial rotation. The dynamic evaluation provided by the wide range of movements allowed by the PKTD in synergy with MRI makes the PKTD a useful tool for objective assessment of the knee ligament injuries. Additionally, it brings new insights to a more detailed anatomical study of the knee, which may be extremely helpful for preoperative planning and postoperative follow-up [24].

3.3.1 Porto-Knee Testing Device: Standard Operation Protocol

The exam starts with the patient supine with the knee flexed at 30° and the foot in neutral position. The first set of images is made without any pressure (Fig. 3.2a). After, it is applied a PA pressure (4 Bar) through a platform containing plunger (activated by pressurized air) at the proximal calf region (Fig. 3.2b). The rotational laxity examination is performed through applying pressure into tibial internal or external rotation by the activation of the rotatory footplate plunger (Fig. 3.2c, d). Whenever possible, this process should be performed also in the contralateral limb to allow side-by-side comparison.

A similar plunger platform may be used superiorly to apply an AP pressure at the proximal third of the tibia, immediately below the tuberosity of the tibia (Fig. 3.3). By this dual approach, it is possible to measure the knee sagittal laxity, assessing both the ACL and the posterior cruciate ligament (PCL).

Placing the knee at 30° of flexion (possible in all MRI machines) and applying a tibial external rotation, the PKTD is able to mimic the dial test for posterolateral corner injuries. This measurement must be compared with the contralateral limb. Additionally, by applying a PA translation, combined with maximum tibial external rotation, it is possible to assess and measure the anteromedial instability.

The measurements are done with sets of 1 mm spacing within the MRI slices. The measurements (in mm) and selection of slices follow the method previously described by Tashiro et al. [25]. The first appearance of the medial portion

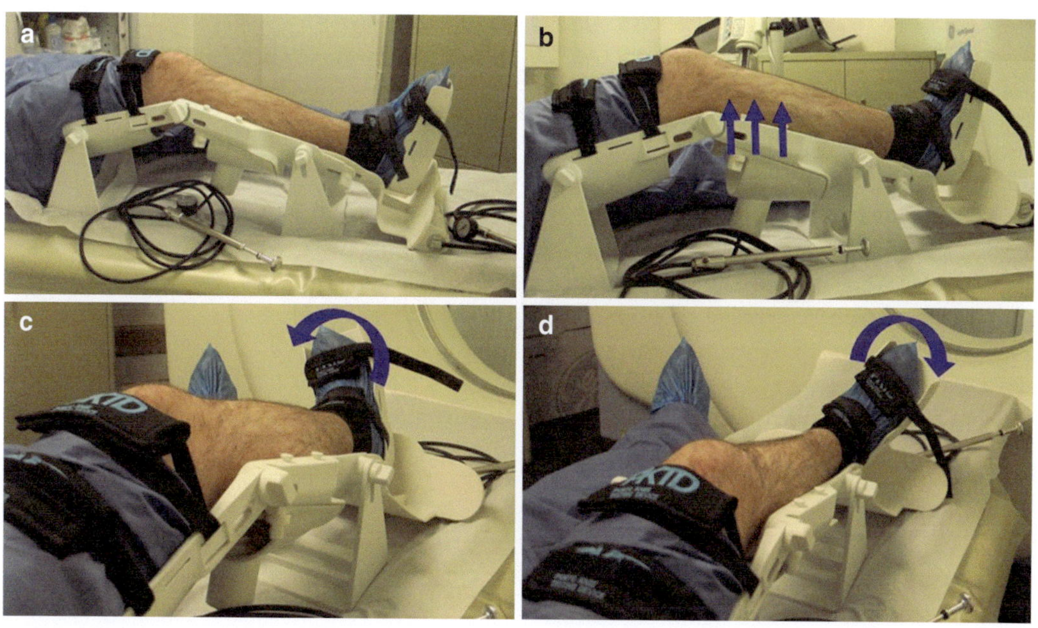

Fig. 3.2 PKTD setting for ACL assessment. The mechanical axis of the device is aligned with the knee joint line, with a 30° angulation. (**a**) Lower limb at rest position (no pressure); (**b**) PA pressure (arrow shows tibial translation); (**c**) tibial internal rotation; and (**d**) tibial external rotation

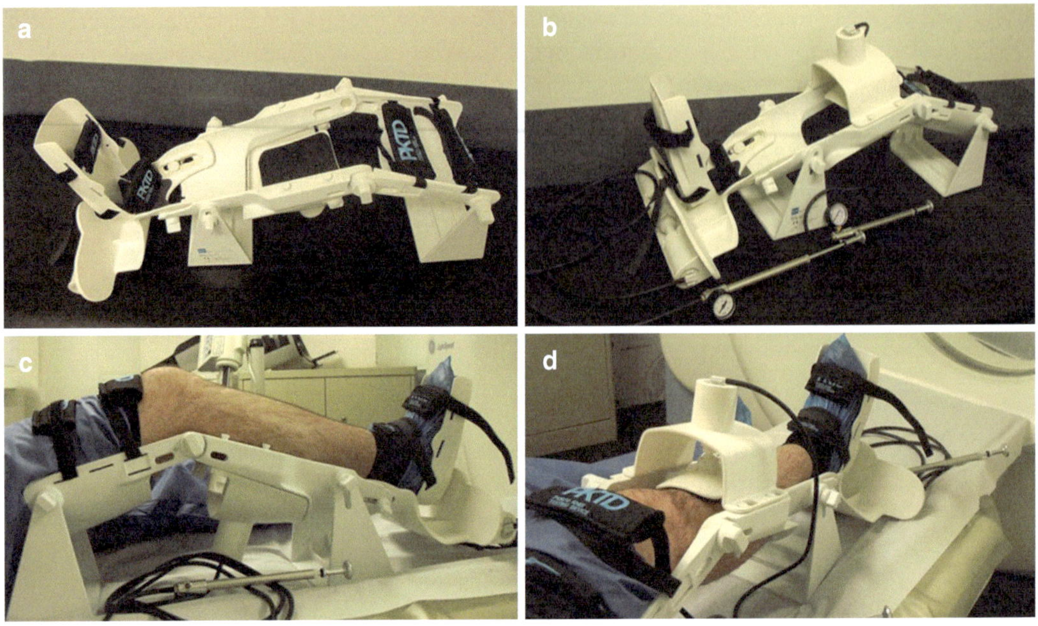

Fig. 3.3 PKTD setting for testing both anterior and posterior cruciate ligaments. (**a**) PKTD setting for testing the ACL; (**b**) By placing a similar plunger platform at the upper part of the device, it is possible to test the PCL; (**c**) PKTD examination with PA translation; and (**d**) PKTD examination with AP translation

of the gastrocnemius proximal insertion determines the reference of the medial plateau. For the lateral plateau, the slice is chosen with reference of the most medial sagittal bone layer of the peroneus. Then, the measurements are performed through a perpendicular line to the tibial slope, crossing the most posterior point of the tibial plateau, and a parallel line, crossing the most posterior point of the femoral condyle. This may be performed to test the presence of ACL, PCL, anteromedial structures, and/or posterolateral corner injuries (Fig. 3.4). The difference between the rest and stress condition determines the amount of tibiofemoral translation. This is measured by the difference between the two drawn parallel lines, as described above.

3.3.2 PKTD Results

PKTD is reliable for sagittal and rotational knee laxity assessment. It showed significant correlation with KT-1000 for PA translation (correlation coefficient = 0.73; $p < 0.05$) and lateral pivot-shift test under anesthesia for rotatory laxity (correlation coefficient = 0.8; $p < 0.05$), with the advantage of evaluation of the knee at any angle of rotation between internal maximum and external maximum tibial rotation [26]. PKTD has shown high sensitivity and specificity in objectively measuring the multiplanar instability, by computing the combined measurements of anterior global translation (PA translation of both medial and lateral tibial plateaus) and global rotation (internal rotation at the lateral tibial plateau plus external rotation at the medial tibial plateau). These measurements showed to be highly specific (anterior global translation, with a cut-off point of 11.1 mm, 93.8%) and sensitive (global rotation, with a cut-off point of 15.1 mm, 92.9%) for total ACL ruptures [27].

3.3.3 PKTD Possible Applications

The PKTD is a valuable medical device for assessing knee multiligament injuries, which should be combined with an accurate clinical examination and MRI evaluation. In this sense,

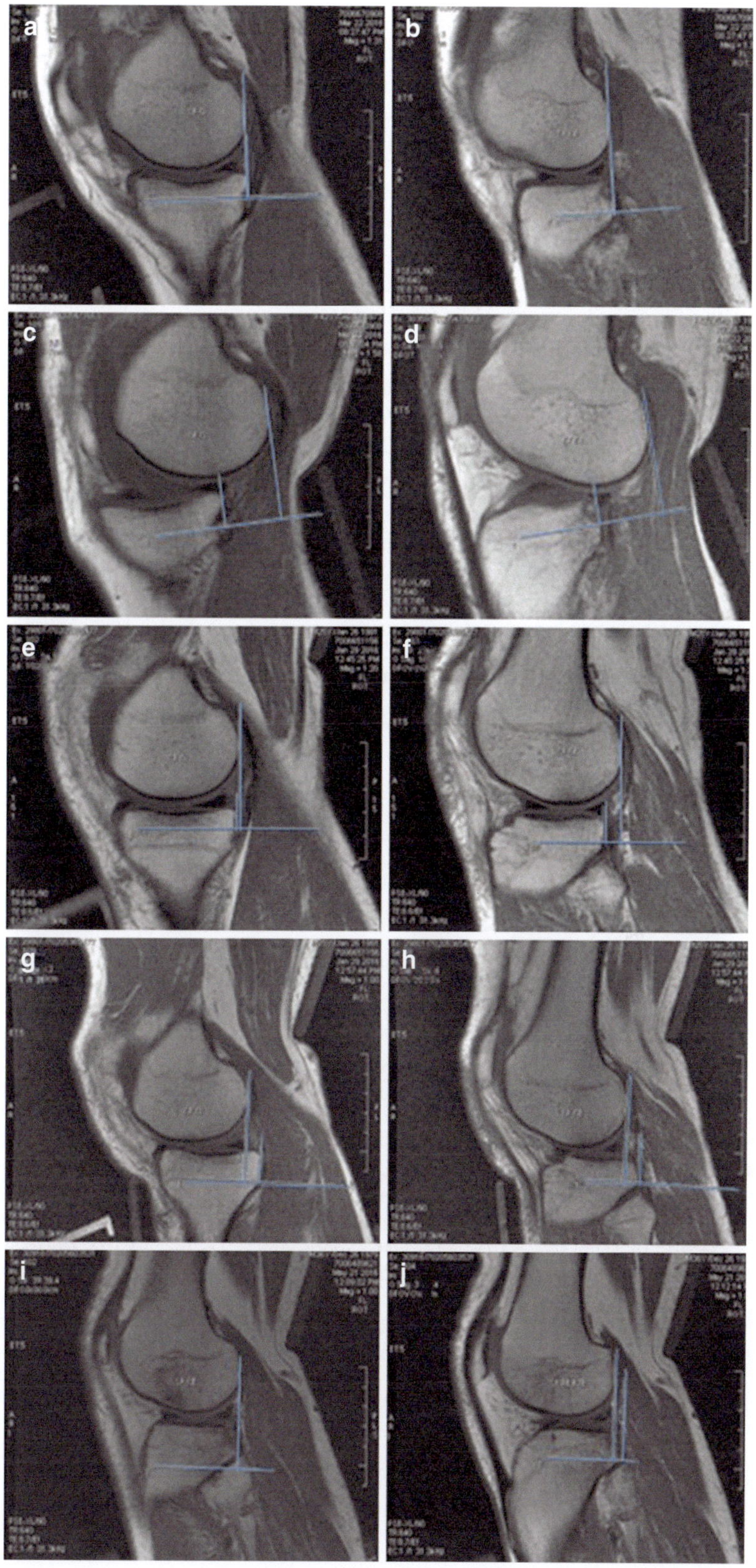

Fig. 3.4 MRI measurements under PKTD examination of an ACL-ruptured patient (**a**–**d**), a PCL-ruptured patient (**e**–**h**), and a posterolateral corner injury (**i**, **j**). (**a**) medial plateau, no stress (−1 mm); (**b**) lateral plateau, no stress (0 mm); (**c**) medial plateau with PA stress (19 mm), the medial tibial plateau translated 20 mm anteriorly; (**d**) lateral plateau PA stress (21 mm), the lateral tibial plateau translated 21 mm anteriorly; (**e**) medial plateau, no stress (1 mm); (**f**) lateral plateau, no stress (8 mm); (**g**) medial plateau with AP stress (−9 mm), the medial tibial plateau translated 10 mm posteriorly; (**h**) lateral plateau AP stress (−7 mm), the lateral tibial plateau translated 15 mm posteriorly; (**i**) lateral plateau, no stress (0 mm); and (**j**) lateral plateau with maximum tibial external rotation (−6 mm), the lateral tibial plateau translated 6 mm posteriorly with the external rotation

the PKTD adds diagnostic value and contributes in the therapeutic decision and surgical planning.

Due to its compatibility with MRI environment, it provides a morphological and functional assessment of the knee ligaments under stressed conditions. Additionally, as it is possible to test both AP and PA translation, in isolation or in combination with tibial rotations, the PKTD is able to test the functional competence of knee sagittal and rotatory restraining structures, which is important in knee multiligament injury evaluation.

In the postoperative follow-up of patients with multiligament knee lesions, the PKTD may be used to evaluate the knee ligamentous laxity and identify any potential residual instability or over-constrain. If it is used concomitantly with CT scanning, it may be useful to evaluate both tibial translations/rotation and the surgical tunnel placement.

In the clinics, this is a very useful tool to perform a 360° evaluation and assessment of knee instability.

References

1. Rihn JA, Cha PS, Groff YJ, Harner CD. The acutely dislocated knee: evaluation and management. J Am Acad Orthop Surg. 2004;12:334–46.
2. Andrade R, Vasta S, Sevivas N, Pereira R, Leal A, Papalia R, et al. Notch morphology is a risk factor for ACL injury: a systematic review and meta-analysis. J ISAKOS. 2016;1:70–81.
3. Fernandes MS, Pereira R, Andrade R, Vasta S, Pereira H, Pinheiro JP, et al. Is the femoral lateral condyle's bone morphology the trochlea of the ACL? Knee Surg Sports Traumatol Arthrosc. 2017;25:207–14.
4. Pereira HFC, Fernandes M, Pereira R, Jones H, Vasconcelos J, Oliveira J, et al. ACL injuries identifiable for pre-participation imagiological analysis: risk factors. In: Doral MN, Karlsson J, editors. Sports injuries: prevention, diagnosis, treatment and rehabilitation: Springer; 2014. p. 1–15.
5. Andrade R, Pereira H, Espregueira-Mendes J. ACL treatment in 2016–controversy and consensus. Asian J Arthrosc. 2016;1:3–10.
6. Pereira H, Gomes S, Silva L, Cunha A, Oliveira JM, Reis RL, et al. Fundamentals on injuries of knee ligaments in footballers. In: Olivera JM, Reis RL, editors. Regenerative strategies for the treatment of knee joint disabilities: Springer; 2017. p. 289–321.
7. Heijink A, Gomoll AH, Madry H, Drobnič M, Filardo G, Espregueira-Mendes J, et al. Biomechanical considerations in the pathogenesis of osteoarthritis of the knee. Knee Surg Sports Traumatol Arthrosc. 2012;20:423–35.
8. Vannini F, Spalding T, Andriolo L, Berruto M, Denti M, Espregueira-Mendes J, et al. Sport and early osteoarthritis: the role of sport in aetiology, progression and treatment of knee osteoarthritis. Knee Surg Sports Traumatol Arthrosc. 2016;24:1786–96.
9. Espregueira-Mendes J, Pereira R, Monteiro A, Pereira H, Sevivas N, Varanda P. Sports and anterior cruciate lesions. Revue de Chirurgie Orthopédique et Traumatologique. 2011;97:S472–S6.
10. Ohashi B, Ward J, Araujo P, Kfuri M, Pereira H, Espregueira-Mendes J, et al. Partial anterior cruciate ligament ruptures: knee laxity measurements and pivot shift. In: Doral MN, Karlsson J, editors. Sports injuries: prevention, diagnosis, treatment and rehabilitation: Springer; 2015. p. 1245–58.
11. Skendzel JG, Sekiya JK, Wojtys EM. Diagnosis and management of the multiligament-injured knee. J Orthop Sports Phys Ther. 2012;42:234–42.
12. Carroll KM, Gregory Cvetanovich M, Heyworth BE, Van de Velde S, Gill TJ IV. Approach to management of the patient with the multiligament-injured knee. Pain. 2013:15.
13. Gimber LH, Scalcione LR, Rowan A, Hardy JC, Melville DM, Taljanovic MS. Multiligamentous injuries and knee dislocations. Skelet Radiol. 2015;44:1559–72.
14. Giaconi JC, Allen CR, Steinbach LS. Anterior cruciate ligament graft reconstruction: clinical, technical, and imaging overview. Top Magn Reson Imaging. 2009;20:129–50.
15. Robertson PL, Schweitzer ME, Bartolozzi AR, Ugoni A. Anterior cruciate ligament tears: evaluation of multiple signs with MR imaging. Radiology. 1994;193:829–34.
16. Tung GA, Davis L, Wiggins M, Fadale P. Tears of the anterior cruciate ligament: primary and secondary signs at MR imaging. Radiology. 1993;188:661–7.
17. Winters K, Tregonning R. Reliability of magnetic resonance imaging of the traumatic knee as determined by arthroscopy. N Z Med J. 2005;118
18. Pereira H, Gomes S, Vasconcelos JC, Soares L, Pereira R, Oliveira JM et al. MRI laxity assessment. In: Musahl V, Karlsson J, Kuroda R, Zaffagnini S. Rotatory knee instability. Springer; 2017. p. 49–61.
19. Behairy NH, Dorgham MA, Khaled SA. Accuracy of routine magnetic resonance imaging in meniscal and ligamentous injuries of the knee: comparison with arthroscopy. Int Orthop. 2009;33:961–7.
20. Rubin DA, Kettering JM, Towers J, Britton C. MR imaging of knees having isolated and combined ligament injuries. AJR Am J Roentgenol. 1998;170:1207–13.
21. Forster I, Warren-Smith C, Tew M. Is the KT1000 knee ligament arthrometer reliable? Bone Joint J. 1989;71:843–7.
22. Graham G, Johnson S, Dent C, Fairclough J. Comparison of clinical tests and the KT1000 in the

diagnosis of anterior cruciate ligament rupture. Br J Sports Med. 1991;25:96–7.
23. Dejour D, Ntagiopoulos PG, Saggin PR, Panisset J-C. The diagnostic value of clinical tests, magnetic resonance imaging, and instrumented laxity in the differentiation of complete versus partial anterior cruciate ligament tears. Arthroscopy. 2013;29:491–9.
24. Pereira H, Sevivas N, Pereira R, Monteiro A, Oliveira JM, Reis R, et al. New tools for diagnosis, assessment of surgical outcome and follow-up. In: Hermoso JAH, Monllau JC, editors. Lesiones ligamentosas de la rodilla; 2012. p. 185–97.
25. Tashiro Y, Okazaki K, Miura H, Matsuda S, Yasunaga T, Hashizume M, et al. Quantitative assessment of rotatory instability after anterior cruciate ligament reconstruction. Am J Sports Med. 2009;37:909–16.
26. Espregueira-Mendes J, Pereira H, Sevivas N, Passos C, Vasconcelos JC, Monteiro A, et al. Assessment of rotatory laxity in anterior cruciate ligament-deficient knees using magnetic resonance imaging with Porto-knee testing device. Knee Surg Sports Traumatol Arthrosc. 2012;20:671–8.
27. Espregueira-Mendes J, Andrade R, Leal A, Pereira H, Skaf A, Rodrigues-Gomes S, et al. Global rotation has high sensitivity in ACL lesions within stress MRI. Knee Surg Sports Traumatol Arthrosc. 2017;25:2993–3003.

Surgical Timing in Combined Ligamentous Injuries

4

Alberto Grassi, Tommaso Roberti di Sarsina, Gian Andrea Lucidi, Federico Raggi, Luca Macchiarola, and Stefano Zaffagnini

4.1 Introduction

Multiligament knee injuries (MLKIs) are a rare condition, making up the 0.02% of the orthopaedic injuries, but are potentially devastating to the patients. The management of such lesions mandates an intimate knowledge of the anatomy on all sides of the joint. In addition to ligamentous injury, the surgeon must also be vigilant for vascular or neurological damage that can often complicate MLKIs.

4.2 Classification

Different classification systems have been proposed for knee dislocations and MLKIs. Kennedy classified knee dislocations (KD) based on the position of the femur relative to the tibia as anterior, posterior, lateral, medial and rotatory with the last ones that are further divided in anteromedial, anterolateral, posteromedial and posterolateral. One limitation of this classification is that it does not consider occult or spontaneously reduced knee dislocation.

The anatomic classification developed by Schenck is more focused on the ligament involved during the injury and ranges from KD-I (tear of one cruciate ligament) to KD-IV (disruption of all four ligaments). If an associated fracture is present, the lesion is defined as KD-V. Neurological (N) and vascular (C) damages are also taken into account.

These classifications are useful to define the prognosis and compare different case series; however, due to the complex pattern of knee injury, it is useful to describe MLKIs based on specific anatomic structures involved and the grade of injury. The treatment strategy should be tailored for each patient, considering the joint kinematics, patient expectations and the healing potential of the damaged structures (Table 4.1).

Table 4.1 Schenck's classification of knee dislocation

Anatomic classification of knee dislocation	
Classification	Description
KD-I	Single ligament injury (ACL or PCL)
KD–II	Bicruciate injury (ACL + PCL)
KD-III	Bicruciate injury and either LCL or MCL
KD-III injuries are classified as KD-III-M if MCL is injured or KD-III-L if the LCL or PLC are injured	
KD-IV	Injury to ACL, PCL, LCL and MCL
KD-V	Multiligamentous injury with periarticular fracture

ACL anterior cruciate ligament, *PCL* posterior cruciate ligament, *LCL* lateral collateral ligament, *MCL* medial collateral ligament, *PLC* posterolateral corner

A. Grassi · T. Roberti di Sarsina · G. A. Lucidi (✉)
F. Raggi · L. Macchiarola · S. Zaffagnini
Department of Orthopaedic Surgery, II Clinic, Rizzoli Institute Bologna, Bologna, BO, Italy
e-mail: gianandrea.lucidi@studio.unibo.it

F. Margheritini et al. (eds.), *Complex Knee Ligament Injuries*,
https://doi.org/10.1007/978-3-662-58245-9_4

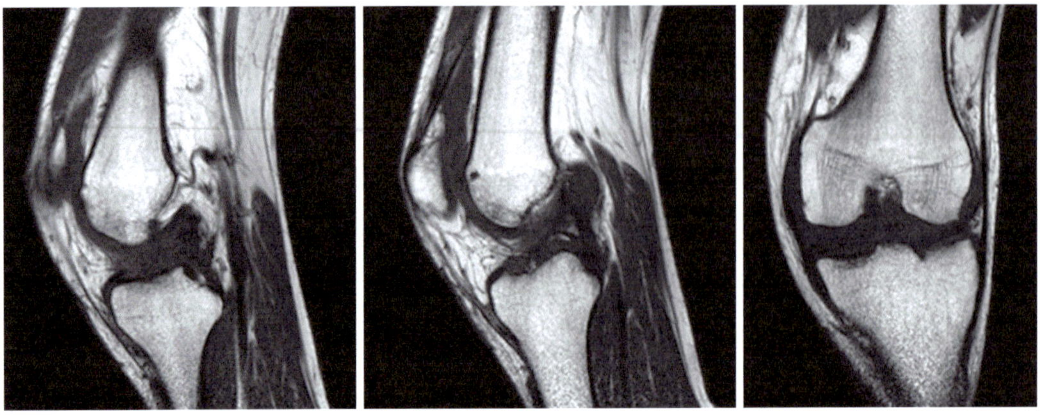

Fig. 4.1 A 30-year-old man with knee dislocation III according to Schenk's classification (ACL, PCL, MCL injury). The patient sustained a high-energy dislocation after a motor vehicle accident

KDs are also divided into high-energy trauma (e.g. motor vehicle collision, falling from heights, etc.) or low-energy trauma (e.g. sports injuries, etc.) and ultralow-velocity injuries (often minor trauma in morbidly obese). The patients of the first group could be polytrauma patients with multiple fractures and more often have neurovascular lesions: these associated pressing injuries could alter the ideal surgical timing (Fig. 4.1).

4.3 Evaluation: Acute Management

In case of polytrauma patients, the initial evaluation follows the ATLS (Advanced Trauma Life Support) protocol: if the patient does not present more pressing injuries and the knee is dislocated, radiographs (with a portable tool) should be taken. In case of major tibia or femur fracture, the surgeon must take into account the risk of further bony fragment dislocation during the manoeuvres. Knee reduction should be attempted in patients under sedation, and subsequent radiographs must be taken to confirm the correct position of the femur relative to the tibia. If the knee remains grossly unstable, the surgeon should apply an articulated external fixator for at least 1 month. The knee should also be inspected for the presence of open injury; in this case, subsequent irrigation and debridement in the operating room are mandatory.

4.4 Vascular Status: Management

After a successful reduction of the knee, attention should be then turned to the vascular status (Fig. 4.2).

In case of acute knee dislocation, the overall incidence of vascular injury is around 20% and is correlated with devastating complication such infection, compartment syndrome and limb amputation. In fact, the anatomic location of the popliteal artery put it at high risk during KD. Posterior dislocation produces shearing forces that cause intimal tearing and arterial transaction, while anterior dislocation causes traction injury. Since it has been shown that the total ischemia time greater than 6–8 h is directly correlated with amputation rate, a prompt identification and management of such lesion are crucial. Some authors advocate routine angiography after KD regardless of pulse examination because of the possibility of subintimal artery damage that can be overlooked. However, a protocol of careful physical examination, ABI (ankle-brachial index) and selective angiography are currently supported by the literature.

The physical examination can show hard signs of ischemia such as pallor, cool skin and delayed capillary refill time. The posterior tibial and dorsalis pedis pulse examination is mandatory and should be compared with the healthy limb. However, the presence of a normal pulse after the

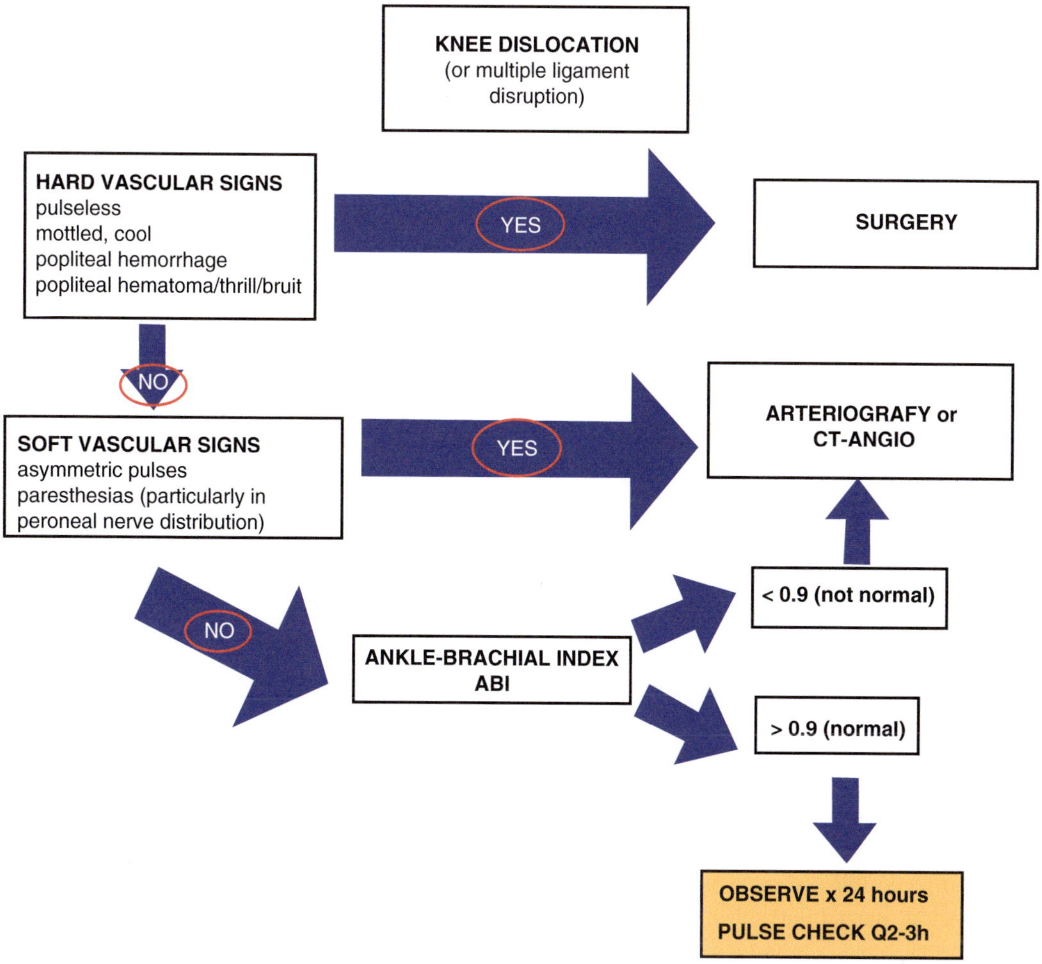

Fig. 4.2 Flowchart for the assessment and treatment of vascular associated lesion in the context of knee dislocation

knee reduction does not rule out vascular injury, and on the contrary, vasospasm is common and can be a pitfall during the examination. Particularly insidious are popliteal artery intimal flap lesion that are at risk for delayed thrombosis [1]. Therefore, ABI should be evaluated in all patients even in the presence of symmetric pulses. Patients with ABI <0.9 warrant selective angiography and, if positive, further vascular surgeon counsel and management. However, if the ABI is greater than 0.9 the physician should continue to check the pulses every 2 h for 24 h.

The decision to perform prophylactic fasciotomy is difficult, but if vascular involvement is confirmed, this surgical procedure is recommended to reduce the risk of compartment syndrome [1].

4.5 Neurologic Status: Management

Attention should be then turned to the neurologic examination. The incidence of nerve injury in the literature ranges from 10% to 40%. Interestingly, the highest nerve injury rate has been found in high-velocity and ultralow-velocity dislocations rather than in low-energy traumas.

Usually, the common peroneal nerve (CPN) is injured; however, in rare conditions, an isolated tibial nerve palsy has been described. The anatomic course of the CPN and the presence of constraints proximally (fibular neck) and distally (arches of the intermuscular septum) that reduces movement compliance put it at high risk during KD. Additionally, anatomical studies have shown the lack of intraneural vessels in the fibular region and therefore a deficient CPN blood supply. In case of CPN involvement, the recovery is usually poor: Niall et al. [2] described full recovery in 21% of patients, partial motor function in 29% and 50% of the patient with neither motor nor sensory function. CPN palsy are more likely to occur during an anterior or lateral dislocation; additionally, the CPN is vulnerable to stretch injury during varus stress, particularly if PLC or PCL tears are present.

The physical examination includes assessment of sensation in the tibial, superficial and deep peroneal nerve distribution. Motor examination includes evaluation of graded motor strength of the flexor and extensor hallucis longus, tibialis anterior and gastrocnemius.

The majority of CPN damage is stretch injury that could be treated with physiotherapy and ankle-foot orthosis to prevent equinus foot. If CPN transection is suspected or directly visualized through open injury, then an acute repair must be performed. Similarly, if the CPN status is gradually deteriorating since the time of injury, an emergent decompression surgery is highly recommended. At the time of multiligament reconstruction, if CPN palsy is still present, neurolysis should be performed in the presence of scar tissue. In cases of chronic CPN palsy, ankle-foot orthosis or tendon transfer surgery are valid options to improve function.

4.6 Imaging

After the rule out of vascular injuries and before physical examination, prereduction radiographs in two planes (anteroposterior and lateral) should be obtained. These are helpful to evaluate associated fractures and the direction of the dislocation. Fractures are associated with KD in 10% to 20% of the cases and, if present, can modify the approach. These fractures can either involve large bony fragments such as tibial plateau and distal femur or can be avulsion fractures such as the arcuate or Segond fracture or tibial spine avulsion. The treatment consists in ligament reconstruction, and if the bony fragment is large enough, it can require internal fixation.

Post-reduction radiographs should then be taken to assess the knee alignment and stability. Stress radiograph is not usually needed in the acute setting but in the preoperative evaluation to assess, objectively, ligamentous instability. If there is concern for intra-articular fracture, a CT scan is recommended to further evaluate the need for surgical management. MRI is also important to elucidate the extent of ligament injuries, menisci involvement and osteochondral damage. For its crucial role, an MRI should be obtained in the acute phase if an external fixation is planned; otherwise, the implant creates artefacts that do not allow a correct imaging evaluation.

4.7 Physical Evaluation

Physical examination in the acute phase is often difficult due to patient pain, knee swelling, muscular contracture and associated injuries; however, gross instability of the main ligaments should be assessed and documented. Intra-articular injection of anaesthetic after aspiration of hemarthrosis can reduce patient discomfort. If the patient still complains about pain, then the evaluation can be performed in the operating room under general anaesthesia (Table 4.2).

The Lachman test and the anterior drawer test are usually performed to evaluate the ACL. The third ACL test, the pivot shift, cannot be performed in the acute setting unless the patient is under anaesthesia.

Varus/valgus stress test, posterior drawer test and posterior sag sign can be useful to evaluate the presence of MCL/LCL or PCL injuries. Other evaluation manoeuvres are the reverse pivot shift test (PCL), dial test (PLC), Apley and McMurray (menisci), but again, in an acute setting, the reliability of these tests is limited.

Table 4.2 Principal tests used for the clinical examination of the knee

Test	Utility
Lachman test	ACL injury (anterior translation increases if combined PLC injury is present)
Pivot shift test	ACL injury
External rotation recurvatum test	Combined ACL and PLC injury
Dial test	10° side-to-side difference at 30° of flexion but not at 90° of flexion: Isolated PLC injury 10° side-to-side difference at both 30° and 90° of knee flexion: Combined PLC and PCL injury
Posterior sag sign	PCL
Posterior drawer test	8 mm side-to-side difference: PCL injury>12 mm side-to-side difference: PCL and PLC injury
Posterolateral drawer test	PLC injury
Valgus stress test	MCL: – 1–2 mm of gap in full extension indicates combined sMCL and ACL injury – gapping at 20° of knee flexion indicates sMCL injury
Varus stress test	LCL: at 20° of knee flexion, increases if PCL is injured

4.7.1 Nonoperative Treatment

The nonoperative treatment has historically represented the standard of care for decades. Current literature advocates surgery in order to improve range of motion, stability, return to daily activity and return to sport. However, in some cases, nonoperative management should be still considered. In polytrauma patients, surgery should be delayed until general health condition is restored and the patients are able to perform postoperative physiotherapy.

The integrity of the soft tissues should also be taken into account, particularly in the presence of blisters, abrasions and degloving injuries. These areas must be avoided until soft tissues have healed properly. In this case, photo documentation is recommended, and the plastic surgeon should be informed as soon as possible.

However, we must remember that because of the intrinsic instability of the lateral side of the knee, due to the lack of congruence between the lateral femoral condyle and the convex tibial plateau, lateral ligament injuries have less tendency to heal nonoperatively if compared to the structure on the medial side.

4.7.2 Surgical Timing

The timing of surgical treatment of MLKIs should be individualized taking into account the ligaments injured, the neurovascular and skin condition and the patient's general health condition. It can be classified in acute, early (within 3 weeks from injury) or delayed. Another classification system is between a single-stage approach, in which all the injured ligaments are repaired or reconstructed together, and a staged approach, in which the medial or lateral structure are treated with or without the PCL (posterior cruciate ligament) in the early period and the ACL (anterior cruciate ligament) is reconstructed in a second surgical time.

Acute surgery is generally not performed. However, there are some conditions that warrant an urgent approach: open knee dislocation, vascular injury and "irreducible" knee dislocation. In this case, the medial femoral condyle is forced through the capsule medially, and the medial joint capsule remains compressed between the articular surfaces; in this setting the knee cannot be reduced manually, and prompt surgery is mandatory. In this setting, if arthroscopy is performed, the surgeon must be aware that the presence of a damaged capsule can lead to fluid extravasation and compartment syndrome, thus contraindicating such procedure.

Some authors perform surgery after a period of 2–3 weeks from injury: this delay allows inflammatory phase to subside and the restoration of the range of motion, reducing the risk of arthrofibrosis. Preoperative deficient ROM (range of motion) can negatively affect the surgical outcome; for this reason it is important to reach an adequate motion before proceeding with surgery.

Other authors advocate an early reconstruction: a systematic review conducted by Levy et al. has reported higher functional outcome,

IKDC and sports activity score in patients treated within 3 weeks. Controversies exist, but it is clear that the timing of surgical treatment should be tailored for each patient taking into account the neurovascular, skin and patient's general health condition as well as ligaments injured.

If we consider an injury of the medial side of the knee, the treatment of choice is bracing and protected weight-bearing followed by cruciate reconstruction; this will allow the MCL (medial collateral ligament) to heal properly. However, attention should be paid in case of tibial side avulsion of the MCL: its close relation with the pes anserinus can potentially lead to a "Stener phenomenon" of the knee. In this case, the presence of a tendon within the damaged MCL prevents the native ligament from healing. In such condition surgery is recommended to repair or reconstruct the avulsed MCL, and concomitant ACL/PCL surgery can also be performed.

Also on the lateral side, there are conditions that require early surgical intervention: high-grade fibular avulsion of the biceps and grade III LCL (lateral collateral ligament) lesions should be treated early in order to avoid excessive scar formation and soft tissue retraction.

4.7.3 Order of Ligament Fixation

Some biomechanical studies can guide the surgeon while deciding which ligament should be tensioned first in the setting of MLKI.

ACL + MCL or PCL (posterolateral Corner) + MCL.

In the contest of MLKIs surgery, if the reconstruction of the MCL is indicated, the author usually performs a single-bundle superficial MCL reconstruction. If MCL and concomitant tear of ACL or PCL are present, Laprade et al. suggest to pass the cruciate graft (ACL or PCL) into the femur and fix them at this point without securing them to the tibia. The second step should be the MCL graft placement in their femoral tunnel, and lastly, the cruciate graft could be secured at the tibial attachment sites (Geeslin and Laprade [3]).

ACL + PLC or PCL + PLC.

If the PLC is injured together with ACL or PCL, varus stress increases the load on the cruciate grafts. For this reason, it is reasonable to repair or reconstruct the PLC together with the ACL or PCL to unload the immature graft. In this setting, the fixation of the PLC graft should be done before the fixation of the ACL graft: this will avoid an external rotation of the tibia.

However, for a combined PCL and PLC injury, the PCL graft should be tensioned and fixed prior to the PLC graft fixation (Wentorf et al. [4]).

ACL + PCL + PLC.

In this setting, the PCL graft needs to be secured first in order to restore the central pivot of the knee, then the ACL is fixed, and lastly the PLC.

4.7.4 Author's Suggested Protocol in Complex Cases (KD-IV and KD-V)

In complex cases, when all the four major ligaments of the knee are injured or when associated lesions, such as knee fractures or neurovascular injuries, coexisted, an external fixator (better if an articulated one) is recommended. Main indications for the external fixator are (1) unstable knee after successful reduction and (2) tenuous vascular repair that needs protection.

In these cases we recommend an open reduction surgery with the standard medial parapatellar arthrotomy and, when possible, a single-bundle PCL reconstruction using hamstring tendons. Concurrently, the authors recommend to reconstruct or repair the lateral and the medial structures if they were severely damaged and internally fixate any associated fractures in the acute setting. After PCL reconstruction and/or caring of the other associated lesions, a dynamic external fixator should be applied (Fig. 4.3). The device used in our institution allows only movements in the sagittal plane with a reduced ROM (0°–100°). However, in certain patients, this protocol could not be applied: (1) in KD-V cases where associ-

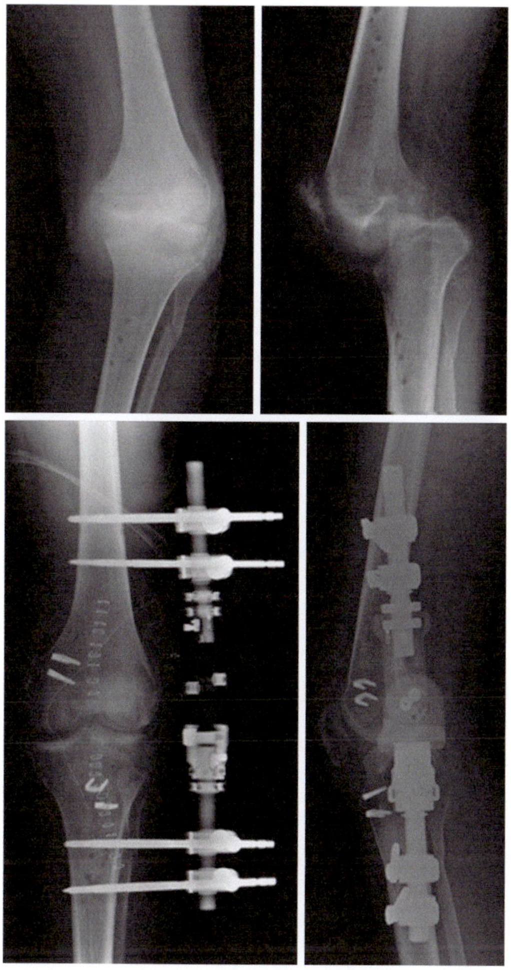

Fig. 4.3 The two pictures above are preoperative of dynamic external fixator used in knee dislocation IV or V: in this case a concomitant PCL reconstruction was performed as illustrated in X-rays below

ated tibial or femoral fractures compromise the ability to perform the tunnels; (2) if there is a wide knee exposure that increase the risk of infection; and (3) in case of severe vascular injury. In these patients, we suggest to surgically treat the associated lesions but to delay the reconstruction of the injured ligaments. Postoperative rehabilitation should start the day after surgery with continuous passive motion for the first week, partial weight-bearing and isometric exercises. For the next 3 weeks, we recommend active ROM with no motion restriction. Patients should begin to walk and perform partial weight-bearing and isometric exercises the day after surgery. We suggest to remove the EF 1 month after surgery and check stability and ROM.

In a series of 8 cases with KD-IV or KD-V treated with this protocol, Marcacci et al. reported Lysholm score of 77, a Tegner level of 4 and a subjective IKDC of 73 at 3 months of follow-up. All patients recovered their preinjury work activity except one unemployed patient. Based on IKDC assessment, stability was normal in one patient, nearly normal in four patients and abnormal in three patients. This surgical approach to complex high-energy knee dislocations resulted in more than 60% of normal or nearly normal knees. These data are similar to those reported in the literature [5]. Moreover, the opportunity to stage surgery while protecting soft tissues and limiting the risk of knee stiffness allowed for later ligament reconstruction to be performed, similar to that performed for isolated ligament injuries.

4.7.5 Clinical Case

A 21-year-old female had ski trauma with knee dislocation: LCP lesion, PLC lesion and bucket handle tear of lateral meniscus. In emergency femoropopliteal bypass was performed due to acute popliteal ischemia, and after 1 day she underwent fasciotomy for compartmental syndrome and external fixation (Fig. 4.4). After 4 weeks the external fixator was removed. After 4 weeks, we performed one-stage surgical reconstruction of PCL and MCL using a single Achilles

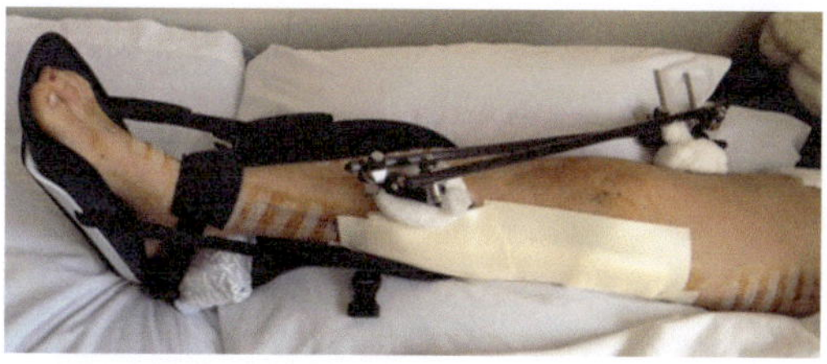

Fig. 4.4 Spanning external fixator was applied in order to stabilize the knee joint and avoid stress on the neovascular graft

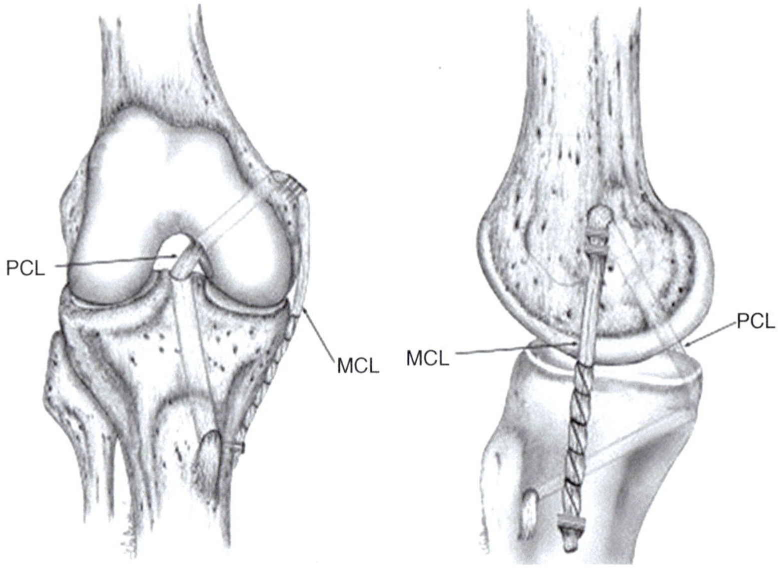

Fig. 4.5 Front and lateral illustrations of the original technique developed by Prof Marcacci and Prof Zaffagnini for treating a combined PCL and MCL lesion. The semintendonous graft is prepared leaving the tibial insertion intact. The graft is than passed through a tunnel inside the joint, passed through a tunnel in the medial femoral condile and then secured on the medial side of the knee

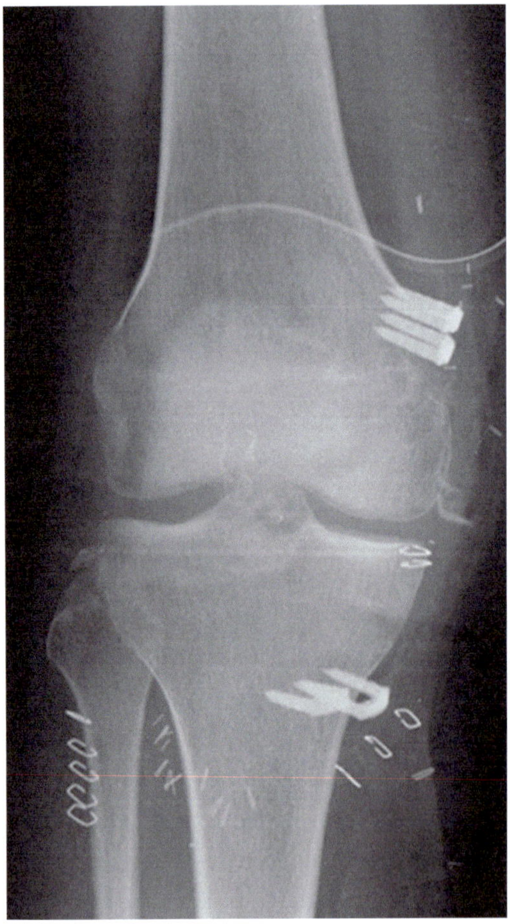

Fig. 4.6 Post-op X-ray of the presented case

tendon allograft that was divided into two parts (Figs. 4.5, 4.6).

References

1. Farber A, Tan TW, Hamburg N, Kalish JA, Joglar F, Onigman T, Rybin D, Doros G, Eberhardt RT. Early fasciotomy in patients with extremity vascular injury is associated with decreased risk of adverse limb outcomes: a review of the National Trauma Data Bank. Injury. 2012;43(9):1486–91.
2. Niall DM1, Nutton RW, Keating JF. Palsy of the common peroneal nerve after traumatic dislocation of the knee. J Bone Joint Surg Br. 2005;87(5):664–7.
3. Geeslin AG, LaPrade RF. Outcomes of treatment of acute grade-III isolated and combined posterolateral knee injuries: a prospective case series and surgical technique. J Bone Joint Surg Am. 2011;93(18):1672–83.
4. Wentorf FA, LaPrade RF, Lewis JL, Resig S. The influence of the integrity of posterolateral structures on tibiofemoral orientation when an anterior cruciate ligament graft is tensioned. Am J Sports Med. 2002;30:796–9.
5. Kowalk DL, Wojtys EM, Loubert JD. Quantitative analysis of the measuring capabilities of the KT-1000 knee ligament arthrometer. Am J Sports Med. 1993;21:744–7.

Part II

Surgical Techniques

Traumatic Knee Injuries

5

Steffen Sauer and Mark Clatworthy

5.1 Patella Dislocation

5.1.1 Background

The patella represents the largest sesamoid bone of the human body and is incorporated into the quadriceps tendon. Patella dislocations are a common sports-related knee injury and defined as the complete disengagement of the patella from the trochlear groove. According to the consistency and associated trauma mechanism, patella dislocations may be subdivided into traumatic, recurrent and habitual dislocations. Traumatic (inaugural/single) dislocations are usually the result of a relevant trauma, typically a pivoting manoeuvre with a twisting movement about the flexed knee [1]. Recurrent (several) patella dislocations usually occur during normal activities and are facilitated by dysplastic changes in the patellofemoral joint [2, 3]. Habitual patella dislocation is defined as the consistent dislocation of the patella whenever the knee is flexed. Predisposing factors of patella dislocation include genu valgum, patella alta, increased distance between the tuberositas tibia and the trochlear groove (TTTG distance) as well as increased internal rotation and anteversion of the femur [1, 4]. The patella usually dislocates laterally, leading to a rupture of the medial patellofemoral ligament (MPFL). Subsequently, the lack of medial retrain supported by the MPFL may lead to patellar instability and recurrent dislocation, especially in cases with associated bony dysplasia or muscle weakness. Spontaneous reposition is usually seen, otherwise emergency reduction is required.

5.1.2 Symptoms

Symptoms arising from patella dislocation are frequently related to the preceding trauma and type of dislocation. Traumatic first-time patella dislocation usually provokes medial para-patellar pain as a result of capsular disruption which is often followed by rapid onset of effusion. However, effusion may be absent, especially in recurrent dislocations where giving way and locking may be the leading symptoms.

5.1.3 Diagnosis

The diagnosis is typically made with the patella reduced as the vast majority of patella dislocations undergo spontaneous reduction. Clinical

S. Sauer (✉)
Department of Sports Traumatology, Aarhus University Hospital, Aarhus, Denmark
e-mail: stefsaue@rm.dk

M. Clatworthy
Department of Orthopaedic Surgery, Middlemore Hospital, Auckland, New Zealand

F. Margheritini et al. (eds.), *Complex Knee Ligament Injuries*,
https://doi.org/10.1007/978-3-662-58245-9_5

examination will usually reveal pain or a depression upon palpation of the medial retinaculum, usually disrupted during the dislocation. Pain during patellofemoral compression or palpation of the lateral condyle is usually present as a result of the patellofemoral collision during the dislocation. A positive apprehension sign when the examiner attempts to manually reproduce the luxation may be present and is thought to be pathognomonic for patella dislocation. In patients with recurrent patella luxation, patellar maltracking may become evident with a positive J-sign when the knee is extended. Massive effusion is typically seen in association with osteochondral lesions.

5.1.4 Imaging

Radiographs may visualize irregularities in the contour of the lateral femoral condyle and/or the medial patella facet consistent with osteochondral fractures. CT scanning should be performed if osteochondral lesions are suspected. MRI is used to visualize bone bruising as a result of the patellofemoral collision (Fig. 5.1) and identify eventual concomitant ligamentous or meniscal lesions. Furthermore, MRI is used to identify the degree of patellofemoral malalignment including the TTTG distance which has implications for the indication of surgical realignment procedures, such as tibial tubercle osteotomies.

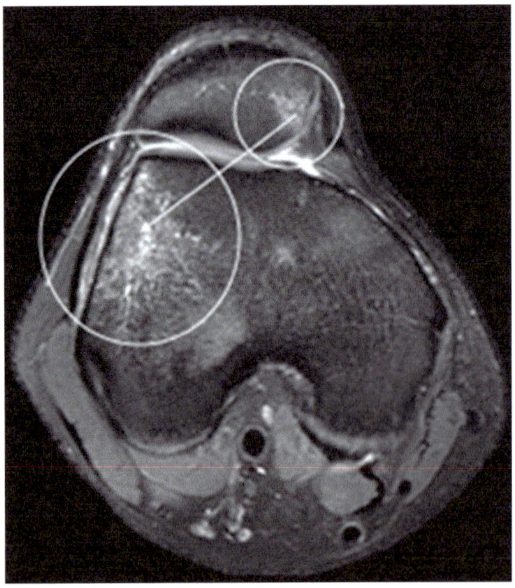

Fig. 5.1 Bone bruising following patellofemoral collision during luxation

5.1.5 Treatment

If the patella is dislocated, emergency reduction in indicated; the knee is hereby extended and the patella is reduced centrally. Following spontaneous or manual reduction of first-time patella dislocation, a conservative treatment approach is indicated [4]. This may entail RICE (rest, ice, compression, elevation), initial knee immobilization and progressive muscle strengthening. Knee arthroscopy may be indicated in the setting of chondral damage or osteochondral lesions that require refixation [1]. In recurrent cases of patella dislocation, surgical stabilization of the patella by either repairing or reconstructing the MPFL is indicated. However, there is no reliable data regarding joint stability or patient satisfaction after either conservative or operative treatment. Procedures that aim for correction of dysplasia as trochleoplasties should be reserved for cases in which basic surgery has failed.

5.1.6 Take-Home Message

The majority of first-time patella dislocations can be treated conservatively. However, acute CT scan is indicated in cases with massive knee effusion to identify eventual osteochondral lesions which are suitable for subacute refixation [1].

5.1.7 Treatment Algorithm

First-time patella dislocation	Conservative treatment
Recurrent patella dislocation	MPFL reconstruction
First-time patella dislocation with osteochondral lesion	Osteochondral refixation if possible and MPFL reconstruction

5.1.8 Facts

- Common injury.
- The vast majority of patella dislocations relocate spontaneously.
- MRI may be useful to identify typical bone bruising from patellofemoral collision when anamnesis is inconclusive.

5.2 Meniscus Injury

5.2.1 Background

Meniscal lesions are among the most common injuries of the knee joint and the most frequent indication for knee arthroscopy. Meniscal lesions are more often degenerative than traumatic in origin and classified after location (medial/lateral, anterior/posterior) and by morphology (longitudinal, radial, horizontal, flap tear type, bucket handle type). Bucket-handle tears are further classified in accordance to location and associated meniscal blood supply from the geniculate artery which has implications for healing potential (white-white zone, red-white zone, red-red zone) [5]. Meniscal lesions of the menisco-capsular junction area (ramp lesions) and the meniscal root area are further classified in accordance to specific injury pattern, which has implications for treatment procedures [6]. The medial meniscus is more frequently injured than the lateral meniscus due to its more rigid tibial and capsular attachment [7]. However, in association with ACL injures, lateral meniscal tears including root injuries are reported to be more frequent compared to medial meniscal tears [8]. The latter, however, may be easily missed during arthroscopy if the posterior menisco-capsular junction area of the medial meniscus is not thoroughly inspected [6]. The medial meniscus does not only account for half of the shock capacity of the medial compartment but does also restrain the tibia from anterior translation [9]. This is the reason why a large number of patients with ACL injuries have concomitant tears of the medial meniscus [7]. The lateral meniscus is more mobile compared to the medial meniscus. As the knee moves, the lateral meniscus moves back and forth across the tibia and is hereby stabilized by menisco-femoral ligaments. As the lateral meniscus can absorb up to 70% of the shock to the lateral compartment of the knee, total lateral meniscectomy is commonly associated with rapid onset of OA. Recently, the role of the lateral meniscus for rotational knee stability has become more evident which has emphasized the importance of meniscal root repairs for better ACLR outcomes [10]. Over time, menisci become more rigid and the incidence of degenerative meniscal tears increases. Especially in association with osteoarthritis, degenerative lesions of the posterior horn of the medial meniscus are frequently seen. There is an emerging body of literature challenging the beneficial effect of partial meniscectomy as a treatment strategy of these lesions [11, 12]. Traumatic meniscal lesions usually arise from a twisting movement about the flexed knee with the ipsilateral foot planted; the resulting compressive and rotational forces cause the meniscus to tear. Degenerative lesions usually show a subtle debut without a history of preceding trauma.

5.2.2 Symptoms

Symptoms arising from meniscal tears are frequently related to location, morphology and origin of the lesion. Purely traumatic meniscal lesions are associated with a sudden onset of focal pain after a rotational knee trauma. However, the degree of instant posttraumatic pain is variable. Patients sustaining small tears without tissue displacement usually proceed with sports activities. Severe tears are associated with more significant pain, and especially in bucket-handle meniscus lesions, hemarthrosis and reduced range of knee motion is usually present. However, a complete bucket-handle lesion may be luxated anteriorly without compromising range of knee motion. Other symptoms of meniscal injury include click sensation, catching and instability due to proprioceptive misinformation caused by the interference of meniscal tissue. Instability may eventually be aggravated by cruciate or collateral ligament injuries. Degenerative lesions often show a subtle debut of diffuse pain without preceding trauma. The ability to squat is usually compromised. A serous effusion and quadriceps atrophy may be encountered.

5.2.3 Diagnosis

The diagnosis of meniscal tears is based on anamnesis followed by clinical examination. Partial, horizontal and anterior meniscal tears without mechanical interference may present without clinical findings. Meniscal injuries are typically associated with pain upon palpation of the respective joint line and may be aggravated by a variety of meniscal provocation tests. The accuracy of the physical examination is dependent on the type of injury and the observer [13]. Among the most important tests are McMurray's test (pain or popping sensation over the joint line during external tibial rotation under repeated passive flexion/extension) [13], the Steinmann I sign (pain during passive knee rotation) and the Thessaly test [14]. The latter has recently been popularized as loading forces on the menisci are simulated; the patient stands hereby on one leg with the knee flexed while actively rotating the knee and body. Pain or locking constitutes a positive test. As no isolated test is highly conclusive, a combination of meniscal provocation tests is recommended, and multiple positive findings with a history of relevant trauma suggest a meniscal injury. A negative test does not exclude a meniscal lesion. Hemarthrosis and reduced range of motion are commonly seen in association with displaced meniscal tears. However, a displaced bucket-handle tear extending into the anterior horn of the meniscus is associated with little or no loss of extension.

5.2.4 Imaging

MRI represents the main imaging modality for the diagnosis of meniscal tears and shows high sensitivity and specificity. Especially when range of knee motion is compromised, MRI should be performed to visualize meniscal injuries that require immediate attention [15]. Generally, however, MRI findings need to be interpreted in relation to clinical findings. Mucoid degeneration of the meniscus, which is associated with an increased signal from the centre of the meniscus, is a common finding and should not be misinterpreted as a traumatic tear. Recently, the role of MRI in the diagnosis of degenerative meniscus injuries has been challenged as consecutive arthroscopic procedures are rarely indicated.

5.2.5 Treatment

The treatment of meniscal tears should depend on location, morphology, origin as well as the correlation of meniscal injuries with clinical symptoms and associated lesions. Other factors affecting treatment procedures include patient age and activity level. In general, treatment of meniscal lesions should always aim to restore the best possible function of the meniscus, consequently reducing pain [9]. Bucket-handle lesions (Fig. 5.2a, b) with high healing potential should be reinserted, regardless of patient age. Different methods are hereby used including all-inside, inside-out and outside-in suturing techniques, which are mostly dependent on lesion accessibility [16, 17]. Isolated meniscal lesions without mechanical symptoms and chondral erosion may initially be treated conservatively. Partial meniscectomy is indicated for cases in which resection of disfunctional meniscal tissue is believed to optimize meniscal pressure distribution by restoring a sharp meniscal rim, e.g. in flap-tear lesions or radial tears. However, it must be kept in mind that the loss of functional meniscal tissue may enhance chondral degeneration [18, 19] (Fig. 5.3). Unstable meniscal lesions that affect the meniscal root or ramp areas should be addressed, especially in the setting of concomitant ACL injury. Meniscal root avulsions should be reattached through a transtibial tunnel [20, 21]. Unstable meniscal ramp lesions are best addressed with an all-inside or inside-out suturing technique through an additional posteromedial portal [22]. In contrast, degenerative lesions with underlying OA without meniscal displacement and mechanical symptoms

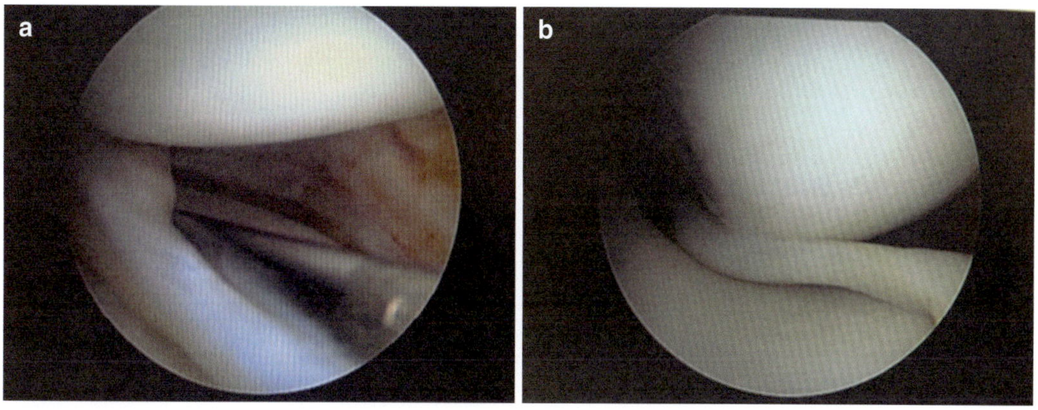

Fig. 5.2 Acute bucket-handle meniscus lesion. (**a**) (left): a small meniscal rim can be seen where the meniscus has been detached from the capsule. (**b**) (right): interfering meniscal tissue lying between the femur and tibia may cause an extension deficit

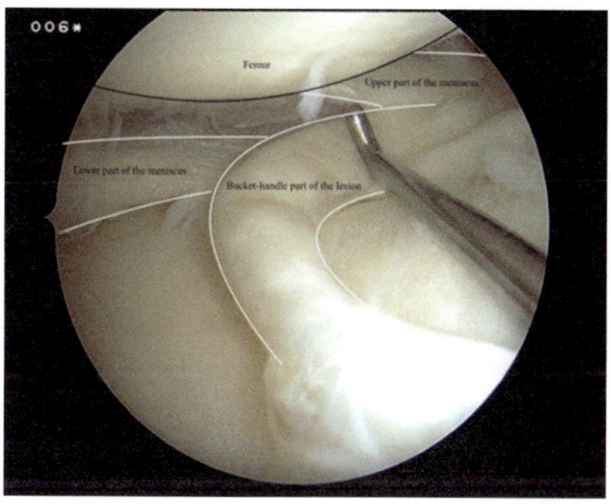

Fig. 5.3 Complex meniscus injury. The central part of the meniscus lies between the femur and tibia as the bucket-handle part of the injury. The peripheral part of the meniscus is torn transversally leaving a lower and upper meniscal portion

should be treated conservatively as no evidence is supporting the beneficial effects of partial meniscectomy [5, 23–26]. Meniscus allograft transplantation is an option for special cases.

5.2.6 Take-Home Message

Patients presenting with the inability to fully extend the knee after a relevant trauma should undergo subacute MRI to identify meniscal injuries that require immediate attention such as bucket-handle lesions.

5.2.7 Diagnosis Algorithm for Acute Meniscal Injuries

Hemarthrosis and reduced range of knee motion	MRI to exclude fracture, patella dislocation, ligament lesions and bucket-handle meniscus injury
Normal range of motion without instability	RICE and re-evaluation after 2–3 weeks

5.2.8 Diagnosis Algorithm for Chronic Meniscal Injuries

Plain radiographs show OA	Conservative treatment
Plain radiographs without OA	MRI to visualize meniscal injuries suitable for surgery

5.2.9 Treatment Algorithm

Degenerative meniscal lesions	Conservative treatment
Bucket-handle meniscal lesions	Subacute arthroscopy and meniscal reinsertion
RAMP lesions	Inside-out or all-inside suture where indicated
Root lesions	Transtibial root refixation

5.2.10 Facts

- The meniscus should always be preserved if possible [15, 27].
- Meniscal surgery is specialist surgery demanding special techniques, especially for root and ramp lesions.
- There is no evidence supporting the beneficial effect of partial meniscectomy in patients with underlying OA.

5.3 ACL Injury

5.3.1 Background

The anterior cruciate ligament (ACL) enables stable knee kinematics by limiting internal tibial rotation and anterior tibial translation. As the ACL has migrated anteriorly during embryologic development to its more central position, it has preserved synovial coverage. The ACL has been thought to be comprised of two distinguishable bundles: an anteromedial and a posterolateral bundle. Recent and revisited anatomical studies, however, have emphasized the ribbon-like structure of the ACL [28], proposing a new nomenclature in which no longer bundles are distinguished but direct from indirect fibres according to their insertional morphology [29]. Acute ACL ruptures are predominantly the result of a non-contact rotational or hyperextensional trauma (Fig. 5.4) [30, 31]. Altered biomechanics of the ACL-deficient knee may cause symptoms of instability, subsequent meniscal and chondral injury as well as osteoarthritis [32, 33]. ACL reconstruction (ACLR) is preformed to improve knee stability and shows overall satisfactory results and low revision rates. The therapeutic approach to ACL injuries has historically been a dynamic process, entailing repair procedures, augmentations, open and arthroscopic reconstructions as well as a variety of graft choices. Even though arthroscopic procedures are currently chosen over open approaches and reconstructions over repair procedures, the optimal graft choice is still controversially discussed. Meta-analysis of studies comparing the outcomes of ACLR depending on graft choice including auto- and allografts and bone-tendon versus pure tendon grafts have not emerged a specific superior graft [34–41]. The reconstruction of both ACL bundles (double-bundle ACLR) has been proposed by some authors [42, 43]. However, its necessity has been challenged as the procedure is technically more demanding without clearly improving patient outcomes [44, 45]. In single-bundle ACLR, graft positioning has been a matter of debate, especially after the transportal ACLR technique has been established as the gold standard [46–48]. Patients with high grade pivot-shift and habitual ligament laxity have shown higher ACL failure rates. In these patients, additional extra-articular stabilizing procedures as the lateral tenodesis or anterior lateral ligament (ALL) reconstruction have currently been popularised and thought to lower ACLR failure and revision rates [49–52]. In general, the susceptibility of ACL lesions is higher among women compared to men engaged in the same pivoting sports [53–55]. Physiological factors such as neuromuscular control and quadriceps-dominant deceleration, the geometrical shape of the knee joint and hormonal factors are thought to be the explanation of this disparity [47, 48, 56–61].

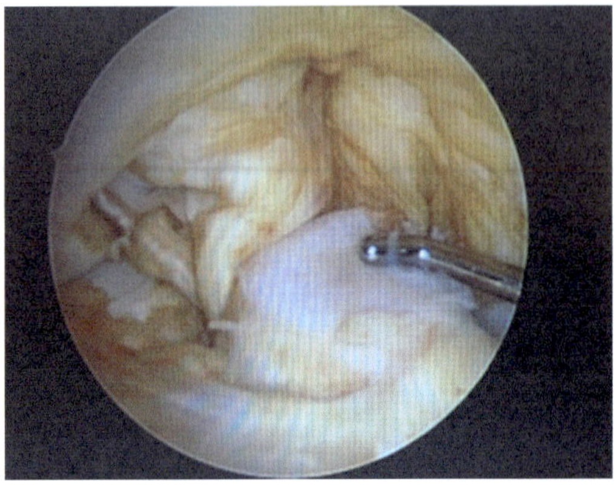

Fig. 5.4 ACL injury: arthroscopic view

5.3.2 Symptoms

Symptoms associated with ACL injury include a hearable snap at the time of injury followed by the inability to continue sports activity and rapid onset of knee effusion. Other symptoms including pain and reduced range of knee motion may be present and are usually aggravated by concomitant meniscal injuries. Subjective instability with or without giving way phenomenon is usually reported. However, subjective instability may first be evident when pain is resolved and the knee is fully loaded.

5.3.3 Diagnosis

Clinical assessment of the knee is best performed shortly after ACL injury before the onset of muscular guarding. The Lachman's test is referred to as the gold standard [62, 63]; the knee is hereby flexed 20–30°, and the amount of anterior tibial translation and the quality of the translation endpoint are evaluated by pulling the lower leg in a forward direction [64]. The test usually induces less pain and muscular guarding than the anterior drawers test in which the knee is flexed 90° or the pivot-shift test, in which a dynamic subluxation of the tibia is induced [65]. Meta-analysis of the efficacy of these tests finds the Lachman test to be the most useful with sensitivity and specificity of 85% and 94%, respectively [62]. Especially regarding the anterior drawers test, PCL injury may mimic ACL insufficiency as the posterior sag will give the impression of increased anterior tibial translation, when in fact the knee is reduced to its neutral position. The clinical examination should include assessment of concomitant injuries that require immediate attention as bucket-handle meniscal lesions, acute patellar dislocations, MCL lesion, rupture of the popliteus tendon as well as PCL lesions. Hemarthrosis may be evacuated by percutaneous aspiration for pain relief.

5.3.4 Imaging

MRI is used to confirm the diagnosis and visualize concomitant injuries. Plain radiographs may visualize an avulsion fracture of the lateral tibial plateau referred to as the Segond fracture which is usually associated with ACL injury [66, 67]. In addition, plain radiographs may visualize fractures of the intercondylar eminentia which may be suitable for ORIF to avoid ACL insufficiency.

5.3.5 Treatment

Acute management of ACL injury include RICE and oral analgesics. Crutches may initially be indicated to avoid full weight-bearing in cases of severe instability. Further management including the necessity and timing of eventual ACL reconstruction is dependent on several factors as patient age and functional level, degree of instability, the condition of the knee and concomitant injuries. In general, patients with concomitant ligament injury or unstable meniscus lesions usually need surgical reconstruction due to increased instability of the knee [68]. Furthermore, patients who experience significant knee instability wishing to resume high-demand sports or occupation usually benefit from ACL reconstruction. Isolated ACL lesions with stable meniscal lesions may be treated conservatively, especially if return to pivoting sports is not desired [69]. As a general rule, ACL surgery is scheduled 6–8 weeks after the injury when normal range of motion is restored and peripheral structures including MCL lesions have healed. Injuries that need immediate surgical attention (e.g. bucket-handle injuries) should be addressed subacutely. Even though evidence is inconclusive, ACL reconstruction is often postponed until normal range of knee motion is restored to avoid complications including arthrofibrosis [70, 71]. However, there is no consensus among knee surgeons regarding optimal timing of ACLR. According to a systematic review of 69 studies including 7556 participants, 90% of patients undergoing ACL reconstruction achieve normal or near normal knee function. However, only 55% of patients resume their preinjury level of competition [72]. This suggests that psychological factors like fear of reinjury may play an important role in the treatment of ACL injury [72, 73]. There is no cutoff age for ACL reconstruction, and based on observational studies, it shows overall satisfactory results in patients over 40 years of age [74]. Even though rigorous prospective studies are rare, ACL deficiency is thought to be associated with increased risk of chondral and meniscal degeneration [75]. It remains a matter of debate how much the initial trauma itself contributes to progressive joint degeneration and to what extend ACL reconstruction may modulate this risk [76–78]. In addition, the severity of the initial trauma, extend of meniscal injury, knee biomechanics and subsequent patient activity level may affect the development of joint degeneration.

5.3.6 Take-Home Message

A relevant knee trauma with early onset of effusion is highly suspicious for ACL injury. Muscular guarding may conceal instability, especially concerning the anterior drawers test.

5.3.7 Treatment Algorithm

If ACLR is indicated	Usually 6–8 weeks after injury when range of motion is normalized
ACL rupture with concomitant bucket-handle meniscal injury and fixed flexion deformity	Subacute meniscal suture if indicated, delayed ACLR until range of motion is normalized

5.3.8 Facts

- Up to seventy-seven percent of patients presenting with traumatic knee hemarthrosis have an ACL injury [79].
- ACLR delay may enhance meniscus and chondral degeneration [80].
- ACL deficiency is associated with increased risk of further injury (e.g. meniscal tear), chronic pain and decreased level of activity.
- OA may develop regardless of treatment approach [76, 81].
- No graft choice has been shown to be superior.
- Geometrical features of the knee joint affect ACL injury and ACL graft failure risk [47].

5.4 PCL Injury

5.4.1 Background

The posterior cruciate ligament (PCL) is the strongest of the intra-capsular ligaments of the knee and primary restrain to posterior tibial translation [82]. As the PCL has migrated anteriorly during embryologic development to its more central position, it has preserved synovial coverage. This extra-synovial location accounts for limited effusion in isolated PCL ruptures. The proximity to the posterior capsule, however, ensures blood supply to the PCL after complete rupture, which allows satisfactory results of primary PCL repair and conservative treatment in some cases [83–85]. The femoral and tibial insertion sites of the PCL are approximately three times larger than its mid-portion diameter. The PCL is inconsistently accompanied by two ligamentous structures that stretch between the medial condyle and posterior horn of the lateral meniscus, referred to as the Humphrey and Wrisberg ligament. PCL ruptures may be classified based on timing (acute versus chronic) and severity (isolated versus multi-ligament). Isolated PCL ruptures are rare and usually the result of a fall onto the flexed knee or forced hyperextension. PCL lesions are more likely found in the setting of complex multi-ligament injuries after high-velocity trauma mechanisms. In these cases, thorough assessment of the knee including the neurovascular status is crucial for satisfactory outcomes [86]. Isolated PCL lesions usually show subtle clinical appearance and may therefore go frequently undetected, leading to chronic insufficiency, a flexion deficit or generalized anterior knee pain [87]. The majority of athletes with isolated PCL injuries may continue to function at a high level [83, 84].

5.4.2 Symptoms

Clinical findings of acute PCL ruptures are highly dependent on the preceding trauma and thereof resulting concomitant injuries. Especially lesions of the posterolateral corner may severely aggravate knee instability. In isolated PCL lesions, effusion is uncommon as the blood usually drains into the posterior soft tissues and lower leg. In addition, muscle guarding may conceal mild instability. Pain in the fossa poplitea may therefore be the only perceptible symptom. A popping sensation is rarely reported, and patients with isolated PCL lesions are usually able to instantly resume sporting activities. In contrast, PCL lesions in the setting of multi-ligament lesions are usually associated with hemarthrosis, severe instability, inability to bear weight as well as reduced range of knee motion. Patients presenting with chronic PCL deficiency suffer from a fixed anterior subluxation of the medial femoral condyle in relation to the tibia, which may cause generalized anterior knee and symptoms related to degeneration of the medial tibiofemoral joint compartment [87, 88].

5.4.3 Diagnosis

Acute and especially isolated PCL lesions may be challenging to diagnose and are frequently overlooked. Spontaneous posterior drawer sign is rare and primarily present with concomitant injury of the posterolateral corner [89]. Anterior-posterior translation is frequently seen in the chronic phase when muscular guarding is overcome [90]. In these cases, a positive posterior drawer test and positive posterior drawer palpation test are typically found (metacarpal joints of the observer's hand react sensitive to hyperextension and may help to identify a spontaneous posterior drawer test). Lesions of the posterolateral corner with rotational instability are assessed with the dial test; the patient is hereby lying prone, and both knees are externally rotated and compared.

5.4.4 Imaging

Plain radiographs may visualize posterior tibial displacement or an avulsion fracture of the tibial PCL insertion site. Subacute MRI is indicated when PCL lesions are suspected. However, MRI does not reveal the functional status of the PCL and degree of instability of the lesion. Treatment is therefore based on anamnesis and clinical findings including the degree of tibial displacement and associated functional instability.

5.4.5 Treatment

Displaced avulsion fractures of the tibial insertion without comminution should undergo ORIF to prevent PCL insufficiency. Arthroscopically assisted procedures and fracture fixation with suspension devises have also shown promising results. Ligamentous lesions should primarily undergo conservative treatment including rehabilitation with a dynamic brace that supports anterior reposition of the tibia during flexion [91]. Results after conservative treatment with mild instability are usually good [84, 92]. PCL reconstruction (PCLR) is indicated in cases of chronic instability [93, 94]. Surgical results after PCLR, especially after severe instability, are worse compared to ACLR outcomes [95–97]. PCL lesions in the setting of a multi-ligament injury should be treated operatively while addressing all injuries in a single operation to ensure early mobilization which is thought to be of paramount importance for satisfactory outcomes [98].

5.4.6 Take-Home Message

Isolated PCL lesions are easily overlooked. Pain in the fossa poplitea after a relevant trauma may be the only symptom.

5.4.7 Treatment Algorithm

Acute isolated PCL	Dynamic bracing
Chronic PCL lesions with mild instability	Physiotherapy
Chronic PCL lesion with distinct instability	PCL reconstruction
PCL injury in the setting of multi-ligament lesions (e.g. PLC)	Multi-ligament reconstruction in a single operation

5.4.8 Facts

- PCL lesions with spontaneous posterior drawer sign are usually associated with lesions of the posterolateral corner (PLC) [89].
- Massive effusion after PCL injury is uncommon as the blood usually drains into the posterior soft tissues and lower leg.
- Isolated PCL lesions show good outcomes when treated conservatively.

5.5 MCL Injury

5.5.1 Background

The medial collateral ligament (MCL) is one of the most commonly injured structures of the knee joint [99, 100]. Partial or complete MCL ruptures are typically the result of a direct valgus trauma, less frequently the result of indirect injury mechanisms including abduction and rotation of the lower leg [101]. MCL injuries usually carry low morbidity, in spite of the complex three-layered medial anatomical structure of the knee [102–104]. The superficial MCL (sMCL) is located within the second layer between the deep MCL and the sartorial facia. The superficial MCL is considered the main static retrain against valgus stress and rotational forces. The deep MCL lies in the third and deepest layer and forms the middle third of the medial capsule [104]. The deep MCL is not ascribed a significant joint-stabilizing function [105]. From the second and third layer originates a conjoint ligamentous structure referred to as the posterior oblique ligament (POL).The deep MCL and posterior oblique ligament have attachments to the medial meniscus which explains why MCL injuries may be associated with medial meniscal tears. MCL injuries are classified into minor stable injuries (grade I), partial injuries with mild instability (grade II) and complete tears with severe instability (grade III). MCL injuries carry low morbidity and tend to heal without complications undergoing the following stages: haemorrhage, inflammation, repair and remodelling. Most patients will resume pre-injury level of competitive sports following conservative treatment. Even though most MCL injuries occur isolated, they may be associated with both ACL and medial meniscus injury, referred to as the unhappy triad. Patients with chronic symptomatic MCL insufficiency should undergo MCL reconstruction [106, 107]. Patients with acute MCL lesions in a severe multi-structural injury setting should undergo repair or reconstruction to ensure early mobilization [106, 108, 109].

5.5.2 Symptoms

Isolated MCL injury is usually associated with pain and periarticular swelling along the course of the MCL. Joint effusion is usually absent and typically indicates concurrent intra-articular structural injury. Concomitant ACL and meniscal injury may aggravate instability and impair range of motion.

5.5.3 Diagnosis

Clinical findings are tenderness along the MCL, predominantly at the femoral insertion site. Instability may be present in 20–30° of flexion indicating MCL insufficiency. Instability in both 20–30° of flexion and extension is usually a sign of combined MCL and ACL injury.

5.5.4 Imaging

Plain radiographs may visualize a bony MCL avulsion. In chronic cases, an osseous irregularity at the femoral insertion site is seen as a result of repetitive trauma, referred to as the Pellegrini-Stieda complex [67, 110]. MRI and ultrasound are used to confirm the diagnosis. Stress radiographs comparing both knees where manual valgus stress is applied may be used to quantify the extent of instability [111, 112].

5.5.5 Treatment

Isolated MCL sprains without valgus instability may be treated conservatively after the RICE principle (rest, ice, compression and elevation) [108]. Early remobilization is encouraged. Grade II and III lesions associated with valgus instability require a coronal stabilizing brace for 5–6 weeks; free range of motion is usually granted. Surgical intervention is rarely indicated as conservative treatment usually shows good results [107]. However, a grade III lesion is often associated with multi-ligament lesions where repair procedures or reconstruction may be indicated in a multi-ligament reconstruction setting [108, 113, 114]. In chronic cases with ongoing instability, MCL reconstruction is usually indicated [100].

5.5.6 Take-Home Message

Even though isolated MCL injury is frequently seen, thorough assessment of the knee is crucial to correctly identify concomitant meniscal or ligamentous injury.

5.5.7 Treatment Algorithm

Grade I	RICE following early remobilization
Grade II	Coronal stabilizing brace with free range of motion for 6 weeks
Grade III	Often associated with multi-ligament lesions where repair procedures or reconstruction may be indicated

5.6 LCL Injury/Posterolateral Corner Injury

5.6.1 Background

The lateral (fibular) collateral ligament (LCL) stretches from the lateral femoral epicondyle to the anterolateral aspect of the fibular head. Due to its tubular shape and the fact that the axial rotational axis of the knee lies within the medial compartment [115], complete injuries of the LCL usually lead to significant instability and poor conservative healing potential. If undetected or untreated, chronic instability is usually seen, frequently associated with a thrust gait [116, 117]. Isolated LCL lesions are rare and the result of a direct varus trauma. Most frequently, LCL lesions are present in the setting of multi-ligament injuries following high-energy trauma mechanisms [118]. The most common associated injuries are the posterior cruciate ligament, the popliteus tendon and the popliteo-fibular ligament [119]. The latter are referred to as the main static stabilizing structures of the posterolateral corner (PLC) in conjunction with the LCL. Other structures forming the posterolateral corner include the lateral capsule and iliotibial band, the biceps tendon and lateral head of the gastrocnemius muscle as well as variable structures as the arcuate and fabello-fibular ligament. Especially following high-energy trauma mechanisms, a fibular avulsion fracture (arcuate fracture) or a common peroneal nerve injury may be present [120].

5.6.2 Symptoms

Pain and swelling along the lateral aspect of the knee is usually found. Complete LCL lesions and associated ACL/PCL or PLC injuries lead to instability near full knee extension [121], typically compounding stair climbing and pivoting manoeuvres.

5.6.3 Diagnosis

Ecchymosis and lateral joint line tenderness may be present and may be aggravated by concomitant meniscal injuries. Coronal stability of the knee is assessed in 20–30° of flexion and extension. Instability in extension and 20–30° of flexion is usually associated with injuries of the posterior capsule and cruciate ligaments. Rotational stability is assessed with the dial test; the patient is hereby lying prone, and both knees are externally rotated at 30 and 90° of flexion. The extent of external rotation is compared to the non-affected side. Rotational asymmetry at 30° but not in 90° indicates an isolated PLC injury. Rotational asymmetry at 30 and 90° indicates a combined PLC and PCL injury. Chronic instability may become evident in a thrust gait.

5.6.4 Imaging

MRI is used to confirm the diagnosis. Plain radiographs may visualize a fibular avulsion fracture of the biceps tendon suitable for subacute refixation. Stress radiographs comparing both knees where manual varus stress is applied may be used to quantify the extent of joint opening and instability.

5.6.5 Treatment

Isolated partial LCL lesions with no varus instability in full knee extension may initially be treated conservatively. This entails RICE (rest, ice, compression, elevation) and functional rehabilitation with a coronal stabilizing brace for 6 weeks. Conservative treatment of complete LCL lesions may result in ongoing varus instability. In these cases, LCL reconstruction is usually indicated. Patients with rotational instability should undergo LCL/PLC reconstruction. Patients with combined ACL/PCL and LCL/PLC insufficiency should undergo multi-ligament reconstruction [118].

5.6.6 Take-Home Message

LCL lesions are frequently associated with lesions of the posterior cruciate ligament and structures of the posterolateral corner (PLC).

5.6.7 Treatment Algorithm

Grade I and II LCL lesion	RICE and coronal stabilizing brace for 6 weeks
Grade III LCL lesion with coronal instability	LCL reconstruction
LCL/PLC lesion with rotational instability	LCL/PLC reconstruction
Multi-ligament setting	Acute reconstruction ±(ACL/PCL/LCL/PCL)

5.7 Multi-Ligament Injury

Multi-ligament injuries are predominantly the result of high-energy trauma mechanisms, and their management require high specialist expertise [122]. Ongoing development in the field of sports traumatology has uncovered a much higher incidence of multi-ligament injuries than initially thought. Thorough assessment of the knee after relevant trauma is crucial to correctly identify the extent of complex multi-ligament injuries [86, 123]. Multi-ligament injuries are typically addressed in a single operation to ensure early mobilization which is thought to be of paramount importance for satisfactory outcomes. In chronic situations, malalignment of the lower limb needs to be addressed before collateral ligament reconstruction is performed. In acute initial management of multi-ligament injuries, the neurovascular status needs to be assessed in accordance to ATLS principles, and CT angiography should always be considered in order to identify vascular injury, especially after knee dislocation [124, 125]. Overlooked vascular injuries are associated with high morbidity and may lead to amputation of the lower limb [120].

5.8 Quadriceps Tendon and Patellar Ligament Rupture

5.8.1 Background

Quadriceps tendon and patellar ligament ruptures may be partial or complete and commonly affect the non-dominant knee of male patients beyond 30 years of age. In younger patients, ruptures are usually the result of a direct trauma. In older patients, the rupture usually represents the final stage of prolonged underlying tendon degeneration. Associated factors which are thought to increase the susceptibility of these ruptures include diabetes, connective tissue disorders, renal failure and the use of intra-articular injections or fluoroquinolone antibiotics [126, 127].

5.8.2 Symptoms

Patients with acute ruptures present with pain and swelling at the rupture site. A popping sensation may be noted at the time of injury, especially in complete ruptures, followed by the inability to continue with sports activity.

5.8.3 Diagnosis

Tenderness and a palpable defect at the rupture site of the quadriceps tendon or patellar ligament is usually found. Knee extension against resistance and a straight leg rise is usually not possible. Quadriceps tendon rupture is associated with reduction of the patella height, while patellar ligament rupture is associated with elevation of the patella height.

5.8.4 Imaging

Ultrasound and MRI are used to confirm the diagnosis. Plain radiographs may show patella alta in patellar ligament ruptures and patella baja in quadriceps tendon ruptures [128].

5.8.5 Treatment

Partial quadriceps tendon and patella ligament ruptures may be treated conservatively with short-term brace immobilization in full extension with a progressive range of motion and weight-bearing protocol. Complete quadriceps tendon and patellar ligament ruptures should undergo primary end-to-end, trans-osseous or suture anchor repair depending on rupture site location. Tendon reconstruction with auto- or allografts may be necessary in special cases. The use of NSAID for pain management after acute tendon rupture is still a matter of controversy as both beneficial and deleterious effects of NSAID on tendon healing have been reported [129, 130].

5.8.6 Treatment Algorithm

Partial ruptures	immobilization with progressive ROM and weight-bearing
Complete ruptures	repair

References

1. Duthon VB. Acute traumatic patellar dislocation. Orthop Traumatol Surg Res. 2015;101:S59–67.
2. Arendt EA, Fithian DC, Cohen E. Current concepts of lateral patella dislocation. Clin Sports Med. 2002;21:499–519.
3. Zaffagnini S, et al. The patellofemoral joint: from dysplasia to dislocation. EFORT Open Rev. 2017;2:204–14.
4. Frosch S, et al. The treatment of patellar dislocation: a systematic review. Z Orthop Unfall. 2011;149:630–45.
5. Mordecai SC, Al-Hadithy N, Ware HE, Gupte CM. Treatment of meniscal tears: an evidence based approach. World J Orthop. 2014;5:233–41.
6. Chahla J, Dean CS, Moatshe G, Mitchell JJ, Cram TR, Yacuzzi C, LaPrade RF. Meniscal ramp lesions. Orthop J Sports Med. 2016;4(7):2325967116657815.
7. Ahn JH, Bae TS, Kang K-S, Kang SY, Lee SH. Longitudinal tear of the medial meniscus posterior horn in the anterior cruciate ligament-deficient knee significantly influences anterior stability. Am J Sports Med. 2011;39:2187–93.
8. Nikolić DK. Lateral meniscal tears and their evolution in acute injuries of the anterior cruciate ligament of the knee. Knee Surg Sports Traumatol Arthrosc. 1998;6(1):26–30.
9. Tscholl PM, Duthon VB, Cavalier M, Menetrey J. Current treatment strategy of meniscal lesions in athletes. Rev Med Suisse. 2016;12:1284–7.
10. Shybut TB, et al. Effect of lateral meniscal root tear on the stability of the anterior cruciate ligament-deficient knee. Am J Sports Med. 2015;43:905–11.
11. Sihvonen R, et al. Arthroscopic partial meniscectomy versus placebo surgery for a degenerative meniscus tear: a 2-year follow-up of the randomised controlled trial. Ann Rheum Dis. 2018;77:188–95.
12. Thorlund JB, Juhl CB, Roos EM, Lohmander LS. Arthroscopic surgery for degenerative knee: systematic review and meta-analysis of benefits and harms. Br J Sports Med. 2015;49:1229–35.
13. Scholten RJ, et al. The accuracy of physical diagnostic tests for assessing meniscal lesions of the knee: a meta-analysis. J Fam Pract. 2001;50:938–44.
14. Karachalios T, Hantes M, Zibis AH, Zachos V, Karantanas AH, Malizos KN. Diagnostic accuracy of a new clinical test (the thessaly test) for early detection of meniscal tears. J Bone Joint Surg Am. 2005;87(5):955–62.
15. Helmark IC, Neergaard K, Krogsgaard MR. Traumatic knee extension deficit (the locked knee): can MRI reduce the need for arthroscopy? Knee Surg Sports Traumatol Arthrosc. 2007;15:863–8.
16. Barber FA, McGarry JE. Meniscal repair techniques. Sports Med Arthrosc Rev. 2007;15:199–207.
17. Fok AWM, Yau WP. Early results of all-inside meniscal repairs using a pre-loaded suture anchor. Hong Kong Med. 2013;J19:124–8.
18. Roemer FW, et al. Partial meniscectomy is associated with increased risk of incident radiographic osteoarthritis and worsening cartilage damage in the following year. Eur Radiol. 2017;27:404–13.
19. van Meer BL, et al. Which determinants predict tibiofemoral and patellofemoral osteoarthritis after anterior cruciate ligament injury? A systematic review. Br J Sports Med. 2015;49:975–83.
20. Bhatia S, LaPrade CM, Ellman MB, LaPrade RF. Meniscal root tears: significance, diagnosis, and treatment. Am J Sports Med. 2014;42:3016–30.

21. LaPrade RF, Matheny LM, Moulton SG, James EW, Dean CS. Posterior meniscal root repairs: outcomes of an anatomic Transtibial pull-out technique. Am J Sports Med. 2017;45:884–91.
22. DePhillipo NN, Cinque ME, Kennedy NI, Chahla J, Geeslin AG, Moatshe G, Engebretsen L, LaPrade RF. Inside-out repair of meniscal ramp lesions. Arthrosc Tech. 2017;6(4):e1315–20.
23. Herrlin S, Hållander M, Wange P, Weidenhielm L, Werner S. Arthroscopic or conservative treatment of degenerative medial meniscal tears: a prospective randomised trial. Knee Surg Sports Traumatol Arthrosc. 2007;15:393–401.
24. Khan M, Evaniew N, Bedi A, Ayeni OR, Bhandari M. Arthroscopic surgery for degenerative tears of the meniscus: a systematic review and meta-analysis. CMAJ. 2014;186:1057–64.
25. Kise NJ, et al. Exercise therapy versus arthroscopic partial meniscectomy for degenerative meniscal tear in middle aged patients: randomised controlled trial with two year follow-up. BMJ. 2016;354:i3740.
26. Ménétrey J, Siegrist O, Fritschy D. Medial meniscectomy in patients over the age of fifty: a six year follow-up study. Swiss Surg. 2002;8:113–9.
27. Stein T, Mehling AP, Welsch F, von Eisenhart-Rothe R, Jäger A. Long-term outcome after arthroscopic meniscal repair versus arthroscopic partial meniscectomy for traumatic meniscal tears. Am J Sports Med. 2010;38:1542–8.
28. Śmigielski R, Zdanowicz U, Drwięga M, Ciszek B, Ciszkowska-Łysoń B, Siebold R. Ribbon like appearance of the midsubstance fibres of the anterior cruciate ligament close to its femoral insertion site: a cadaveric study including 111 knees. Knee Surg Sports Traumatol Arthrosc. 2015;23(11):3143–50.
29. Moulton SG, Steineman BD, Haut Donahue TL, Fontboté CA, Cram TR, LaPrade RF. Direct versus indirect ACL femoral attachment fibres and their implications on ACL graft placement. Knee Surg Sports Traumatol Arthrosc. 2017;25(1):165–71.
30. Alentorn-Geli E, et al. Prevention of non-contact anterior cruciate ligament injuries in soccer players. Part 1: mechanisms of injury and underlying risk factors. Knee Surg Sports Traumatol Arthrosc. 2009;17:705–29.
31. Koga H, et al. Mechanisms for noncontact anterior cruciate ligament injuries: knee joint kinematics in 10 injury situations from female team handball and basketball. Am J Sports Med. 2010;38:2218–25.
32. Lohmander LS, Englund PM, Dahl LL, Roos EM. The long-term consequence of anterior cruciate ligament and meniscus injuries: osteoarthritis. Am J Sports Med. 2007;35:1756–69.
33. Mihelic R, Jurdana H, Jotanovic Z, Madjarevic T, Tudor A. Long-term results of anterior cruciate ligament reconstruction: a comparison with non-operative treatment with a follow-up of 17-20 years. Int Orthop. 2011;35:1093–7.
34. Carey JL, Dunn WR, Dahm DL, Zeger SL, Spindler KP. A systematic review of anterior cruciate ligament reconstruction with autograft compared with allograft. J Bone Joint Surg Am. 2009;91:2242–50.
35. Cavaignac E, et al. Is quadriceps tendon autograft a better choice than hamstring autograft for anterior cruciate ligament reconstruction? A comparative study with a mean follow-up of 3.6 years. Am J Sports Med. 2017;45:1326–32.
36. Dopirak RM, Adamany DC, Steensen RN. A comparison of autogenous patellar tendon and hamstring tendon grafts for anterior cruciate ligament reconstruction. Orthopedics. 2004;27:837–42; quiz 843–844.
37. Foster TE, Wolfe BL, Ryan S, Silvestri L, Kaye EK. Does the graft source really matter in the outcome of patients undergoing anterior cruciate ligament reconstruction? An evaluation of autograft versus allograft reconstruction results: a systematic review. Am J Sports Med. 2010;38:189–99.
38. Goldblatt JP, Fitzsimmons SE, Balk E, Richmond JC. Reconstruction of the anterior cruciate ligament: meta-analysis of patellar tendon versus hamstring tendon autograft. Art Ther. 2005;21:791–803.
39. Hu J, Qu J, Xu D, Zhou J, Lu H. Allograft versus autograft for anterior cruciate ligament reconstruction: an up-to-date meta-analysis of prospective studies. Int Orthop. 2013;37:311–20.
40. Laoruengthana A, Pattayakorn S, Chotanaputhi T, Kosiyatrakul A. Clinical comparison between six-strand hamstring tendon and patellar tendon autograft in arthroscopic anterior cruciate ligament reconstruction: a prospective, randomized clinical trial. J Med Assoc Thail. 2009;92:491–7.
41. Xie X, et al. A meta-analysis of bone-patellar tendon-bone autograft versus four-strand hamstring tendon autograft for anterior cruciate ligament reconstruction. Knee. 2015;22:100–10.
42. Li X, Xu C, Song J, Jiang N, Yu B. Single-bundle versus double-bundle anterior cruciate ligament reconstruction: an up-to-date meta-analysis. Int Orthop. 2013;37:213–26.
43. Siebold R, Branch TP, Freedberg HI, Jacobs CA. A matched pairs comparison of single- versus double-bundle anterior cruciate ligament reconstructions, clinical results and manual laxity testing. Knee Surg Sports Traumatol Arthrosc. 2011;19(Suppl 1):S4–S11.
44. Kondo E, Yasuda K, Azuma H, Tanabe Y, Yagi T. Prospective clinical comparisons of anatomic double-bundle versus single-bundle anterior cruciate ligament reconstruction procedures in 328 consecutive patients. Am J Sports Med. 2008;36:1675–87.
45. Murawski CD, van Eck CF, Irrgang JJ, Tashman S, Fu FH. Operative treatment of primary anterior cruciate ligament rupture in adults. J Bone Joint Surg Am. 2014;96:685–94.
46. Brophy RH, et al. Changes in the length of virtual anterior cruciate ligament fibers during stability testing: a comparison of conventional single-bundle reconstruction and native anterior cruciate ligament. Am J Sports Med. 2008;36:2196–203.

47. Sauer S, English R, Clatworthy M. The ratio of tibial slope and meniscal bone angle for the prediction of ACL reconstruction failure risk. Surg J. 2018;04(03):e152–9.
48. Clatworthy M, Sauer S, Roberts T. Transportal central femoral tunnel placement has a significantly higher revision rate than transtibial AM femoral tunnel placement in hamstring ACL reconstruction. Knee Surg Sports Traumatol Arthrosc. 2018; https://doi.org/10.1007/s00167-018-5036-x.
49. Guenther D, et al. The role of extra-articular Tenodesis in combined ACL and anterolateral capsular injury. J Bone Joint Surg Am. 2017;99:1654–60.
50. Ramesh R, Von Arx O, Azzopardi T, Schranz PJ. The risk of anterior cruciate ligament rupture with generalised joint laxity. J Bone Joint Surg Br. 2005;87:800–3.
51. Slette EL, et al. Biomechanical results of lateral extra-articular Tenodesis procedures of the knee: a systematic review. Art Ther. 2016;32:2592–611.
52. Weber AE, et al. Lateral augmentation procedures in anterior cruciate ligament reconstruction: anatomic, biomechanical, imaging, and clinical evidence. Am J Sports Med. 2018:363546517751140. https://doi.org/10.1177/0363546517751140.
53. Mountcastle SB, Posner M, Kragh JF, Taylor DC. Gender differences in anterior cruciate ligament injury vary with activity: epidemiology of anterior cruciate ligament injuries in a young, athletic population. Am J Sports Med. 2007;35:1635–42.
54. Prodromos CC, Han Y, Rogowski J, Joyce B, Shi K. A meta-analysis of the incidence of anterior cruciate ligament tears as a function of gender, sport, and a knee injury-reduction regimen. Art Ther. 2007;23:1320–5.e6.
55. Toth AP, Cordasco FA. Anterior cruciate ligament injuries in the female athlete. J Gend Specif Med. 2001;4:25–34.
56. Hewett TE, Myer GD, Zazulak BT. Hamstrings to quadriceps peak torque ratios diverge between sexes with increasing isokinetic angular velocity. J Sci Med Sport. 2008;11:452–9.
57. Hewett TE, Zazulak BT, Myer GD. Effects of the menstrual cycle on anterior cruciate ligament injury risk: a systematic review. Am J Sports Med. 2007;35:659–68.
58. LaPrade RF, Burnett QM. Femoral intercondylar notch stenosis and correlation to anterior cruciate ligament injuries. A prospective study. Am J Sports Med. 1994;22:198–202; discussion 203.
59. Shelbourne KD, Davis TJ, Klootwyk TE. The relationship between intercondylar notch width of the femur and the incidence of anterior cruciate ligament tears. A prospective study. Am J Sports Med. 1998;26:402–8.
60. Wordeman SC, Quatman CE, Kaeding CC, Hewett TE. In vivo evidence for tibial plateau slope as a risk factor for anterior cruciate ligament injury: a systematic review and meta-analysis. Am J Sports Med. 2012;40:1673–81.
61. Sauer S, Clatworthy M. The effect of medial tibial slope on anterior tibial translation and short-term ACL reconstruction outcome. Surg J. 2018;04(03):e160–3.
62. Benjaminse A, Gokeler A, van der Schans CP. Clinical diagnosis of an anterior cruciate ligament rupture: a meta-analysis. J Orthop Sports Phys Ther. 2006;36:267–88.
63. van Eck CF, van den Bekerom MPJ, Fu FH, Poolman RW, Kerkhoffs GMMJ. Methods to diagnose acute anterior cruciate ligament rupture: a meta-analysis of physical examinations with and without anaesthesia. Knee Surg Sports Traumatol Arthrosc. 2013;21:1895–903.
64. König DP, Rütt J, Kumm D, Breidenbach E. Diagnosis of anterior knee instability. Comparison between the Lachman test, the KT-1,000 arthrometer and the ultrasound Lachman test. Unfallchirurg. 1998;101:209–13.
65. Lane CG, Warren R, Pearle AD. The pivot shift. J Am Acad Orthop Surg. 2008;16:679–88.
66. Goldman AB, Pavlov H, Rubenstein D. The Segond fracture of the proximal tibia: a small avulsion that reflects major ligamentous damage. AJR Am J Roentgenol. 1988;151:1163–7.
67. Lee CH, et al. Osseous injury associated with ligamentous tear of the knee. Can Assoc Radiol. 2016;J67:379–86.
68. Lorbach O, et al. The influence of the medial meniscus in different conditions on anterior tibial translation in the anterior cruciate deficient knee. Int Orthop. 2015;39:681–7.
69. Monk AP, et al. Surgical versus conservative interventions for treating anterior cruciate ligament injuries. Cochrane Database Syst Rev. 2016;4:CD011166.
70. Duquin TR, Wind WM, Fineberg MS, Smolinski RJ, Buyea CM. Current trends in anterior cruciate ligament reconstruction. J Knee Surg. 2009;22:7–12.
71. Mayr HO, Weig TG, Plitz W. Arthrofibrosis following ACL reconstruction--reasons and outcome. Arch Orthop Trauma Surg. 2004;124:518–22.
72. Ardern CL, Taylor NF, Feller JA, Webster KE. Fifty-five per cent return to competitive sport following anterior cruciate ligament reconstruction surgery: an updated systematic review and meta-analysis including aspects of physical functioning and contextual factors. Br J Sports Med. 2014;48:1543–52.
73. Czuppon S, Racette BA, Klein SE, Harris-Hayes M. Variables associated with return to sport following anterior cruciate ligament reconstruction: a systematic review. Br J Sports Med. 2014;48: 356–64.
74. Legnani C, Terzaghi C, Borgo E, Ventura A. Management of anterior cruciate ligament rupture in patients aged 40 years and older. J Orthop Traumatol. 2011;12:177–84.
75. Sri-Ram K, Salmon LJ, Pinczewski LA, Roe JP. The incidence of secondary pathology after

anterior cruciate ligament rupture in 5086 patients requiring ligament reconstruction. Bone Joint J. 2013;95-B:59–64.
76. Barenius B, et al. Increased risk of osteoarthritis after anterior cruciate ligament reconstruction: a 14-year follow-up study of a randomized controlled trial. Am J Sports Med. 2014;42:1049–57.
77. Frobell RB, et al. Treatment for acute anterior cruciate ligament tear: five year outcome of randomised trial. Br J Sports Med. 2015;49:700.
78. Gillquist J, Messner K. Anterior cruciate ligament reconstruction and the long-term incidence of gonarthrosis. Sports Med. 1999;27:143–56.
79. Hardaker WT, Garrett WE, Bassett FH. Evaluation of acute traumatic hemarthrosis of the knee joint. South Med J. 1990;83(6):640–4.
80. Anderson AF, Anderson CN. Correlation of meniscal and articular cartilage injuries in children and adolescents with timing of anterior cruciate ligament reconstruction. Am J Sports Med. 2015;43:275–81.
81. Culvenor AG, et al. Accelerated return to sport after anterior cruciate ligament reconstruction and early knee osteoarthritis features at 1 year: an exploratory study. PM R. 2017;10(4):349–56. https://doi.org/10.1016/j.pmrj.2017.09.005.
82. Wind WM, Bergfeld JA, Parker RD. Evaluation and treatment of posterior cruciate ligament injuries: revisited. Am J Sports Med. 2004;32:1765–75.
83. Agolley D, Gabr A, Benjamin-Laing H, Haddad FS. Successful return to sports in athletes following non-operative management of acute isolated posterior cruciate ligament injuries: medium-term follow-up. Bone Joint J. 2017;99-B:774–8.
84. Parolie JM, Bergfeld JA. Long-term results of non-operative treatment of isolated posterior cruciate ligament injuries in the athlete. Am J Sports Med. 1986;14:35–8.
85. Patel DV, Allen AA, Warren RF, Wickiewicz TL, Simonian PT. The nonoperative treatment of acute, isolated (partial or complete) posterior cruciate ligament-deficient knees: an intermediate-term follow-up study. HSS J. 2007;3:137–46.
86. Woodmass JM, et al. Poly-traumatic multi-ligament knee injuries: is the knee the limiting factor? Knee Surg Sports Traumatol Arthrosc. 2017;26(9):2865–71. https://doi.org/10.1007/s00167-017-4784-3.
87. Logan M, Williams A, Lavelle J, Gedroyc W, Freeman M. The effect of posterior cruciate ligament deficiency on knee kinematics. Am J Sports Med. 2004;32:1915–22.
88. Allen CR, Kaplan LD, Fluhme DJ, Harner CD. Posterior cruciate ligament injuries. Curr Opin Rheumatol. 2002;l14:142–9.
89. Sekiya JK, Whiddon DR, Zehms CT, Miller MD. A clinically relevant assessment of posterior cruciate ligament and posterolateral corner injuries. Evaluation of isolated and combined deficiency. J Bone Joint Surg Am. 2008;90:1621–7.
90. Rosenthal MD, Rainey CE, Tognoni A, Worms R. Evaluation and management of posterior cruciate ligament injuries. Phys Ther Sport. 2012;13:196–208.
91. Jansson KS, Costello KE, O'Brien L, Wijdicks CA, Laprade RF. A historical perspective of PCL bracing. Knee Surg Sports Traumatol Arthrosc. 2013;21:1064–70.
92. Fowler PJ, Messieh SS. Isolated posterior cruciate ligament injuries in athletes. Am J Sports Med. 1987;15:553–7.
93. Bedi A, Musahl V, Cowan JB. Management of Posterior Cruciate Ligament Injuries: an evidence-based review. J Am Acad Orthop Surg. 2016;24:277–89.
94. Lopez-Vidriero E, Simon DA, Johnson DH. Initial evaluation of posterior cruciate ligament injuries: history, physical examination, imaging studies, surgical and nonsurgical indications. Sports Med Arthrosc Rev. 2010;18:230–7.
95. Hammoud S, Reinhardt KR, Marx RG. Outcomes of posterior cruciate ligament treatment: a review of the evidence. Sports Med Arthrosc Rev. 2010;18:280–91.
96. Pierce CM, O'Brien L, Griffin LW, Laprade RF. Posterior cruciate ligament tears: functional and postoperative rehabilitation. Knee Surg Sports Traumatol Arthrosc. 2013;21:1071–84.
97. Voos JE, Mauro CS, Wente T, Warren RF, Wickiewicz TL. Posterior cruciate ligament: anatomy, biomechanics, and outcomes. Am J Sports Med. 2012;40:222–31.
98. Harner CD, Höher J. Evaluation and treatment of posterior cruciate ligament injuries. Am J Sports Med. 1998;26:471–82.
99. Craft JA, Kurzweil PR. Physical examination and imaging of medial collateral ligament and posteromedial corner of the knee. Sports Med Arthrosc Rev. 2015;23:e1–6.
100. Duffy PS, Miyamoto RG. Management of medial collateral ligament injuries in the knee: an update and review. Phys Sportsmed. 2010;38:48–54.
101. Schein A, et al. Structure and function, injury, pathology, and treatment of the medial collateral ligament of the knee. Emerg Radiol. 2012;19:489–98.
102. Lundberg M, Messner K. Long-term prognosis of isolated partial medial collateral ligament ruptures. A ten-year clinical and radiographic evaluation of a prospectively observed group of patients. Am J Sports Med. 1996;24:160–3.
103. Lundberg M, Messner K. Ten-year prognosis of isolated and combined medial collateral ligament ruptures. A matched comparison in 40 patients using clinical and radiographic evaluations. Am J Sports Med. 1997;25:2–6.
104. Warren LF, Marshall JL. The supporting structures and layers on the medial side of the knee: an anatomical analysis. J Bone Joint Surg Am. 1979;61:56–62.
105. Narvani A, Mahmud T, Lavelle J, Williams A. Injury to the proximal deep medial collateral ligament: a problematical subgroup of injuries. J Bone Joint Surg Br. 2010;92:949–53.
106. Fanelli GC, Harris JD. Surgical treatment of acute medial collateral ligament and posteromedial

corner injuries of the knee. Sports Med Arthrosc Rev. 2006;14:78–83.
107. Menzer H, Treme G, Wascher D. Surgical treatment of medial instability of the knee. Sports Med Arthrosc Rev. 2015;23:77–84.
108. Smyth MP, Koh JL. A review of surgical and nonsurgical outcomes of medial knee injuries. Sports Med Arthrosc Rev. 2015;23:e15–22.
109. Stannard JP. Medial and posteromedial instability of the knee: evaluation, treatment, and results. Sports Med Arthrosc Rev. 2010;18:263–8.
110. Wang JC, Shapiro MS. Pellegrini-Stieda syndrome. Am J Orthop. 1995;24:493–7.
111. Kurzweil PR, Kelley ST. Physical examination and imaging of the medial collateral ligament and posteromedial corner of the knee. Sports Med Arthrosc Rev. 2006;14:67–73.
112. Laprade RF, Bernhardson AS, Griffith CJ, Macalena JA, Wijdicks CA. Correlation of valgus stress radiographs with medial knee ligament injuries: an in vitro biomechanical study. Am J Sports Med. 2010;38:330–8.
113. Bollier M, Smith PA. Anterior cruciate ligament and medial collateral ligament injuries. J Knee Surg. 2014;27:359–68.
114. Jiang KN, West RV. Management of Chronic Combined ACL medial posteromedial instability of the knee. Sports Med Arthrosc Rev. 2015;23:85–90.
115. Blaha JD, Mancinelli CA, Simons WH, Kish VL, Thyagarajan G. Kinematics of the human knee using an open chain cadaver model. Clin Orthop Relat Res. 2003;410:25–34.
116. Lunden JB, Bzdusek PJ, Monson JK, Malcomson KW, Laprade RF. Current concepts in the recognition and treatment of posterolateral corner injuries of the knee. J Orthop Sports Phys Ther. 2010;40:502–16.
117. Ranawat A, Baker CL, Henry S, Harner CD. Posterolateral corner injury of the knee: evaluation and management. J Am Acad Orthop Surg. 2008;16:506–18.
118. Malone AA, Dowd GSE, Saifuddin A. Injuries of the posterior cruciate ligament and posterolateral corner of the knee. Injury. 2006;37:485–501.
119. Davies H, Unwin A, Aichroth P. The posterolateral corner of the knee. Anatomy, biomechanics and management of injuries. Injury. 2004;35:68–75.
120. Johnson ME, Foster L, DeLee JC. Neurologic and vascular injuries associated with knee ligament injuries. Am J Sports Med. 2008;36:2448–62.
121. Frank JB, Youm T, Meislin RJ, Rokito AS. Posterolateral corner injuries of the knee. Bull NYU Hosp Jt Dis. 2007;65:106–14.
122. Helgeson MD, Lehman RA, Murphy KP. Initial evaluation of the acute and chronic multiple ligament injured knee. J Knee Surg. 2005;18:213–9.
123. Tay AKL, MacDonald PB. Complications associated with treatment of multiple ligament injured (dislocated) knee. Sports Med Arthrosc Rev. 2011;19:153–61.
124. Peskun CJ, et al. Diagnosis and management of knee dislocations. Phys Sportsmed. 2010;38:101–11.
125. Seroyer ST, Musahl V, Harner CD. Management of the acute knee dislocation: the Pittsburgh experience. Injury. 2008;39:710–8.
126. Kim BS, Kim YW, Song EK, Seon JK, Do Kang K, Kim HN. Simultaneous bilateral quadriceps tendon rupture in a patient with chronic renal failure. Knee Surg Relat Res. 2012;24(1):56–9.
127. Omar M, Haas P, Ettinger M, Krettek C, Petri M. Simultaneous bilateral quadriceps tendon rupture following long-term low-dose nasal corticosteroid application. Case Rep Orthop. 2013;2013:1–5.
128. Hockings M, Cameron JC. Patella baja following chronic quadriceps tendon rupture. Knee. 2004;11(2):95–7.
129. Hanson CA, Weinhold PS, Afshari HM, Dahners LE. The effect of analgesic agents on the healing rat medial collateral ligament. Am J Sports Med. 2005;33:674–9.
130. Warden SJ, et al. Low-intensity pulsed ultrasound accelerates and a nonsteroidal anti-inflammatory drug delays knee ligament healing. Am J Sports Med. 2006;34:1094–102.

ACL + Anterolateral Capsular Injuries: Extra-articular Procedures in Combination with ACL Reconstruction

6

Simone Cerciello, Sebastian Orduna, Nadrr Darvich, and Philippe Neyret

6.1 Introduction

Anterior cruciate ligament (ACL) injury is one of the most frequent injuries in sportsmen with a reported prevalence of around 68.6/100,000 per year [1]. ACL reconstruction (ACLR) is one of the most commonly performed orthopedic procedures. An ACL-deficient knee shows an anterior laxity and a variable degree of associated rotational instability. A variable injury to the lateral capsulo-ligamentous structures has been hypothesized in the onset of rotational laxity. Historically, anterior laxity in ACL-deficient knees was surgically treated with isolated extra-articular tenodesis, as described by Lemaire or MacIntosh. This procedure was effective in reducing the rotation of the tibial plateau relative to the femur; however, isolated extra-articular reconstructions provided only moderate control of anterior laxity. In addition the overall long-term results of these procedures were poor, and only few patients reported good to excellent results. The main drawback of these techniques is that they do not restore the function of the ACL in preventing anterior tibial translation in the medial compartment. These procedures were largely abandoned when single-bundle intra-articular ACL reconstruction emerged as the gold standard surgical treatment of ACL tear. However, traditional transtibial ACLR had the disadvantage of interrelated tunnel preparation. This may lead to a vertical femoral tunnel, with insufficient pivoting control. In fact the most common problem after ACLR is the residual rotational instability, which has been described in 11–30% [2–4].

More anatomic single-bundle procedures (e.g., the femoral tunnel performed through an anteromedial portal) have the advantage of more horizontal graft with better rotational stability [5–7]. More recently double-bundle technique has been proposed to achieve better anatomy and biomechanics of the native knee. Unfortunately up to date there is no clear evidence of better control of rotational laxity [8–10]. Rotational instability has been also related to the injury and loss of function of the anterolateral structures [11, 12] with the anterolateral complex receiving increasing interest in recent years. The anterolateral capsular injury is frequently associated with ACL tears; the capsular avulsion is termed a Segond fracture when associated with bony avulsion of the lateral tibial plateau but does not always include an osseous fragment.

S. Cerciello
Casa Di Cura Villa Betania, Rome, Italy

Marrelli Hospital, Crotone, Italy

S. Orduna
Abu Dhabi Knee and Sports Medicine Centre, Healthpoint Hospital, Abu Dhabi, UAE

N. Darvich · P. Neyret (✉)
Burjeel Orthopedic and Sports Medicine Centre, Abu Dhabi, UAE
e-mail: philippe.neyret@chu-lyon.fr

F. Margheritini et al. (eds.), *Complex Knee Ligament Injuries*,
https://doi.org/10.1007/978-3-662-58245-9_6

This lesion has been shown by some authors and references to be present in the vast majority of acute ACL injuries, and its presence is associated with significantly increased rotational knee laxity [13]. In order to improve the control of pivoting phenomenon in patients with anterolateral capsule injury, some surgeons have started using the addition of a lateral extra-articular tenodesis to the standard intra-articular ACL reconstruction (ACLR). Nevertheless the place and indication of ALL complex augmentation are still a matter of concern.

6.2 Anatomy and Biomechanics

The anterolateral ligament (ALL) takes origin near the popliteus tendon insertion and inserts into the lateral meniscus and tibial plateau 5 mm distal to the articular surface and slightly posterior to Gerdy's tubercle [14, 15] (Fig. 6.1). The average width of this relatively flat structure is 8.2 ± 1.5 mm, and the average length is 34.1 ± 3.4 mm. Histologic analysis shows a fibrous core surrounded by synovium; additional peripheral nervous innervation and mechanoreceptors have also been showed. Biomechanics studies have shown that ALL section resulted in a significant increase in ATT at 60° and IR at 30°, 45°, and 60° [16]. Therefore it was postulated that damage of the ALL after knee sprain could be related to the pivot shift phenomenon. On the contrary the role of ALL in meniscal stability and in the onset of meniscal pathology remains unclear.

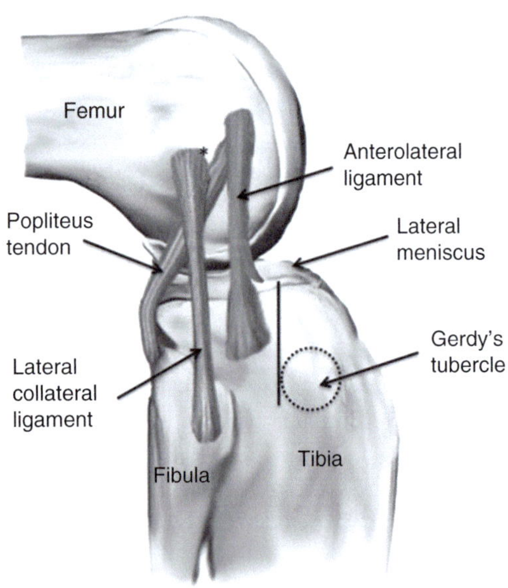

Fig. 6.1 The ALL has close interaction with the popliteus tendon and the iliotibial band

6.3 Indications and Contraindications

6.3.1 Indications

Extra-articular procedures should be considered in cases where the expected failure rate is increased. Therefore the primary indication for an extra-articular tenodesis is a 3+ pivot shift during physical examination or severe anterior tibial translation of the lateral compartment. In these situations, isolated intra-articular reconstruction may not completely control excessive anterior tibial translation and internal rotation in the lateral compartment. Other indication is in the case of patients with generalized hyperlaxity. Extra-articular augmentation is also indicated in patients who plan to return to collision or pivot sports and in female patients playing contact sports. The additional constraint may help to protect these knees from the high loads seen in these sports and may decrease the re-rupture rate. Extra-articular tenodesis should also be considered in patients younger than 20 years of age. It has been shown that these patients are at an increased risk of re-rupture of an isolated intra-articular graft. Finally, these augmentations should be performed in revision cases when no technical error of the initial procedure has been found.

6.3.2 Contraindications

The addition of an extra-articular reconstruction is contraindicated in ACL-deficient knees with an associated posterolateral corner injury. In this situation, the lateral augmentation may fix the tibia in a posterolaterally subluxed position. The extra-articular reconstruction should also be carefully considered and therefore modified in skeletally immature patients because of the risk of injury to the femoral physis. Older studies have shown increased risk of lateral tibiofemoral degeneration after an isolated extra-articular reconstruction when a previous medial meniscectomy had been performed. This may have been a result of overtensioning of the graft leading to overconstraint of the lateral compartment or may have been related to the 4–6 weeks of postoperative immobilization.

6.4 The History of Extra-articular Procedures

Segond was the first to describe a reinforcement of the lateral joint capsule by fibers of the iliotibial band [17]; in addition this structure showed increased tension during forced internal rotation. Terry and LaPrade referred to this reinforcement as the "capsulo-osseous layers" of the iliotibial band and associated its injury with increasingly abnormal Lachman, pivot shift, and anterior drawer tests [18, 19]. LaPrade and colleagues described the same structure as the "mid-third lateral capsular ligament" [19]. Campos and colleagues called it the "lateral capsular ligament," and Vieira and colleagues referred to it as the anterolateral ligament [20]. Vincent and All in 2012 reported its constant presence. This is a true and strong ligament better seen during a medial arthrotomy as during TKA. Claes on year later uses the same terminology to describe a more superficial and shiner structure. It explains some confusion and misunderstanding in the description of the anatomy of this anterolateral complex.

6.4.1 Isolated Extra-articular Procedures

These operations were proposed as isolated procedures in anterior cruciate-deficient knees.

1967 Lemaire procedure [21]: A strip of iliotibial band was harvested detaching it proximally. The strip was prepared and then passed deep to the fibular collateral ligament (FCL), through a femoral tunnel at the attachment point of the head of the lateral gastrocnemius. The graft was then passed deep to the FCL a second time and fixed with sutures to the iliotibial band with the knee flexed to 30° and held in external rotation.

1976 MacIntosh procedure [22]: A strip of iliotibial band was detached proximally and passed deep to the FCL. The strip was then passed through an osteoperiosteal tunnel prepared posterior to the FCL femoral attachment. The graft was then looped through the lateral intermuscular septum and sutured back onto itself at Gerdy's tubercle with the knee flexed to 90° and held in external rotation.

1978 Losee procedure [23]: An iliotibial band graft was detached proximally and passed through a femoral tunnel that originated at the attachment point of the lateral gastrocnemius and ended anterodistal to the FCL femoral insertion site. The graft was then sutured at Gerdy's tubercle with the knee flexed to 30° and held in external rotation.

1979 Arnold and Coker procedure [24]: A strip of iliotibial band was detached proximally, passed beneath the FCL and popliteus tendon, and sutured to Gerdy's tubercle with the knee flexed to 90–100° and the foot held in external rotation.

1979 Ellison procedure [25]: A distally detached strip of iliotibial band with a bone flake was passed deep to the FCL and anchored in a bone trough slightly anterior to its original harvest site at Gerdy's tubercle with the knee flexed at 90° and held in external rotation. The capsular structures were reefed deep to the FCL.

1982 Benum procedure [26]: The lateral one-third of the patellar tendon was harvested proximally with a patellar bone block, passed deep to the FCL, and fixed with a staple within a bony groove deep to the femoral origin of the FCL with the knee flexed to 45° and held in external rotation.

1982 Andrews procedure [27]: Two strips of iliotibial band were detached proximally and sutured and tubulized at their proximal ends. Then, the sutures were passed through two parallel tunnels, which originated at the lateral femoral condyle and exited at the medial femoral condyle. After passing through the tunnels in the lateral-to-medial direction, the sutures were tied together over the adductor tubercle. The grafts were fixed with the knee flexed to 90° and held in external rotation. In addition, the grafts were fixed to ensure that the anterior bundle was taut in flexion and the posterior bundle was taut in extension.

1983 Müller procedure [28]: A strip of iliotibial band was detached proximally and fixed with two cancellous screws to a point anterior to the junction of the femoral shaft and lateral femoral condyle with the knee held in external rotation.

1990 Modified Andrews procedure [27]: The iliotibial band was divided, and a 20-mm-wide portion of the band was detached proximally. The strip of iliotibial band was fixed with a soft-tissue fixation screw and washer at the distal insertion of the lateral muscular septum on the linea aspera, just anterior to the posterior femoral cortex.

1990 Wilson and Scranton procedure [29]: A strip of iliotibial band was detached proximally, passed deep to the FCL and lateral gastrocnemius tendon, and sutured back onto itself with the knee flexed to 60° and the foot held in external rotation. This extra-articular reconstruction was used in conjunction with an intra-articular ACL semitendinosus graft reconstruction.

6.4.2 Combined Extra-articular Procedures

These operations were proposed in addition to ACLR to increase stability and achieve better control of pivot shift phenomenon.

1978 Dejour procedure [30]: This procedure has been described in 1978 and then published in 1988. It is an open reconstruction of the ACL through a parapatellar approach using the middle third of the patellar tendon associated with a Lemaire procedure. The Lemaire procedure is performed through a 15–20 cm incision. A 7/8 mm strip of the ITB is harvested on its upper portion. A 3 mm femoral tunnel is prepared having one end between the insertion of the LCL and the lateral gastrocnemius and the other one just superior and posterior to the condylar tubercles slightly anterior to the intermuscular septum. A second, short tunnel is prepared at the level of Gerdy's tubercle. The ITB strip is passed under the LCL to the femoral tunnel, where it is fixed with some sutures, back under the LCL to the tibial tunnel where it is fixed with other sutures holding the knee at 30° of flexion.

1979 Marshall procedure [31]: It was described as a modification of the original MacIntosh procedure to address both the ACL insufficiency and the lateral structure damage. The central third of the entire extensor mechanism was harvested including part of the prepatellar aponeurotic tissue. The tibial tunnel was prepared in a standard fashion and location; the graft was then passed through this tunnel, into the joint, and over the top of the lateral femoral condyle to be fixed on Gerdy's tubercule.

1985 Combined MacIntosh procedure [32]: It is variation of the previous isolated extra-articular tenodesis to perform combined ACLR and lateral tenodesis. A 25 cm × 4 cm ITB strip was obtained keeping the distal insertion in place. The graft was passed underneath the LCL and through a subperiosteal tunnel to exit anterior to the condylar attachment of the lateral intermuscular septum. The strip was then retrieved in the joint and passed in the tibial tunnel and finally through another tunnel running deep from the insertion of the patellar tendon back to Gerdy's tubercle. The fixation with nonabsorbable suture was performed at three levels: the femoral attachment of the LCL, the exit of the subperiosteal tunnel, and the medial aspect of the tibial tuberosity and at Gerdy's tubercle.

1986 Zarins and Rowe procedure [33]: The semitendinosus tendon was detached proximally and passed through an obliquely oriented tibial tunnel, across the knee joint, and over the lateral femoral condyle. After passing it over the lateral femoral condyle, the graft was passed deep to the FCL and sutured onto the iliotibial band. Similarly, the iliotibial band was passed deep to the FCL and over the superior aspect of the lateral femoral condyle. After passing over the lateral femoral condyle, the graft was passed across the knee joint, through the same obliquely oriented tibial tunnel as the semitendinosus tendon, and fixed with sutures to the semitendinosus tendon with the knee flexed to 60° and held in external rotation.

1987 Lerat procedure [34]: The lateral third of the patellar tendon with an attached 10–12 cm strip of quadriceps tendon was harvested. The tibial tunnel was created in a standard fashion, and the femoral tunnel emerged just proximal to the LCL insertion. An additional tunnel was then created at the level of Gerdy's tubercle. The patellar bone graft was shaped in order to obtain a press-fit fixation in the femoral tunnel, while the tibial bone block was retrieved from the tibial tunnel, tensioned with a metallic wire, and fixed over a screw. With the knee at 60° of flexion, the quadriceps tendon was passed underneath the LCL, through the tunnel under Gerdy's tubercle, and sutured to itself.

1989 Ekstrand procedure [35]: It is a personal modification of the combined MacIntosh procedure. A femoral tunnel was prepared to host the graft instead of the "over the top" option.

1998 Marcacci and Zaffagnini procedure [36]: The semitendinosus and gracilis tendons were harvested proximally, sutured together, and passed through a tibial ACL reconstruction tunnel. The graft exited the tibial tunnel intra-articularly and was passed through the posterior aspect of the femoral notch and over the top of the lateral femoral condyle. The graft was then passed deep to the iliotibial band and over the FCL and was fixed distal to Gerdy's tubercle with the knee flexed to 90° and held in external rotation.

2011 Colombet procedure [37]: A 21 cm hamstring graft was prepared after detachment of the tibial insertion. The femoral and tibial tunnels were drilled in a standard manner, while an additional tunnel was drilled from Gerdy's tubercle to the hamstring origin. In the case of sufficient length, a four-strand intra-articular portion (9 cm) was used to replace the ACL, and two-strand extra-articular part (12 cm) was prepared to perform the lateral tenodesis. In the case of insufficient length, both the intra- and extra-articular portions were prepared in a two-strand fashion. The graft was then fixed with two screws at the level of tibial and femoral tunnel. The extra-articular portion was passed under the ITB but superficial to the LCL, into the tunnel in Gerdy's tubercle, and finally fixed with an interference screw.

2013 Neyret procedure [38]: This technique was introduced in the 1990s; it predicts an "out-in" ACLR using a 9 mm central third bone-patellar tendon-bone graft. The tibial bone block, used on the femoral tunnel, was wider (around 11–12 mm) to host a 4.5 mm drill hole. The femoral tunnel was drilled just posterior and proximal to the origin of the LCL. An additional tunnel was created at the level of Gerdy's tubercle. The gracilis tendon, which was prepared for the extra-articular tenodesis, was passed through the tibial bone block hole to obtain two strands of the same length. The patellar tendon graft was introduced into the knee through the femoral tunnel. The tibial bone block was impacted into the femoral tunnel to achieve a press-fit fixation, securing at the same time the gracilis into the bone tunnel. Tibial fixation was achieved with an interference screw. The two ends of gracilis were passed underneath the LCL and in opposite directions through a bony tunnel created in Gerdy's tubercle. Final fixation was obtained suturing the ends to each other with the knee held at 30° of flexion.

6.4.3 Anterolateral Ligament Reconstruction

2015 Smith procedure [39]: This technique uses both hamstring tendons. The semitendinosus is used for an "all-inside" ACLR, the gracilis to reconstruct the ALL. Two 4.5 mm by 25 mm tunnels are created, one just anterior and superior to the femoral insertion of the LCL and the second halfway between Gerdy's tubercle and the fibular head, around 1 cm below the joint line. A whipstitch is placed in the proximal end of the gracilis tendon, which is then passed into the femoral tunnel and secured with an absorbable fully threaded knotless anchor. The graft is then passed underneath the ITB and into the tibial tunnel.

Final fixation is performed with another fully threaded knotless anchor.

2015 Helito procedure [40]: It is a combined procedure involving tripled semitendinosus and single-strand gracilis in order to obtain a four-strand ACL and single-strand ALL. Under fluoroscopic control, a 5 mm metal suture anchor is placed at the ALL femoral attachment (3–4 mm distal to the halfway point on Blumensaat's line). ACL femoral tunnel is performed in an out-in fashion and the tibial tunnel in a standard manner. The graft is retrieved from distal to proximal in order to have the four strands in the joint. Femoral fixation is performed first, with a line-to-line absorbable screw. Tibial fixation is the achieved with a +1 absorbable screw holding the knee at 30° of flexion and neutral rotation. The gracilis is fixed on the femur using the metal anchor. Tibial fixation is achieved with a second suture anchor positioned at the anatomic insertion halfway between Gerdy's tubercle and the fibular head, 5–10 mm below the joint line. The graft is then passed under the ITB and is fixed with the second anchor sutures at 60–90° of flexion.

2016 Sonnery-Cottet procedure [41]: It is a similar technique, with pediculate hamstring graft. The tibial tunnel is performed in a standard fashion. Two stab incisions are performed to create an additional 3.2 mm tunnel connecting the superolateral corner of Gerdy's tubercle, and the site of the Segond fracture (more proximal and lateral) is created. The ACL femoral tunnel emerged at the ALL isometric point. ACL graft was fixed with absorbable screws. The remaining part of the gracilis tendon is passed deep to the ITB but superficial to the LCL, through the ALL tibial tunnel and then back through the femoral tunnel in order to create a Y-shaped ALL construct. The ALL graft is fixed with an interference screw in extension and neutral rotation and secured at the ACL femoral tunnel with the ACL graft traction sutures.

2016 Wagih procedure [42]: It is a percutaneous technique of ALL reconstruction using a polyester tape. A 5 mm transverse skin incision is performed at the level of femoral insertion of the ALL (just anterior and distal to the lateral femoral condyle). A 4.5 mm tunnel is drilled over a 2.7 mm passing pin. In a similar way, two 4.5 mm transverse tunnels are drilled just proximal to the midpoint between the head of the fibula and Gerdy's tubercle leaving a 1 cm bony bridge. A polyester tape of 4 mm diameter and 60 mm length is loaded over a cortical suspensory fixation button, which is retrieved from the medial femoral tunnel. The two free hands of the tape are passed deep to the ITB and retrieved on the lateral aspect of the proximal tibia. Finally the two strands are passed through the tibial tunnels and tied together over the 1 cm bone bridge with the knee in 30° of flexion.

6.5 Personal Technique

Lateral extra-articular tenodesis (LET) technique was developed to improve the anterolateral capsular structure deficiency. The patient is set in supine position under femoral block anesthesia. Physical examination is performed to assess the degree of knee laxity with the Lachman test, anterior drawer and pivot shift tests, and varus-valgus stress test at 0°–30°–90° of flexion. Surgery begins by drawing the approach line over the lateral area of the knee (Fig. 6.2). Tourniquet is positioned but not inflated.

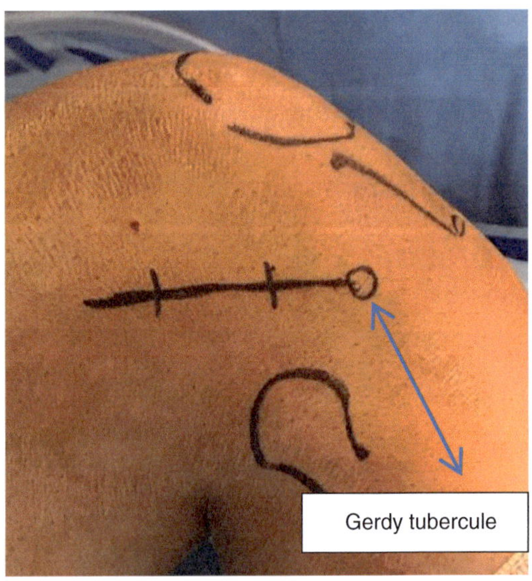

Fig. 6.2 With the knee at 90° of flexion, the incision line is drawn

We perform 4–5 cm incision from Gerdy's tubercle along the fascia lata. After soft-tissue dissection, the iliotibial band is identified. With the aid of three retractors, a fascia lata graft of approximately 2 cm width and 10 cm length is prepared (Fig. 6.3).

The graft is prepared and released proximally leaving the distal end inserted on Gerdy's tubercle (Figs. 6.4 and 6.5).

A white cottony tape is then used to augment the graft and make strong Krackow suture in the end of the graft (Fig. 6.6).

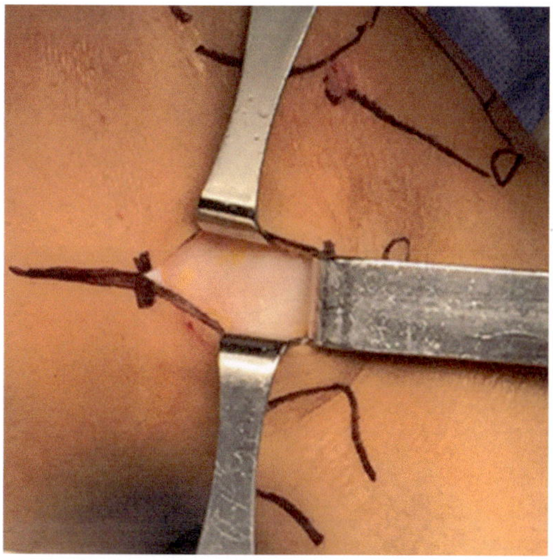

Fig. 6.3 Exposure iliotibial band after soft-tissue release

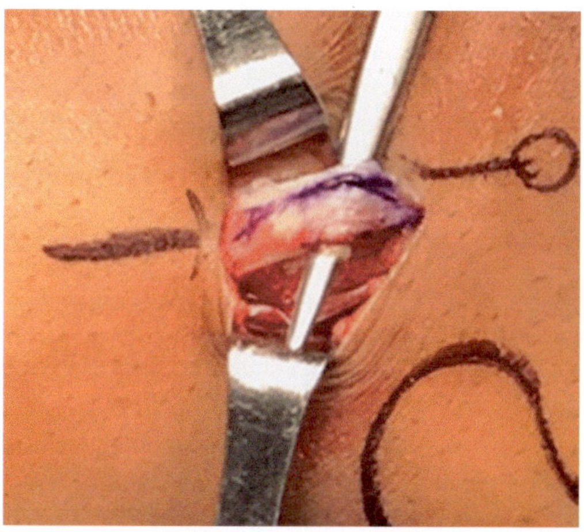

Fig. 6.4 Harvesting the iliotibial band

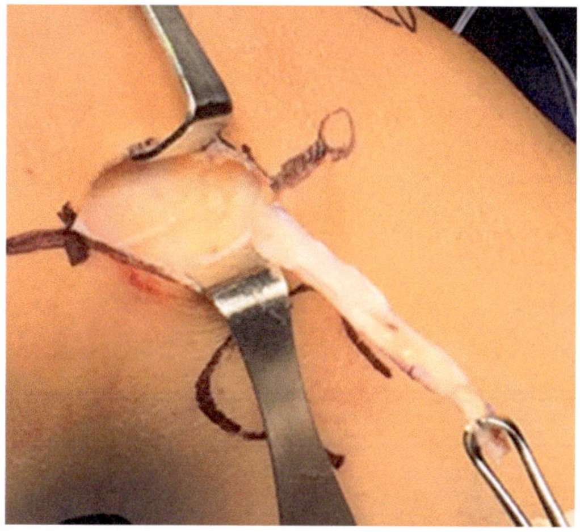

Fig. 6.5 2 cm × 10 cm iliotibial graft with the distal end pediculated at Gerdy's tubercle

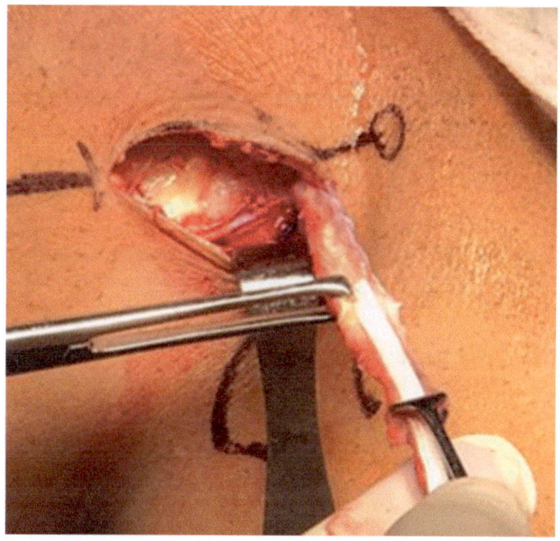

Fig. 6.6 Cotton tape augmentation

The LCL is identified after blunt dissection. The graft is then passed under the LCL using a right-angle pincer (Figs 6.7 and 6.8).

After the graft is passed under the LCL, the femoral tunnel is performed. Its location is situated 2 mm posterior and 2 mm superior from the lateral epicondyle (Fig. 6.9).

A Kirschner wire is passed through both condyles. The graft size is then measured, and a tunnel of approximately 6–7 mm in diameter and 6 cm in length is drilled to host the graft (Fig. 6.10).

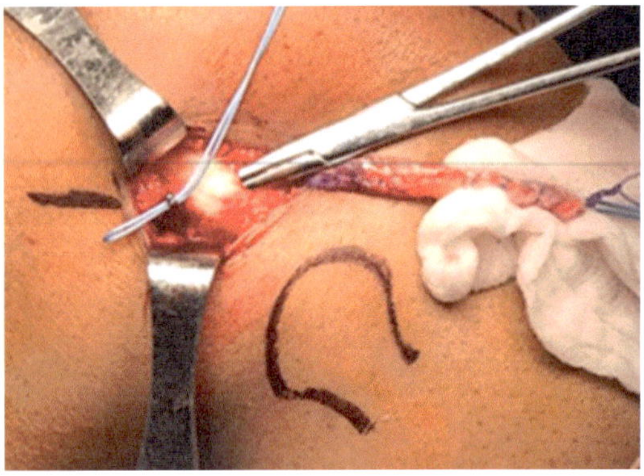

Fig. 6.7 Right-angle pincer under the LCL

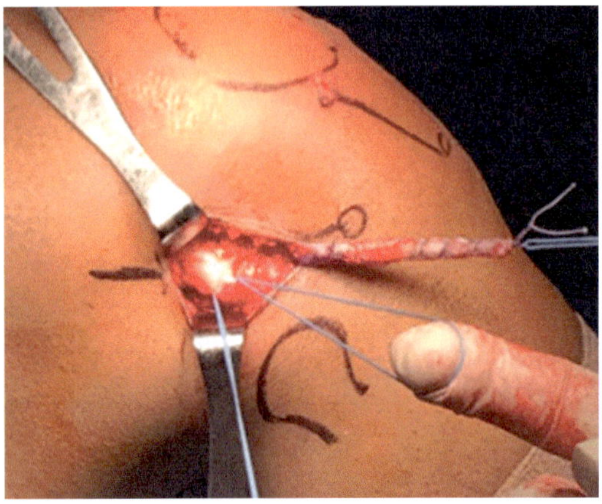

Fig. 6.8 Passage of the graft under the LCL

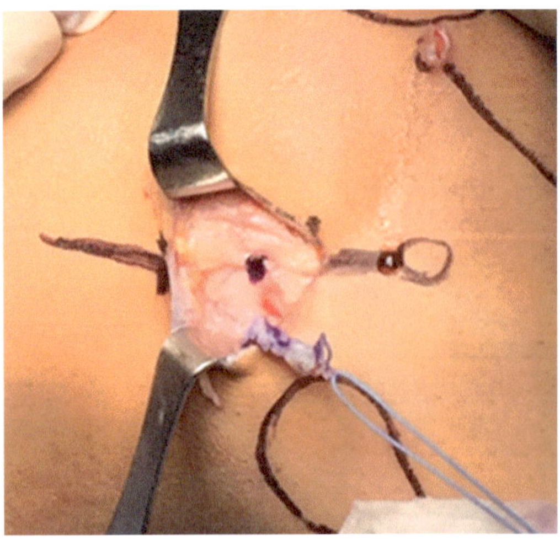

Fig. 6.9 The graft lays under the LCL, and the femoral tunnel has been drilled 2 mm posterior and 2 mm superior to the lateral epicondyle

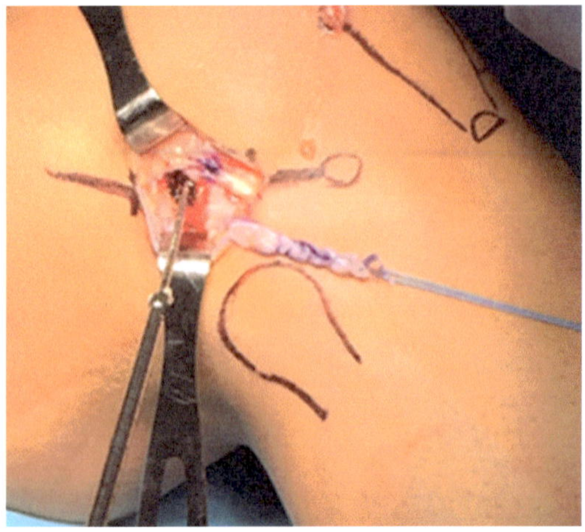

Fig. 6.10 A Kirschner wire is used to drill a 6 mm tunnel

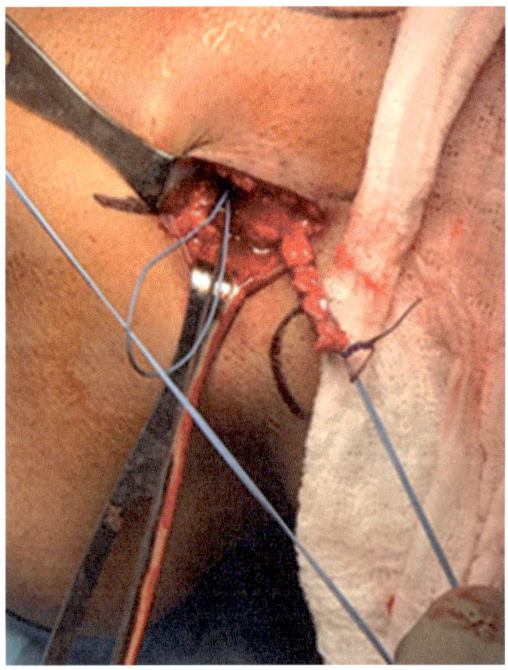

Fig. 6.11 The wire loop is inside the tunnel and is used as a shuttle to pull the graft on the tunnel

A K-wire is used as a shuttle to pass the graft through the tunnel (Fig. 6.11).

The graft is passed through the tunnel, and it is fixed temporarily to perform knee stability tests, to confirm the full range of motion of the knee

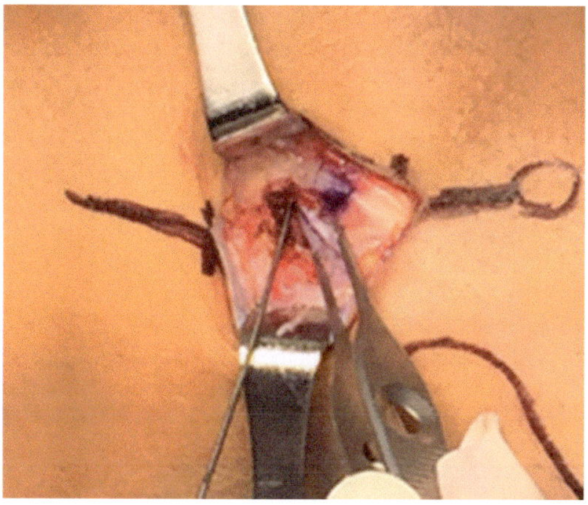

Fig. 6.12 The graft is inside the tunnel. The correct tension is assessed through the whole ROM

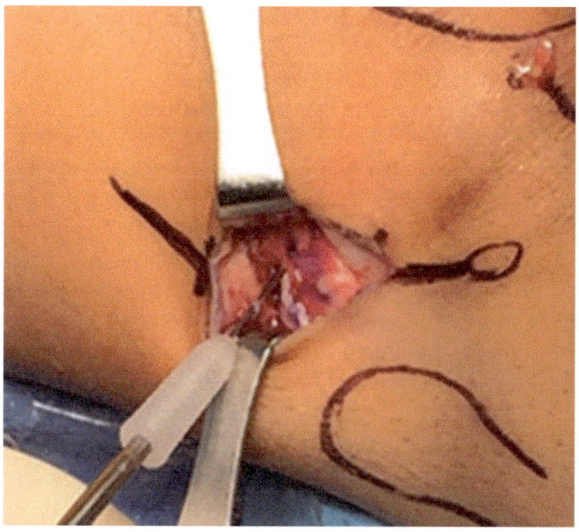

Fig. 6.13 Bioabsorbable interferential screw is used to fix the graft with the knee in full extension

and the proper graft tension through the whole ROM (Fig. 6.12).

The graft is fixed with an interferential bioabsorbable screw in full extension and neutral rotation of the foot (Fig. 6.13).

The iliotibial band is carefully closed avoiding overtightening since it is source of pain in the first post-op period (Fig. 6.14). A drainage is held for the first 24 h. A brace is used for 4 weeks. Passive 0–90° motion is allowed 48 h after surgery.

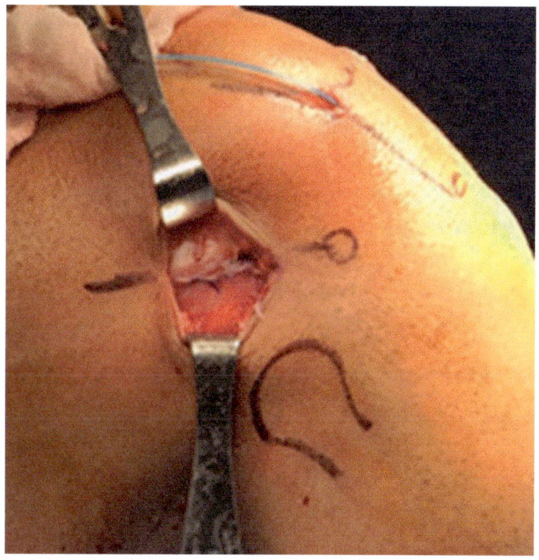

Fig. 6.14 Iliotibial band fascia closure

6.6 Conclusions

ACLR is a successful procedure both in terms of patients' satisfaction and daily life activities. Return to full sports activities is less satisfactory, and persistent instability and re-rupture rates are still a concern. Anatomic and biomechanics studies have investigated the role of the structures of the lateral and anterolateral aspect of the knee. They contribute to the rotatory stability of the knee, thus preventing the pivot shift phenomenon. Imaging studies have shown high rate of injuries of these structures in patients who have been diagnosed as affected by isolated ACL rupture. It seems therefore reasonable to address the damage of the anterolateral structures in the setting of an ACLR at least in specific situations. Historic extra-articular procedures associated to intra-articular ACL reconstruction has proven to be efficient for a long time but was abandoned for many years. Recently there has been a new interest for these techniques, supported by the new anatomical and biomechanical findings and the new minimally invasive techniques. However there is still some debate about the ideal indication and the best surgical technique: for some surgeons it must be an anatomical reconstruction, for the others it is considered as a functional lateral augmentation of the ACL graft. These different considerations may explain the controversy that still exists regarding its indications.

References

1. Sanders TL, Maradit Kremers H, Bryan AJ, et al. Incidence of anterior cruciate ligament tears and reconstruction: a 21-year population-based study. Am J Sports Med. 2016;44(6):1502–7. https://doi.org/10.1177/0363546516629944.
2. Anderson AF, Snyder RB, Lipscomb AB Jr. Anterior cruciate ligament reconstruction. A prospective randomized study of three surgical methods. Am J Sports Med. 2001;29:272–9.
3. Kocher MS, Steadman JR, Briggs K, et al. Determinants of patient satisfaction with outcome after anterior cruciate ligament reconstruction. J Bone Joint Surg Am. 2002;84:1560–72.
4. Sonnery-Cottet B, Thaunat M, Freychet B, et al. Outcome of a combined anterior cruciate ligament and anterolateral ligament reconstruction technique with a minimum 2-year follow-up. Am J Sports Med. 2015;43:1598–605.
5. Bedi A, Feeley BT, Williams RJ. Management of articular cartilage defects of the knee. J Bone Joint Surg Am. 2010;92:994–1009.
6. Markolf KL, Jackson SR, McAllister DR. A comparison of 11 o'clock versus oblique femoral tunnels in the anterior cruciate ligament reconstructed knee: knee kinematics during a simulated pivot test. Am J Sports Med. 2010;38:912–7.
7. Kato Y, Maeyama A, Lertwanich P, et al. Biomechanical comparison of different graft positions for single-bundle anterior cruciate ligament reconstruction. Knee Surg Sports Traumatol Arthrosc. 2012;21:816–23.
8. Meredick RB, Vance KJ, Appleby D, et al. Outcome of single-bundle versus double-bundle reconstruction of the anterior cruciate ligament: a meta-analysis. Am J Sports Med. 2008;36:1414–21.
9. Muneta T, Hara K, Ju YJ, et al. Revision anterior cruciate ligament reconstruction by double-bundle technique using multi-strand semitendinosus tendon. Arthroscopy. 2010;26:769–81.
10. Zaffagnini S, Signorelli C, Lopomo N, et al. Anatomic double-bundle and over-the-top single-bundle with additional extra-articular tenodesis: an in vivo quantitative assessment of knee laxity in two different ACL reconstructions. Knee Surg Sports Traumatol Arthrosc. 2012;20:153–9.
11. Matsumoto H, Seedhom BB. Treatment of the pivot-shift intra-articular versus extra-articular or combined reconstruction procedures: a biomechanical study. Clin Orthop Relat Res. 2004;299:298–304.
12. Bull AMJ, Amis A. The pivot-shift phenomenon: a clinical and biomechanical perspective. Knee. 1998;5(1):141–58.
13. Claes S, Bartholomeeusen S, Bellemans J. High prevalence of anterolateral ligament abnormalities in magnetic resonance images of anterior cruciate ligament injured knees. Acta Orthop Belg. 2014;80:45–9.
14. Claes S, Vereecke E, Maes M, et al. Anatomy of the anterolateral ligament of the knee. J Anat. 2013;223(4):321–8.
15. Vincent JP, Magnussen RA, Gezmez F, et al. The anterolateral ligament of the human knee: an anatomic and histologic study. Knee Surg Sports Traumatol Arthro. 2012;20(1):147–52.
16. Monaco E, Ferretti A, Labianca L, et al. Navigated knee kinematics after cutting of the ACL and its secondary restraint. Knee Surg Sports Traumatol Arthrosc. 2012;20:870–7.
17. Ségond P. Recherches cliniques et expérimentales sur les épanchements sanguins du genou par entorse. Prog Med. 1879;7:297–9. 319–21, 340–1.
18. Terry GC, Hughston JC, Norwood LA. The anatomy of the iliopatellar band and iliotibial tract. Am J Sports Med. 1986;14:39–45.
19. LaPrade RF, Gilbert TJ, Bollom TS, et al. The magnetic resonance imaging appearance of individual structures of the posterolateral knee. A prospective study of normal knees and knees with surgically verified grade III injuries. Am J Sports Med. 2000;28:191–9.
20. Campos JC, Chung CB, Lektrakul N, et al. Pathogenesis of the Segond sracture: anatomic and MR imaging evidence of an iliotibial tract or anterior oblique band avulsion. Radiology. 2001;219:381–6.
21. Lemaire M. Ruptures anciennes du ligament croise anterieur du genou. J Chir. 1967;93:311–20.
22. Macintosh D, Darby T. Lateral substitution reconstruction. In: Proceedings of the Canadian Orthopaedic Association. J Bone Joint Surg Br. 1976;58(1):142.
23. Losee RE, Johnson TR, Southwick WO. Anterior subluxation of the lateral tibial plateau. A diagnostic test and operative repair. J Bone Joint Surg Am. 1978;60:1015–30.
24. Arnold JA, Coker TP, Heaton LM, et al. Natural history of anterior cruciate tears. Am J Sports Med. 1979;7:305–13.
25. Ellison AE. Distal iliotibial-band transfer for anterolateral rotatory instability of the knee. J Bone Joint Surg Am. 1979;61:330–7.
26. Benum P. Anterolateral rotary instability of the knee joint. Results after stabilization by extraarticular transposition of the lateral part of the patellar ligament. A preliminary report. Acta Orthop Scand. 1982;53(4):613–7.
27. Andrews JR, Sanders R. A "mini-reconstruction" technique in treating anterolateral rotatory instability (ALRI). Clin Orthop Relat Res. 1983;172:93–6.
28. Muller W. The knee form, function, and ligament reconstruction. New York, NY: Springer; 1983. p. 253–7.

29. Wilson WJ, Scranton PE Jr. Combined reconstruction of the anterior cruciate ligament in competitive athletes. Bone Joint Surg Am. 1990;72(5): 742–8.
30. Dejour H, Walch G, Neyret P, Adeleine P. Results of surgically treated chronic anterior laxities. Apropos of 251 cases reviewed with a minimum follow-up of 3 years. Rev Chir Orthop Reparatrice Appar Mot. 1988;74(7):622–36.
31. Marshall JL, Warren RF, Wickiewicz TL, et al. The anterior cruciate ligament: a technique of repair and reconstruction. Clin Orthop Relat Res. 1979;143:97–106.
32. Bertoia JT, Urovitz EP, Richards RR, et al. Anterior cruciate reconstruction using the MacIntosh lateral-substitution over-the-top repair. J Bone Joint Surg Am. 1985;67:1183–8.
33. Zarins B, Rowe CR. Combined anterior cruciate-ligament reconstruction using semitendinosus tendon and iliotibial tract. J Bone Joint Surg Am. 1986;68:160–77.
34. Lerat JL, Duprã La Tour L, Herzberg G, et al. Review of 100 patients operated on for chronic anterior laxity of the knee by a procedure derived from the Jones and MacIntosh methods. Value of dynamic radiography for the objective analysis of the results. Rev Chir Orthop Reparatrice Appar Mot. 1987;73(Suppl 2):201–4.
35. Ekstrand J. Reconstruction of the anterior cruciate ligament in athletes, using a fascia lata graft: a review with preliminary results of a new concept. Int J Sports Med. 1989;10:225–32.
36. Marcacci M, Zaffagnini S, Iacono F, et al. Arthroscopic intra- and extra-articular anterior cruciate ligament reconstruction with gracilis and semitendinosus tendons. Knee Surg Sports Traumatol Arthrosc. 1998;6:68–75.
37. Colombet PD. Navigated intra-articular ACL reconstruction with additional extraarticular tenodesis using the same hamstring graft. Knee Surg Sports Traumatol Arthrosc. 2011;19:384–9.
38. Duthon VB, Magnussen RA, Servien E, et al. ACL reconstruction and extra-articular tenodesis. Clin Sports Med. 2013;32:141–53.
39. Smith JO, Yasen SK, Lord B, et al. Combined anterolateral ligament and anatomic anterior cruciate ligament reconstruction of the knee. Knee Surg Sports Traumatol Arthrosc. 2015;23:3151–6.
40. Helito CP, Bonadio MB, Gobbi RG, et al. Combined intra- and extra-articular reconstruction of the anterior cruciate ligament: the reconstruction of the knee anterolateral ligament. Arthrosc Tech. 2015;4:239–44.
41. Sonnery-Cottet B, Daggett M, Helito CP, et al. Combined anterior cruciate ligament and anterolateral ligament reconstruction. Arthrosc Tech. 2016;5(6):e1253–9. https://doi.org/10.1016/j.eats.2016.08.003.
42. Wagih AM, Elguindy AM. Percutaneous reconstruction of the anterolateral ligament of the knee with a polyester tape. Arthrosc Tech. 2016;5(4):691–7.

Clinical Applications for Combined MCL and PCL Injury

7

Mitchell I. Kennedy, Zachary S. Aman, and Robert F. LaPrade

7.1 Introduction

The most common injuries to the knee are of the medial knee stabilizers, especially the medial collateral ligament (MCL) [1]. The incidence of posterior cruciate ligament (PCL) injuries in isolation is uncommon, but rather more regularly found with concurrent injuries of the anterior cruciate ligament (ACL), MCL, or posterolateral corner (PLC) [2].

Grade III PCL tears are reported to occur between 3% and 37% of patients with knee ligament injuries [3], and its prevalence is more closely associated with multiligamentous injuries (MLIs) [1]. One study reports trauma-based MLIs involving the PCL in as many as 79% of cases [4]. Literature shows that in the trauma setting, PCL injuries occur concomitantly with the ACL, MCL, and PLC in 46%, 31%, and 62% of cases, respectively [3]. The occurrence of isolated PCL injuries is much lower, representing 18% of all PCL injuries, with car accidents the predominant cause of PCL injuries, reportedly accounting for 57% of injuries [3, 5].

Due to the high rate of occurrence these injuries portray, diagnostic procedures are essential for determining the structures requiring attention and the subsequent means for treatment. Current methods for approaching reconstruction of the PCL following injury reside between the single-bundle (SB) and double-bundle (DB) approaches. Recent literature has reported on the comparable outcomes of each respective treatment and found more favorable outcomes among the more anatomically correlated DB procedure. Lack of outcomes research following variable MCL treatments clouds our ability to select the most favorable procedure, but the predominant focus for future direction is upon the selection between repair and reconstruction. With most studies reinforcing the idea of anatomic reconstructions for properly restoring the knee to its native kinematics, this chapter will address the anatomic and biomechanical features of both the MCL and PCL, further leading into precise diagnosis, the most efficient means of treatment, and concluding with reported outcomes.

7.2 Anatomy

An extensive understanding of the anatomical characteristics of each ligament in the knee is vital to assure proper graft placement for reconstructions, because most surgical solutions are transitioning to anatomic reconstruction techniques [6]. Current literature shows consistent data on the specificity of attachment sites and ligamentous characteristics, which is beneficial

M. I. Kennedy · Z. S. Aman (✉)
Steadman Philippon Research Institute, Vail, CO, USA
e-mail: Zaman@sprivail.org

R. F. LaPrade
Twin Cities Orthopaedics, Minnepaolis, MN, USA

F. Margheritini et al. (eds.), *Complex Knee Ligament Injuries*,
https://doi.org/10.1007/978-3-662-58245-9_7

for surgical intervention to restore the native anatomy and subsequently to restore native knee joint kinematics.

7.2.1 The Medial Collateral Ligament

The MCL, spanning between the medial aspect of the femur and tibia, consists of the superficial medial (tibial) collateral ligament (sMCL) and deep medial collateral ligament (dMCL), also referred to as the mid-third medial capsular ligament [7]. The anatomic characteristics of the sMCL have been variable across multiple studies, while evaluations of the dMCL are fairly consistent (Fig. 7.1).

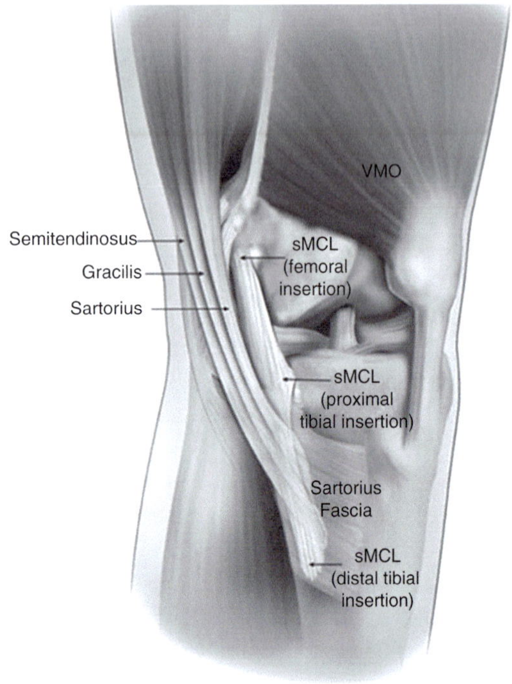

Fig. 7.1 Illustration of the intact superficial medial collateral ligament (sMCL) depicting the proximal femoral and distal tibial attachment locations. Also shown is the sartorius fascia, superior to the distal tibial attachment of the sMCL. The sartorius, gracilis, and semitendinosus tendons run next to the sMCL, inserting anteriorly to the distal sMCL attachment site on the tibia. *VMO* vastus medialis oblique. *Reprinted with permission of SAGE Publications, Inc. from Wijdicks CA, Michalski MP, Rasmussen MT, Goldsmith MT, Kennedy NI, Lind M, Engebretsen L, LaPrade RF: Superficial medial collateral ligament anatomic augmented repair versus anatomic reconstruction: an in vitro biomechanical analysis. Am J Sports Med 2013, 41:2858–66*

The sMCL is the largest structure coursing across the medial aspect of the knee, with its overall length consistently reported between 10 and 12 cm [7–10]. Anatomic studies show the proximal attachment of the sMCL to be oval shaped and centered in a small depression slightly proximal and posterior to the center of the medial epicondyle, approximately 3.2 and 4.8 mm, respectively [7]. However, other studies report the sMCL to attach directly to the medial epicondyle (ME) [8–10]. The sMCL was found coursing distally until two distinct tibial attachments, proximal and distal [7]. The proximal tibial attachment primarily attached to soft tissue, rather than directly to bone [7]. The soft tissue deep to this proximal attachment primarily consists of the anterior arm of the semimembranosus tendon, which itself attaches directly to bone [7]. Just anterior to the posteromedial crest of the tibia, the distal tibial sMCL attachment is found within the pes anserine bursa [7]. Also, the posterior tibial attachments seemingly blend with the posterior oblique ligament, along the tibial expansion of its distal aspect [7].

The dMCL courses roughly parallel to the anterior aspect of the sMCL and is most notably characterized as a thickening of the medial joint capsule that is deep and firmly adherent to, but separable from, the sMCL [7]. The dMCL consists of both a meniscofemoral and meniscotibial section; the meniscofemoral portion attaches distal and deep to the femoral attachment of the sMCL, and the meniscotibial portion attaches distal to the edge of the articular cartilage of the medial tibial plateau [7, 8].

7.2.2 Posterior Cruciate Ligament

The PCL is the largest intra-articular ligament with an approximate length of 38 mm and width of 13 mm [11]. The PCL courses from the medial femoral condyle (MFC) to the posterior aspect of the tibia and has relations to many surrounding structures of the posterior knee including the

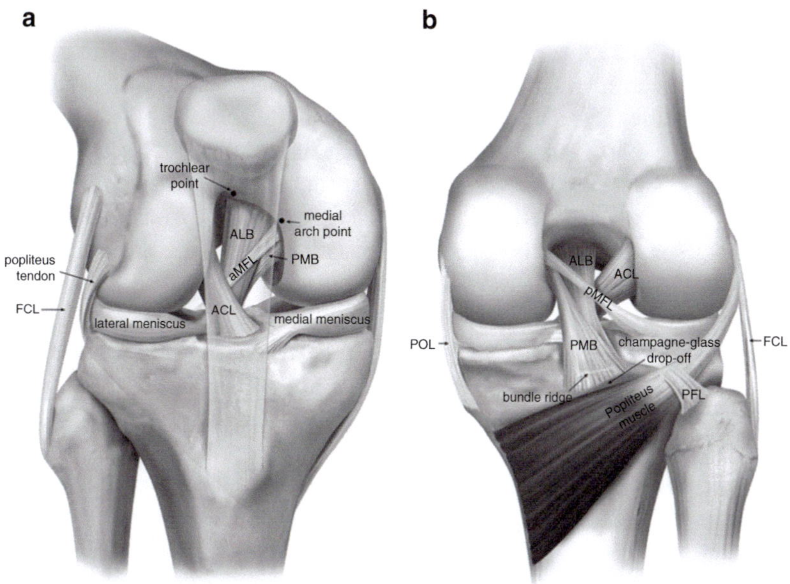

Fig. 7.2 (**a**) Anterior and (**b**) posterior views of the posterior cruciate ligament (PCL). Illustration depicts the femoral and tibial attachment sites of the posteromedial bundle (PMB) and the anterolateral bundle (ALB) and identifiable bony landmarks. Anterior cruciate ligament (ACL), anterior meniscofemoral ligament (aMFL), fibular collateral ligament (FCL), popliteofibular ligament (PFL), posterior meniscofemoral ligament (pMFL), posterior oblique ligament (POL). *Reprinted with permission of SAGE Publications, Inc, from Kennedy NI, Wijdicks CA, Goldsmith MT, Michalski MP, Devitt BM, Aroen A, Engebretsen L, LaPrade RF: Kinematic analysis of the posterior cruciate ligament, part 1: the individual and collective function of the anterolateral and posteromedial bundles. Am J Sports Med 2013, 41:2828–38*

ACL, menisci, and the major neurovascular structures of the leg [11]. Consisting of two bundles, the larger anterolateral bundle (ALB) and smaller posteromedial bundle (PMB) are distinct yet inseparable, each with individually identifiable tibial and femoral attachments (Fig. 7.2) [11].

In respect to the femoral attachments of each PCL bundle, the center of the ALB is triangulated between the trochlear point, the medial arch point, and the medial bifurcate prominence, while the PMB is consistently bordered by the medial intercondylar ridge proximally and the ALB anteriorly [12]. The distance measured between the femoral centers of each bundle averaged 12.1 mm [12].

Below the articular surface of the tibia, in a sulcus (PCL facet) that lies between the posterior aspects of the medial and lateral tibial plateaus, the tibial attachment of the PCL is located [12]. The PMB footprint is noted to envelope the medial and posterior sides of the ALB, with the thickest portion of the PMB posteromedial to the ALB [12]. Anteromedial to the ALB and distal to the posterior root attachment fibers of the posterior horn of the medial meniscus, the shiny white fibers of the posterior horn of the medial meniscus represent a notable landmark in the PCL facet [12]. In addition, the "champagne glass drop-off," a prominent ridge at the most posterior aspect of the tibial plateau, provides a useful arthroscopic landmark as it consistently marks the distal border of the PMB [5]. The distance between the centers of the PMB and ALB attachments of the tibia is 8.9 mm [12].

7.3 Biomechanics

Understanding the biomechanics of the knee is beneficial for clinical examinations and restoration of knee kinematics, especially in determining the hierarchy of ligamentous structures for restraint of abnormal knee motion, to significantly improve anatomic repairs and reconstructions [13, 14]. Many factors affect the success/outcomes following reconstructions/repairs of ligamentous knee structures. Due to the immense complexity of the knee and its ensuing soft tissue composition, a diverse range of variables may affect the efficacy of surgical intervention in respect to characteristics of structure-specific loading across variable flexion angles, which ultimately can disturb native internal/external rotation, anterior/posterior translation, or varus/valgus motions [13].

7.3.1 Medial Collateral Ligament

The sMCL consists of two divisions, proximal and distal, that each contribute to the stability of the medial aspect of the knee [6, 7]. Griffith et al. determined the functionality of each and found the proximal division provided primary static stabilization from valgus motion at all tested angles of flexion (0°, 20°, 30°, 60°, and 90°) and secondary stabilization to external rotation at knee flexion angles greater than 90° and internal rotation at flexion angles of 0°, 30°, and 90° [13]. The distal division of the MCL provided primary stabilization for external rotation at 30° and internal rotation at all tested angles of flexion, while also providing secondary stabilization to external rotation at 0°, 20°, and 60° of flexion [13]. This data shows that the load response for the distal division of the sMCL is dependent upon varying angles of knee flexion, while no significant load difference was noted for the proximal division upon angle variation [13]. Additionally, the distal division was found to have an indirect role in preventing abnormal valgus motion [13].

The dMCL also has various stabilizing functions dependent on the meniscotibial and meniscofemoral portions, with the meniscofemoral portions having a greater role in providing stabilization [13]. The meniscotibial portion provides secondary stabilization for internal rotation at 0°, 30°, and 90° and valgus restraint at 60° for knee flexion [13]. The meniscofemoral portion likewise provides secondary valgus stabilization at all tested flexion angles and secondary stabilization for internal rotation at 0° and 30° of knee flexion but also provides primary stabilization for internal rotation at 20°, 60°, and 90° and secondary stability for external rotation at 30° and 90° of knee flexion [13].

Structural properties of the MCL were previously reported by Wijdicks et al., in which mean loads at failure were determined. A detachment of the proximal tibial attachment resulted in load of 87.6 ± 36.1 N at failure, and detachment of the distal division resulted in a load of 557.1 ± 55.4 N at failure, which is comparable to a similar study by Robinson et al. in which they reported the sMCL had a mean load at failure of 534 N [6, 15]. However, the failure load for the dMCL was less consistent, with findings of 101 N and 194 N, while the most common means of failure occurred at the meniscofemoral portion (Fig. 7.3) [6, 15].

7.3.2 Posterior Cruciate Ligament

The PCL, composed of two bundles (ALB and PMB), is the strongest of the intra-articular knee ligaments and provides its stabilizing features predominantly as the primary restraint to posterior tibial translation and secondary restraint to external and internal tibial rotation at flexion angles greater than 90° [11, 16, 17]. Posterior translation and rotational stability are attributed to its tensile strength and the complex fiber orientation [11]. The ALB is the major contributor in tensile strength, measuring approximately 1620 N, compared with the smaller PMB, failing around 258 N [18, 19]. As the knee enters increasing flexion angles, the PCL takes on a greater role in posterior translational restraint, amounting for 95% between 30° and 90° [20].

A more recent study by Kennedy et al. elucidated specified stabilization by the PCL with individual analysis of the ALB and PMB and found that each plays a specific role throughout the full range of knee flexion, in the absence of the other. Between the flexion angles of 15° and 90°, the ALB provides the predominant resistance to posterior translation, with the PMB providing supplemental restraint [16]. Resistance to internal rotation beyond 90° of knee flexion

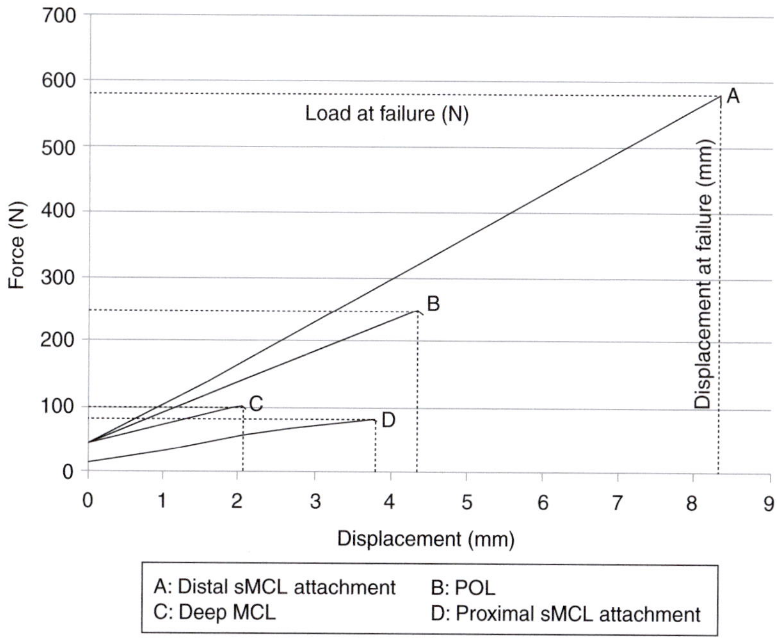

Fig. 7.3 Load-displacement curve for determining load-at-failure (N), displacement-at-failure (mm), and stiffness (N/mm). When a change in displacement no longer exhibited concomitant load increases, failure and displacement were determined. Stiffness was calculated as slope of the linear region just before failure on the force-versus-displacement curve, as the steepest straight-line tangent to the curve. *sMCL* superficial medial collateral ligament, *POL* posterior oblique ligament, *MCL* medial collateral ligament. *Reprinted with permission of SAGE Publications, Inc, from Wijdicks CA, Ewart DT, Nuckley DJ, Johansen S, Engebretsen L, Laprade RF: Structural properties of the primary medial knee ligaments. Am J Sports Med 2010, 38:1638–46*

specifically was derived from the PMB, while restraint of external rotation was significantly lessened from the sectioning of either bundle [16]. In addition, the role of each bundle in restraint to external and internal rotation was relatively small, yet still significant, most profoundly beyond 90° of knee flexion [16]. Overall, from the few differences noted above, the ALB and PMB seemingly have a codominant role in PCL functionality and restraint to abnormal translation/rotation (Fig. 7.4) [16].

7.4 Diagnosis

Management of MCL and PCL injuries begins with an integrated physical examination. The posterior drawer test, quadriceps active test, and valgus stress test are beneficial in determining presence of either an isolated MCL or concomitant cruciate injury. Application of a valgus stress load at 0° or 20° of flexion determines the severity of medial compartment gapping [21]. At 20° of flexion, valgus stress testing isolates the sMCL in determining its specific injury classification. In the occurrence of an isolated grade III sMCL tear, medial gapping of 1–2 mm at full extension relative to the contralateral knee is expected [21, 22]. A concomitant cruciate injury is potentially present upon greater gapping of the medial compartment [14, 22].

PCL deficiency is evaluated by the posterior sag sign, the quadriceps active test, and the posterior drawer test [23]. The PCL sag sign, seen from the lateral view in supine positioning, and compared to the contralateral knee, is indicated by an abnormal contour located on the proximal anterior tibia [24]. The quadriceps active test indicates a PCL tear from posterior tibial subluxation of at least 2 mm [25]. The posterior drawer test compares posterior tibial laxity between contralateral knees, with a greater laxity indicating a

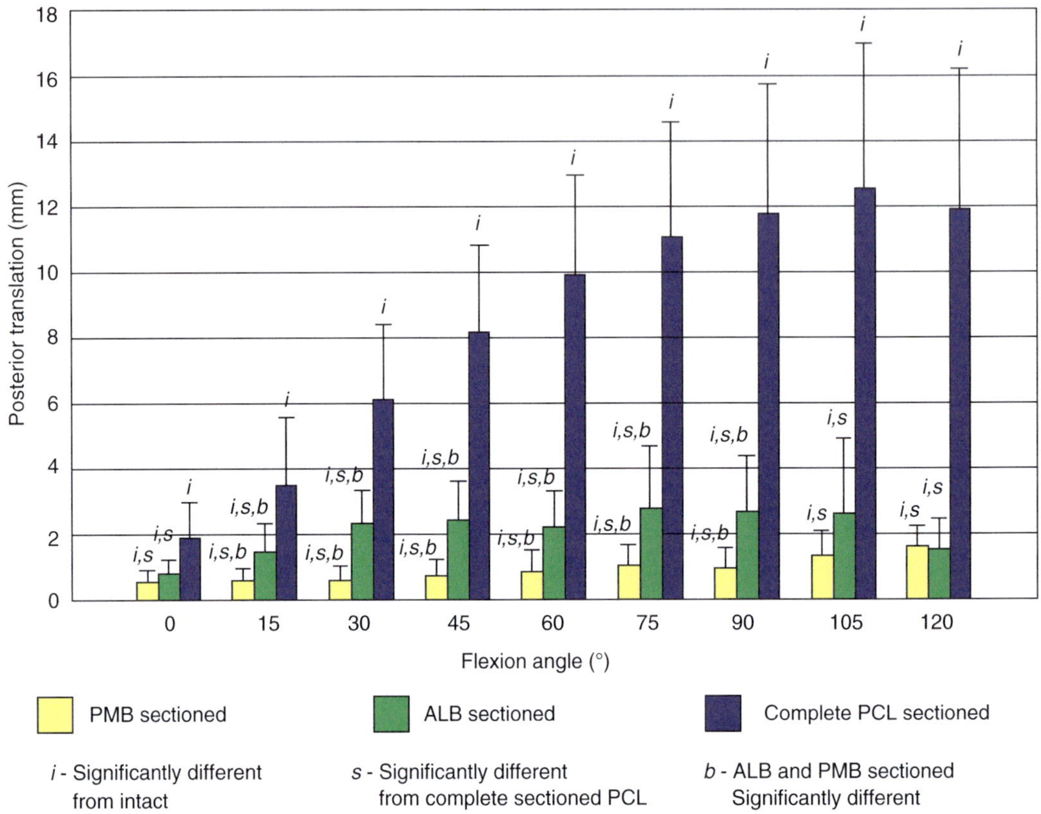

Fig. 7.4 Measured posterior tibial translation (mm) mean increases in response to 134 N posterior tibial force, following isolated sectioning of the posteromedial bundle (PMB) or anterolateral bundle (ALB), and by the complete sectioning of the posterior cruciate ligament (PCL). *Reprinted with permission of SAGE Publications, Inc., from Kennedy NI, Wijdicks CA, Goldsmith MT, Michalski MP, Devitt BM, Aroen A, Engebretsen L, LaPrade RF: Kinematic analysis of the posterior cruciate ligament, part 1: the individual and collective function of the anterolateral and posteromedial bundles. Am J Sports Med 2013, 41:2828–38*

PCL injury. However, this test can be highly subjective and should be followed by posterior knee stress imaging (Fig. 7.5) [23].

In the occurrence of combined PCL and MCL tears, magnetic resonance imaging (MRI) can detect lateral compartment bone bruises which are indicative of this type of injury [26]. Although MRI is highly accurate for the overall diagnosis of acute PCL tears (97–100% sensitivity), chronic injuries can be masked by the healing processes following injury [27]. Therefore, kneeling and telos posterior knee stress radiographs are recommended for more accurate and objective diagnosis [27].

Kneeling stress radiographs are increasingly more popular from its superior reproducibility in evaluating the presence of PCL tears by assessing tibial translation between injured and uninjured knees [2, 28]. The telos stress device is also commonly used for the diagnosis of PCL tears, producing an adjustable, quantifiable, and reproducible posterior force for knee analysis [28]. When comparing side-to-side posterior tibial translation (PTT), the presence of 8–12 mm of increased PTT is indicative of an isolated complete PCL tear, while ≥12 mm of PTT is indicative of a combined complete PCL tear (Fig. 7.6) [28].

7.5 Treatment

Because of the intrinsic ability of the MCL to attenuate self-healing, non-operative treatment of an isolated MCL tear with the use of a hinged

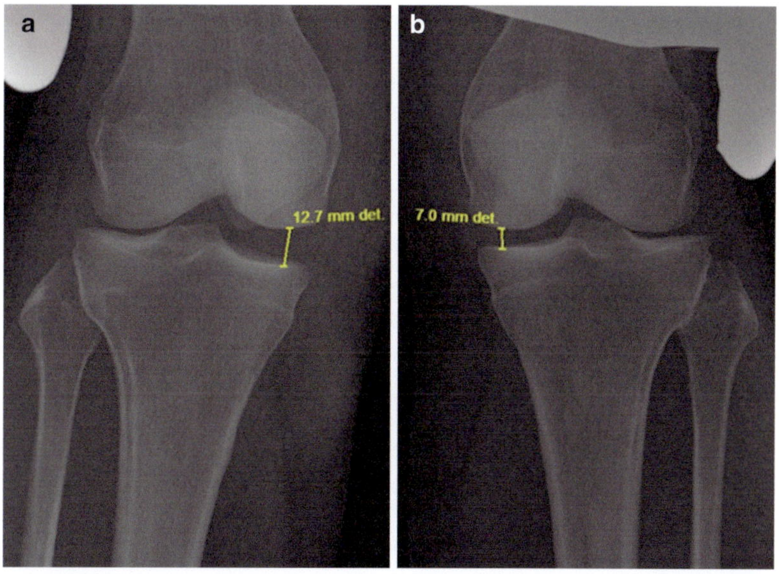

Fig. 7.5 Bilateral valgus stress radiographs to detect medial-sided instability when comparing the injured (**a**) and uninjured knee; (**b**) this case shows a 5.7 mm increase in medial compartment gapping relative to the uninjured knee, indicating a complete sMCL tear

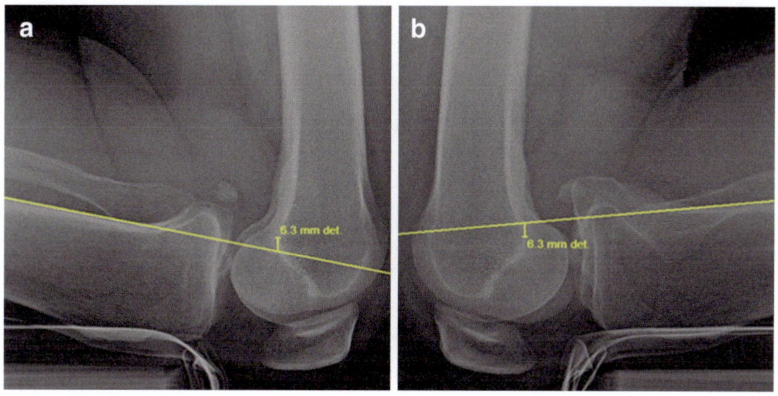

Fig. 7.6 Kneeling stress radiographs for evaluating posterior tibial translation (PTT) in the injured knee (**b**) compared to the uninjured knee (**a**). This case displays PTT of 12.6 mm, indicating a combined complete PCL tear

knee brace usually allows for sufficient recovery and results in similar comparative outcomes to reconstructive and reparative surgical interventions [29]. However, in the case of grade III MCL lesions concomitant with a cruciate ligament tear, especially MCL tears displaying valgus gapping in full extension, MCL reconstructive techniques should be opted for as posteromedial instability can lead to high rates of PCL and ACL graft failure [30].

Surgical techniques utilizing combined MCL and PCL injuries commonly encounter the obstacle of femoral tunnel convergence [31]. With two tunnels reamed in the medial femoral condyle, tunnel directionality and location are delicate [31]. Two recent studies have identified surgical techniques evading this issue [30, 31].

Camarda et al. evaluated axial and coronal angulations of femoral tunnels for MCL reconstruction. A coronal angulation between 0° and 20° yielded a tunnel convergence rate of 62.5%, while at an angulation of 40°, this rate decreased to 0% [30]. However, the PCL reconstruction (PCLR) used in this study did not involve a DB technique. Recent literature reports that DB PCLR better restores the native kinematics of the knee and therefore should be implemented for multi-ligament reconstructions [32]. Furthermore, Moatshe et al. report that aiming the sMCL femoral tunnel anterior and proximally at 40° in axial and coronal planes assures the sMCL tunnel and two femoral PCL tunnels will avoid collision [33].

For sMCL anatomic augmented repair or anatomic reconstruction, a 16 cm long semitendinosus or gracilis graft should be harvested, initially fixed in a 7 mm tibial tunnel reamed 6 cm distal to the medial joint line, and passed deep to the sartorius fascia [34]. For both anatomical techniques, the graft can then be fixed at 20° of flexion into the femoral tunnel, at the femoral sMCL attachment site located 12 mm distal and 8 mm anterior to the adductor tubercle [34]. The proximal sMCL attachment site is then fixed with a suture anchor 12 mm from the joint line [34]. Literature suggests that both anatomic augmented repair and reconstruction techniques are not significantly different in restoring native kinematics of the knee, although both significantly reduce laxity in the knee when compared to preoperative laxity measurements (Fig. 7.7) [34].

Due to the evidence of improved functional and objective outcomes of the DB PCLR technique, it is recommended that two femoral tunnels should be reamed to reproduce the normal femoral footprints of the PCL [32]. A study by Johannsen et al. reports that in the anteroposterior (AP) femoral view, the centers of the ALB and PMB footprints are 34.1 ± 3.0 mm and 29.2 ± 3.0 mm lateral to the most MFC, respectively [35]. Using the lateral femur view and the Blumensaat reference line, Johannsen et al. also reported that the ALB and PMB centers are located 17.4 ± 1.7 mm and 23.9 ± 2.7 mm posteroproximal to a line perpendicular to the reference line, which intersects the anterior margin of the MFC cortex [35].

For tibial tunnel placement, AP tibial radiographic images showed the center of the ALB and PMB attachment sites were 0.2 ± 2.1 mm proximally and 4.9 ± 2.9 mm distally to proximal joint line, respectively [35]. Additionally, lateral tibial radiography found that the ALB and PMB

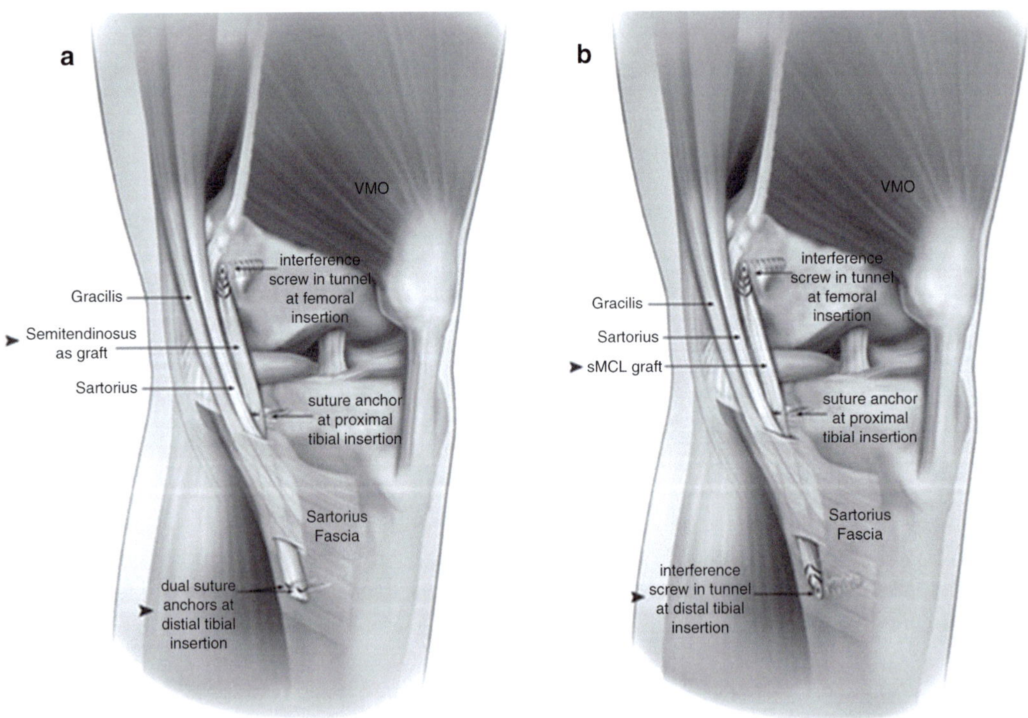

Fig. 7.7 Anatomic augmented sMCL repair using a semitendinosus graft (**a**) and anatomic sMCL reconstruction (**b**). Grafts are fixated at the femoral and tibial insertions with interference screws, replicating the native attachment sites of the sMCL. *sMCL* superficial medial collateral ligament, *VMO* vastus medialis oblique. *Reprinted with permission of SAGE Publications, Inc, from Wijdicks CA, Michalski MP, Rasmussen MT, Goldsmith MT, Kennedy NI, Lind M, Engebretsen L, LaPrade RF: Superficial medial collateral ligament anatomic augmented repair versus anatomic reconstruction: an in vitro biomechanical analysis. Am J Sports Med 2013, 41:2858–66*

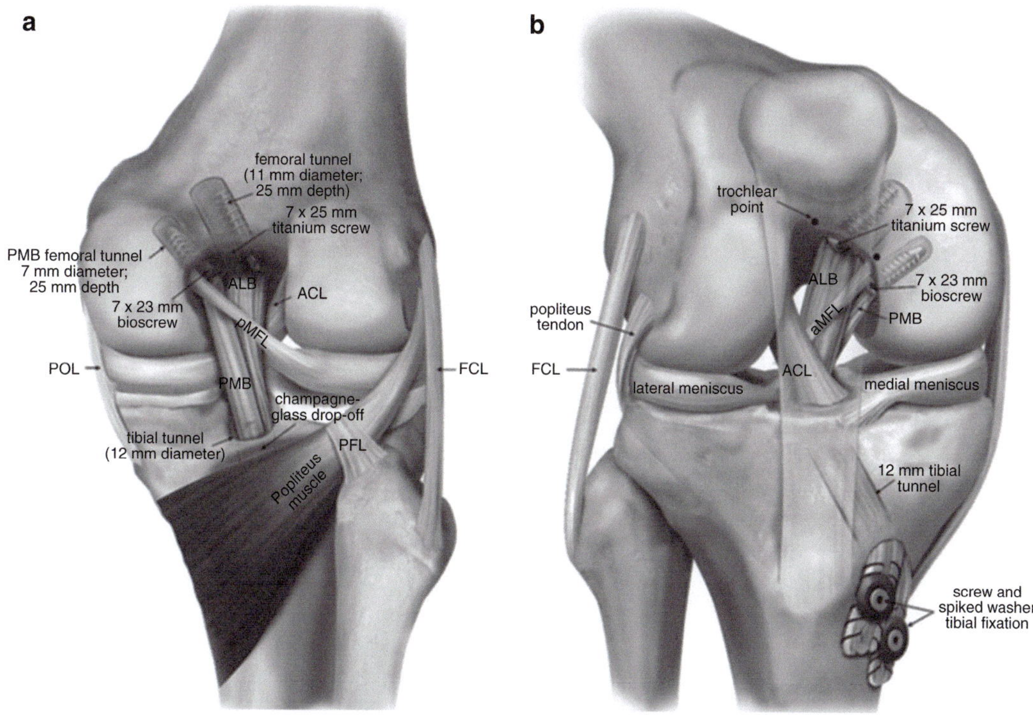

Fig. 7.8 (**a**) Posterior and (**b**) anterior view diagrams of an anatomic double-bundle PCL reconstruction. The illustrations depict femoral and tibial tunnels with interference screw fixation regarding size, shape, and location. *ACL* anterior cruciate ligament, *PMB* posteromedial bundle, *ALB* anterolateral bundle, *FCL* fibular collateral ligament, *PFL* popliteofibular ligament, *pMFL* posterior meniscofemoral ligament, *POL* posterior oblique ligament. *Reprinted with permission of SAGE Publications, Inc, from Wijdicks CA, Kennedy NI, Goldsmith MT, Devitt BM, Michalski MP, Aroen A, Engebretsen L, LaPrade RF: Kinematic analysis of the posterior cruciate ligament, part 2: a comparison of anatomic single- versus double-bundle reconstruction. Am J Sports Med 2013, 41:2839–48*

centers were located 8.4 ± 1.8 and 2.5 ± 1.5 mm superior to the champagne-glass drop-off, respectively. In combination, the overall center of the PCL attachment site is 5.5 ± 1.5 mm superior to the same osseous landmark, and a singular tibial tunnel is used [32]. In the case of a concomitant MCL lesion, the femoral tunnels should be reamed in accordance to the angles previously suggested, to avoid tunnel convergence. Radiographic imaging is important for location of bony landmarks to assure correct tunnel placement and provide a repeatable approach for intraoperative assessments (Fig. 7.8) [35].

An Achilles tendon graft can be used for the ALB and a semitendinosus or tibialis anterior graft for the PMB, with the ALB graft being fixed at 90° flexion and the PMB graft being fixed at full extension [35–37]. By reconstructing both the MCL and PCL to their anatomic attachment sites, surgical intervention is capable of restoring native kinematics to the knee joint, relieving contact pressures, and reducing the progression of osteoarthritis (OA) in long-term scenarios [32, 37, 38].

7.6 Clinical Outcomes

7.6.1 PCL Isolated

Isolated PCL tears significantly alter joint kinematics and can lead to high rates of osteoarthritis (OA) progression or concomitant injury [38]. Hermans et al. reported that isolated SB PCLR procedures have the ability to nearly restore normal subjective function (in 75% of patients) and significantly improve posterior knee laxity [39]. However, although subjective IKDC scores were favorable, the study reported 60% presenting evidence of OA progression and ultimately failed to restore normal knee kinematics [39].

Emerging updates of the DB PCLR technique are promising for long-term clinical outcomes following the analysis of several short-term outcome reports [2]. In one such study, after a mean time of 2.5 years postoperative for isolated PCL lesions, Cincinnati scores significantly improved, with the average scores increasing from 49.0 ± 18.4 preoperatively to 87.4 ± 18.0 postoperatively [5]. Additionally, average IKDC subjective outcome scores significantly increased from 53.5 ± 12.2 preoperatively to 88.3 ± 14.6 postoperatively [5]. Lastly, DB PCLR significantly reduced average PTT from 10.4 ± 1.6 to 0.7 ± 1.1 mm, as indicated by preoperative and postoperative stress radiographs [5]. With DB PCLR being a relatively new and upcoming technique, longer postoperative outcome studies are needed to determine long-term efficacy [32]. However, short-term clinical outcome scores show DB PCLR lead to improved subjective and objective scores with full restoration of native kinematics of the knee joint through anatomic reconstruction [32]. Therefore, for isolated PCL tears, it is believed that long-term outcomes will be significantly improved and the prevalence of OA will be reduced (Fig. 7.9) [32].

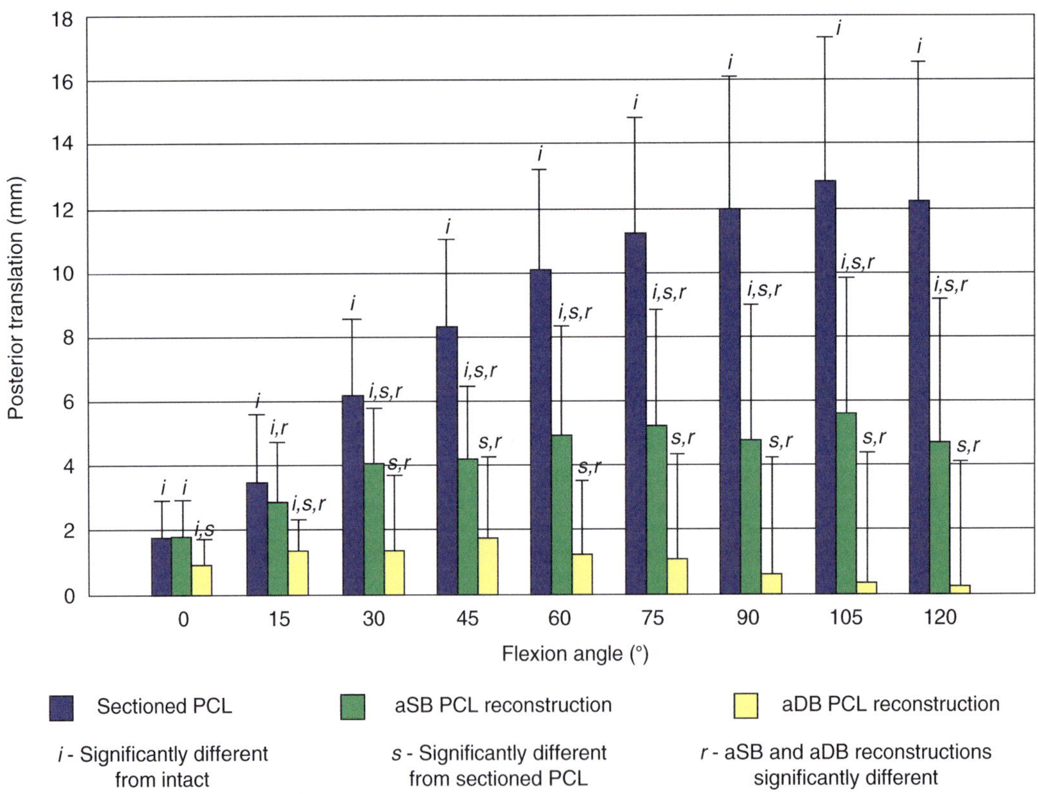

Fig. 7.9 Measurement of posterior translation (mm) following complete sectioning of the posterior cruciate ligament (PCL), as well as anatomic single-bundle (aSB) PCL reconstruction and anatomic double-bundle (aDB) PCL reconstruction. Relative to the intact PCL knee, mean average increases of posterior translation were reported in response to a 134 N posterior tibial force. *Reprinted with permission of SAGE Publications, Inc, from Wijdicks CA, Kennedy NI, Goldsmith MT, Devitt BM, Michalski MP, Aroen A, Engebretsen L, LaPrade RF: Kinematic analysis of the posterior cruciate ligament, part 2: a comparison of anatomic single- versus double-bundle reconstruction. Am J Sports Med 2013, 41:2839–48*

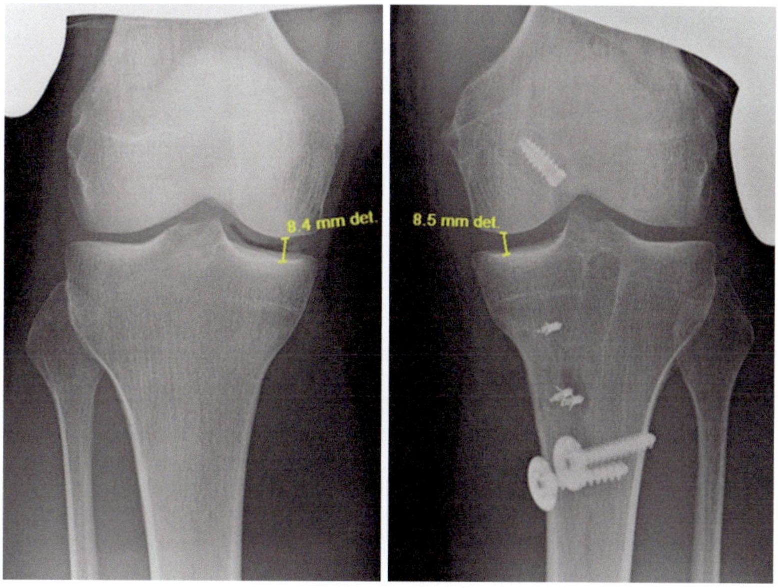

Fig. 7.10 Postoperative valgus stress radiograph for a case following superficial medial collateral ligament (sMCL) and double-bundle (DB) posterior cruciate ligament reconstruction (PCLR). Medial gapping has been restored to normative expectations, relative to the contralateral knee

7.6.2 PCL Combined

The most common reason for graft failure in PCLRs is unaddressed concomitant injuries that result in residual instability of the knee joint [33]. Therefore, it is essential that all pathologies be attended to concurrently with PCLRs, as PCL tears are most frequently observed with concomitant injuries [5, 33] In a study reported by Spiridonov et al., 32 patients with combined injury had significantly increased Cincinnati scores with an improvement from 33.6 ± 22.3 preoperatively to 67.5 ± 28.0 postoperatively [5]. Average IKDC scores and posterior translation also improved from 37.7 ± 19.0 to 69.3 ± 23.5 and 16.1 ± 3.7 mm to 0.8 ± 1.1 mm, respectively [5]. At 6-year follow-up, Mygind-Klavsen et al. compared outcomes between isolated and combined PCL injuries and found nearly no significant difference in outcomes between each cohort, with an exception to the KOOS subscore of sport [40]. However, the results included a mix of SB and DB PCLR procedures (89% DB), requiring further clinical investigation [40].

Unfortunately, there is relative paucity in objective and functional outcomes of MCL injuries associated with concomitant cruciate ligament lesions. Combined MCL and PCL injuries are grouped into the KD-III-M and KD-IV cohorts of the Schenck classification system of knee dislocations. However, these cohorts include injury to the ACL and therefore must be considered while presenting combined PCL-MCL clinical outcomes. Because of the complexity of multiligament injuries, it is often difficult to measure the isolated significance of the MCL lesion and its role in long-term recovery. Therefore, it is important that clinicians document cases that involve solely combined PCL and MCL injury. Increased understanding on treatment of these injuries and expected outcomes can significantly enhance the care for patients that present PCL and MCL combined lesions (Fig. 7.10).

7.7 Conclusions

The occurrence of concomitant sMCL and PCL injuries is relatively low, and many factors play into long-term patient outcomes and success of surgery. Obstacles like femoral tunnel convergence and/or failure to diagnose concomitant injuries may result in failure of restoring the knee to its natural state. For treatment, current literature reinforces anatomic reconstruction techniques in reestablishing kinematics of the knee joint. Failure may result in graft failure, damage to neighboring structures, or the onset of

OA. DB PCLRs are popularized for reproducing both bundles of the PCL, and a significant difference between repair and reconstruction of the sMCL has yet to come to light; further studies are required to display outcomes at longer follow-ups and success among current surgical procedures.

References

1. Miyasaka KC, Daniel DM, Stone ML. The incidence of knee ligament injuries in the general population. Am J Knee Surg. 1991;4:43–8.
2. LaPrade CM, Civitarese DM, Rasmussen MT, LaPrade RF. Emerging updates on the posterior cruciate ligament: a review of the current literature. Am J Sports Med. 2015;43:3077–92.
3. Fanelli GC, Edson CJ. Posterior cruciate ligament injuries in trauma patients: part II. Arthroscopy. 1995;11:526–9.
4. Becker EH, Watson JD, Dreese JC. Investigation of multiligamentous knee injury patterns with associated injuries presenting at a level I trauma center. J Orthop Trauma. 2013;27:226–31.
5. Spiridonov SI, Slinkard NJ, LaPrade RF. Isolated and combined grade-III posterior cruciate ligament tears treated with double-bundle reconstruction with use of endoscopically placed femoral tunnels and grafts: operative technique and clinical outcomes. J Bone Joint Surg Am. 2011;93:1773–80.
6. Wijdicks CA, Ewart DT, Nuckley DJ, Johansen S, Engebretsen L, Laprade RF. Structural properties of the primary medial knee ligaments. Am J Sports Med. 2010;38:1638–46.
7. LaPrade RF, Engebretsen AH, Ly TV, Johansen S, Wentorf FA, Engebretsen L. The anatomy of the medial part of the knee. J Bone Joint Surg Am. 2007;89:2000–10.
8. De Maeseneer M, Van Roy F, Lenchik L, Barbaix E, De Ridder F, Osteaux M. Three layers of the medial capsular and supporting structures of the knee: MR imaging-anatomic correlation. Radiographics. 2000;20:S83–9.
9. Loredo R, Hodler J, Pedowitz R, Yeh LR, Trudell D, Resnick D. Posteromedial corner of the knee: MR imaging with gross anatomic correlation. Skelet Radiol. 1999;28:305–11.
10. Warren LF, Marshall JL. The supporting structures and layers on the medial side of the knee: an anatomical analysis. J Bone Joint Surg Am. 1979;61:56–62.
11. Bowman KF Jr, Sekiya JK. Anatomy and biomechanics of the posterior cruciate ligament, medial and lateral sides of the knee. Sports Med Arthrosc. 2010;18:222–9.
12. Anderson CJ, Ziegler CG, Wijdicks CA, Engebretsen L, LaPrade RF. Arthroscopically pertinent anatomy of the anterolateral and posteromedial bundles of the posterior cruciate ligament. J Bone Joint Surg Am. 2012;94:1936–45.
13. Griffith CJ, LaPrade RF, Johansen S, Armitage B, Wijdicks C, Engebretsen L. Medial knee injury: part 1, static function of the individual components of the main medial knee structures. Am J Sports Med. 2009;37:1762–70.
14. Griffith CJ, Wijdicks CA, LaPrade RF, Armitage BM, Johansen S, Engebretsen L. Force measurements on the posterior oblique ligament and superficial medial collateral ligament proximal and distal divisions to applied loads. Am J Sports Med. 2009;37:140–8.
15. Robinson JR, Bull AM, Amis AA. Structural properties of the medial collateral ligament complex of the human knee. J Biomech. 2005;38:1067–74.
16. Kennedy NI, Wijdicks CA, Goldsmith MT, Michalski MP, Devitt BM, Aroen A, Engebretsen L, LaPrade RF. Kinematic analysis of the posterior cruciate ligament, part 1: the individual and collective function of the anterolateral and posteromedial bundles. Am J Sports Med. 2013;41:2828–38.
17. Moulton SG, Cram TR, James EW, Dornan GJ, Kennedy NI, LaPrade RF. The supine internal rotation test: a pilot study evaluating tibial internal rotation in grade III posterior cruciate ligament tears. Orthop J Sports Med. 2015;3:2325967115572135.
18. Kennedy JC, Hawkins RJ, Willis RB, Danylchuck KD. Tension studies of human knee ligaments. Yield point, ultimate failure, and disruption of the cruciate and tibial collateral ligaments. J Bone Joint Surg Am. 1976;58:350–5.
19. Race A, Amis AA. The mechanical properties of the two bundles of the human posterior cruciate ligament. J Biomech. 1994;27:13–24.
20. Butler DL, Noyes FR, Grood ES. Ligamentous restraints to anterior-posterior drawer in the human knee. A biomechanical study. J Bone Joint Surg Am. 1980;62:259–70.
21. Laprade RF, Wijdicks CA. The management of injuries to the medial side of the knee. J Orthop Sports Phys Ther. 2012;42:221–33.
22. Laprade RF, Bernhardson AS, Griffith CJ, Macalena JA, Wijdicks CA. Correlation of valgus stress radiographs with medial knee ligament injuries: an in vitro biomechanical study. Am J Sports Med. 2010;38:330–8.
23. Kopkow C, Freiberg A, Kirschner S, Seidler A, Schmitt J. Physical examination tests for the diagnosis of posterior cruciate ligament rupture: a systematic review. J Orthop Sports Phys Ther. 2013;43:804–13.
24. Lubowitz JH, Bernardini BJ, Reid JB 3rd. Current concepts review: comprehensive physical examination for instability of the knee. Am J Sports Med. 2008;36:577–94.
25. Daniel DM, Stone ML, Barnett P, Sachs R. Use of the quadriceps active test to diagnose posterior cruciate-ligament disruption and measure posterior laxity of the knee. J Bone Joint Surg Am. 1988;70:386–91.

26. Mair SD, Schlegel TF, Gill TJ, Hawkins RJ, Steadman JR. Incidence and location of bone bruises after acute posterior cruciate ligament injury. Am J Sports Med. 2004;32:1681–7.
27. Jackman T, LaPrade RF, Pontinen T, Lender PA. Intraobserver and interobserver reliability of the kneeling technique of stress radiography for the evaluation of posterior knee laxity. Am J Sports Med. 2008;36:1571–6.
28. James EW, Williams BT, LaPrade RF. Stress radiography for the diagnosis of knee ligament injuries: a systematic review. Clin Orthop Relat Res. 2014;472:2644–57.
29. Indelicato PA. Non-operative treatment of complete tears of the medial collateral ligament of the knee. J Bone Joint Surg Am. 1983;65:323–9.
30. Camarda L, Grassedonio E, Lauria M, Midiri M, D'Arienzo M. How to avoid collision between PCL and MCL femoral tunnels during a simultaneous reconstruction. Knee Surg Sports Traumatol Arthrosc. 2016;24:2767–72.
31. Moatshe G, Slette EL, Engebretsen L, LaPrade RF. Intertunnel relationships in the tibia during reconstruction of multiple knee ligaments: how to avoid tunnel convergence. Am J Sports Med. 2016;44:2864–9.
32. Chahla J, Moatshe G, Engebretsen L, LaPrade RF. Anatomic double-bundle posterior cruciate ligament reconstruction. Arthrosc Tech. 2017;7:e4.
33. Moatshe G, Chahla J, LaPrade RF, Engebretsen L. Diagnosis and treatment of multiligament knee injury: state of the art. J ISAKOS. 2017;2:152–61.
34. Wijdicks CA, Michalski MP, Rasmussen MT, Goldsmith MT, Kennedy NI, Lind M, Engebretsen L, LaPrade RF. Superficial medial collateral ligament anatomic augmented repair versus anatomic reconstruction: an in vitro biomechanical analysis. Am J Sports Med. 2013;41:2858–66.
35. Johannsen AM, Anderson CJ, Wijdicks CA, Engebretsen L, LaPrade RF. Radiographic landmarks for tunnel positioning in posterior cruciate ligament reconstructions. Am J Sports Med. 2013;41:35–42.
36. Kennedy NI, LaPrade RF, Goldsmith MT, Faucett SC, Rasmussen MT, Coatney GA, Engebretsen L, Wijdicks CA. Posterior cruciate ligament graft fixation angles, part 2: biomechanical evaluation for anatomic double-bundle reconstruction. Am J Sports Med. 2014;42:2346–55.
37. Wijdicks CA, Kennedy NI, Goldsmith MT, Devitt BM, Michalski MP, Aroen A, Engebretsen L, LaPrade RF. Kinematic analysis of the posterior cruciate ligament, part 2: a comparison of anatomic single- versus double-bundle reconstruction. Am J Sports Med. 2013;41:2839–48.
38. Skyhar MJ, Warren RF, Ortiz GJ, Schwartz E, Otis JC. The effects of sectioning of the posterior cruciate ligament and the posterolateral complex on the articular contact pressures within the knee. J Bone Joint Surg Am. 1993;75:694–9.
39. Hermans S, Corten K, Bellemans J. Long-term results of isolated anterolateral bundle reconstructions of the posterior cruciate ligament: a 6- to 12-year follow-up study. Am J Sports Med. 2009;37:1499–507.
40. Mygind-Klavsen B, Nielsen TG, Lind MC. Outcomes after posterior cruciate ligament (PCL) reconstruction in patients with isolated and combined PCL tears. Orthop J Sports Med. 2017;5:2325967117700077.

8 Management of Complex Knee Injuries: How to Manage Combined Posterior Cruciate Ligament and Posterolateral Corner Injuries

Carola F. van Eck and Mohsen Hussein

8.1 Introduction

Multi-ligament knee injuries present a wide spectrum of pathology. They can involve one cruciate and one or both of the collaterals or both cruciates and the collateral(s). The latter is consistent with a knee dislocation pattern. Injuries to the ligaments can be partial (grade I or II) or complete (grade III). Partial injuries can heal, especially when they concern the posterior cruciate ligament (PCL).

This chapter will focus specifically on combined PCL and posterolateral corner (PLC) injuries. It will briefly discuss the anatomy, function, history, physical exam findings, and indicated diagnostic tests. A classification guiding management will be introduced. Surgical management will be the focus of this chapter with a detailed description of the authors' preferred surgical technique with illustrations to each of the steps. The aim is to prepare the reader for (surgical) management of PCL-PLC injuries.

C. F. van Eck
Department of Orthopaedic Surgery, University of Pittsburgh, Pittsburgh, PA, USA

M. Hussein (✉)
Artros Center for Orthopaedic Surgery and Sports Medicine, Ljubljana, Slovenia
e-mail: mhussein@artros.si

F. Margheritini et al. (eds.), *Complex Knee Ligament Injuries*,
https://doi.org/10.1007/978-3-662-58245-9_8

8.2 Anatomy

The PCL arises from the posterior tibial sulcus, just below the articular surface. It attaches to the femur on the anterolateral aspect of the medial femoral condyle. It has a broad, crescent-shaped footprint. The main function of the PCL is to prevent posterior tibial displacement. It sees the highest forces in flexion [1]. The PLC is comprised of several distinct anatomic structures: the fibular (or lateral) collateral ligament (FCL/LCL), the popliteus tendon (PT), and the popliteofibular ligament (PFL). Secondary contributing structures include the lateral capsule, arcuate ligament, and fabellofibular ligament. Lastly, there are dynamic stabilizers such as the biceps femoris, popliteus muscle, iliotibial tracts (ITT), and the lateral head of the gastrocnemius muscle. The posterolateral corner serves several roles: the popliteus works with the PCL to control external rotation and varus and posterior translation, the popliteus and popliteofibular ligaments resist external rotation during knee flexion, and the LCL is the primary restraint to varus stress at lower knee flexion angles [2].

8.3 Patient History

Evaluation of a patient with a combined PCL-PLC injury starts with the physical examination. There are generally two distinct types of multiple ligament injured knee patients.

Perhaps the most common, or well-known, is the young athlete with a high-energy sports injury resulting in a knee dislocation. This usually involves contact sports such as football. Symptoms will include pain and the inability to bear weight following the trauma. In this situation on-the-field management is critical, which involves prompt reduction, immobilization, and a check of the neurovascular status, followed by transfer to a level I trauma center [3]. Management will be discussed in more detail below.

The second group of patients involves low-energy injury mechanisms in the older population. This can appear to be a relative minor injury such as stepping off a curb. Due to this and to the sometimes more obese patient body habitus, a knee dislocation may easily be missing. However, these patients require the same thorough management as high-energy injuries [3]. Otherwise the injury can be limb threatening.

8.4 Physical Examination

Physical examination is extremely important in the evaluation of knee dislocations. Initial examination should include a thorough neurovascular examination. The dorsalis pedis and posterior tibial pulse should be palpated, an ankle-brachial index should be performed, and sensation to the foot should be tested. Approximately 25% of patients will have some form of peroneal nerve dysfunction. This may range from altered sensation to the dorsum of the foot to a complete foot drop. Also, in the setting of a polytrauma patient, the ABCs of trauma should always be employed first: check the airway, breathing, and circulation to ensure the patient is stable before proceeding with a musculoskeletal exam. It is advised for a level 1 trauma center to have an algorithm in place in collaboration with trauma team to treat these patients [3].

Although PCL-PLC injuries may present more often in the acute setting, they can also be seen in the chronic setting when initially missed or not properly addressed. In the chronic setting, when patients present to the office, physical examination shoulder include a gait exam to look for a varus of hyperextension thrust.

Further exam maneuvers should involve varus stress: varus laxity at 0° indicates both LCL and cruciate injury; varus laxity at 30° points to an isolated LCL injury. In addition, a dial test should be performed: >10° external rotation asymmetry at 30° only is consistent with isolated PLC injury, while >10° external rotation asymmetry at 30° and 90° points to a combined PLC and PCL injury. Other potential exams for instability include the posterolateral drawer test (combined posterior drawer and external rotation force) and the reverse pivot shift test (going from knee flexion, external rotation, and valgus to extension). Examination under anesthesia may reveal that the injured extremity falls into external rotation and recurvatum when the legs are suspended by the toes with the patient supine.

8.5 Diagnostics Studies

Several diagnostic studies can be considered based on the clinical scenario. Initial evaluation starts with plain radiographs. If the knee is not reduced, a reduction should be performed as soon as possible, and radiographs should be repeated to confirm (Fig. 8.1). If there is any concern for a vascular injury based on the ankle-brachial index or peripheral pulse examination, angiography should be performed (Fig. 8.2). This can be done on the operating room by a consulting vascular surgeon, or as part of a computed tomography (CT) angiogram in the emergency department, based on the availability and further treatment plan. After the knee is reduced and immobilized with a splint, brace or external fixator and neurovascular issues addressed, a magnetic resonance imaging (MRI) study should be obtained to evaluate the ligamentous injury in more detail (Fig. 8.3) [4].

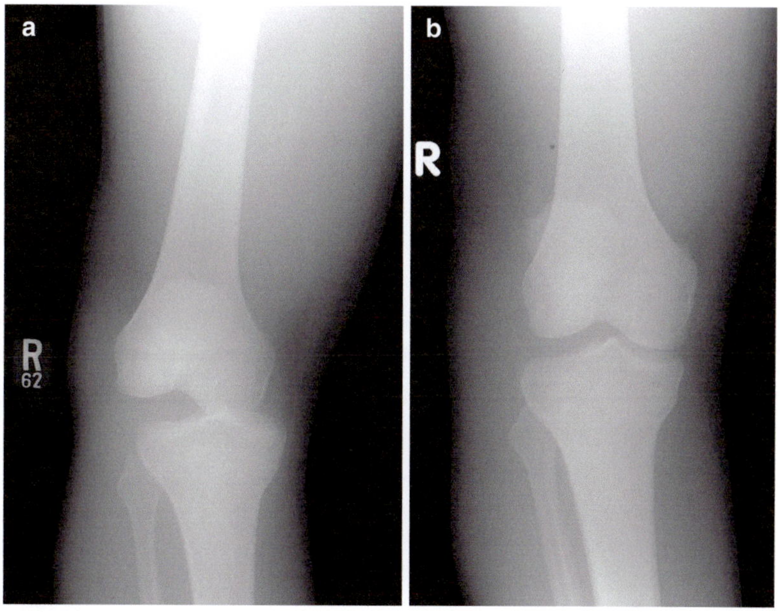

Fig. 8.1 Plain radiograph of a right knee dislocation. (**a**) Prereduction. (**b**) Postreduction, note there is still widening of the lateral joint space as compared to the medial side indicated of a lateral-sided injury

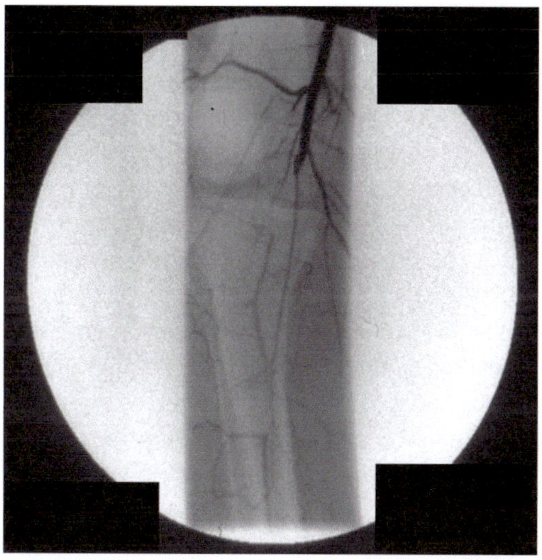

Fig. 8.2 Angiography image or a right knee showing a vascular occlusion as the result of a knee dislocation

8.6 Classification

Multi-ligament knee injuries can be classified several different ways. However, for the purpose of management, important aspect of the injury are the timing, anatomic structures involved, and concomitant injuries that may dictate management (Table 8.1) [5]. Associate injuries can involve meniscal tears, cartilage lesion, (avulsion) fractures, and tibiofibular joint dislocation. The reported incidence of proximal tibiofibular joint instability is 9% [6].

8.7 Treatment

When it comes to management of combined PCL-PLC injuries, treatment will depend on the classification of the injury (Table 8.1). Treatment will most often be surgical unless the patient has significant contraindications to undergoing surgery. In that case, bracing to keep the tibia from posteriorly subluxation and physical therapy to strengthen the quadriceps can be considered. With regard to surgery, consideration should include the timing of surgery, repair versus reconstruction of the PLC, one-stage versus staged treatment, and graft type.

Timing is still a topic of discussion when it comes to management of the multi-ligament injured knee. Both acute and delayed or staged management are good options and each has their

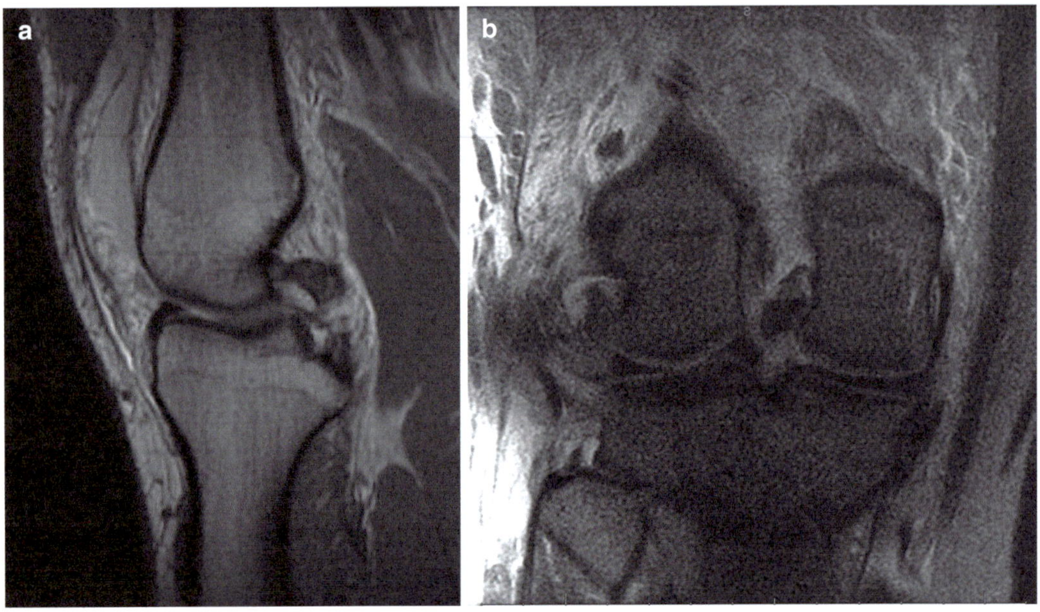

Fig. 8.3 MRI of a right knee. (**a**) T1 sagittal image showing complete midsubstance tear of the PCL. (**b**) T2 coronal image showing a sleeve avulsion of the posterolateral corner structures of the tibial/fibular side

Table 8.1 Multi-ligament knee injury classification

Timing	Anatomic structures	Associated injuries
Acute	Cruciates	Tendon
Chronic	Collaterals	Bone
	Meniscus	Neurovascular

own indications [7]. The authors prefer acute management (within 1–3 weeks after the injury) in the setting of a sleeve-type avulsion of the posterolateral corner structures where there is an option for repair, either with or without augmentation with a graft. In this setting the authors perform the reconstruction of the PCL at the same time. However, this can also be done staged. In the setting of more chronic injuries or when repair is not an option, reconstruction of the PLC is preferred. In this scenario the PCL reconstruction is performed in a staged fashion, about 2–3 months after such that the patient can work on improving range of motion and strengthen the quadriceps [1]. Both methods have been shown to result in good outcomes [7].

The authors' preferred technique for acute PLC repair and PCL reconstruction is described below. The patient is placed supine on the operating room table. After general anesthesia is introduced, an exam under anesthesia is performed. A thigh tourniquet is placed, but not inflated. An L bar is used to allow 90° of flexion with the foot on it and hyperflexion with the entire foot behind it. A side post is placed to allow support of the leg in 90° as well as to administer valgus stress. The leg is then prepped and draped in routine sterile fashion. A diagnostic arthroscopy is performed using a standard anterolateral and anteromedial as well as accessory posteromedial portal. The PCL remnant is removed and the insertion sites are marked for anatomic tunnel placement (Fig. 8.4). An accessory posteromedial portal may aid in debriding and marking the tibial PCL insertion site. The authors prefer single-bundle PCL reconstruction with a transtibial tunnel technique in the setting of a multi-ligament injured knee [8]. A 2–3 cm incision is placed over the anteromedial tibial adjacent to the pes anserine to be used for tibial tunnel placement. The tibial PCL tunnel is drilled first using a drill guide with a guide pin (Fig. 8.4). This is then over-reamed to a 9 or 10 mm tunnel. The femoral PCL tunnel is drilled free hand from the anterolateral portal with a guide pin and also over-reamed to a 9 or 10 mm tunnel to a depth of approximately 20–25 mm (Fig. 8.5). The cortex

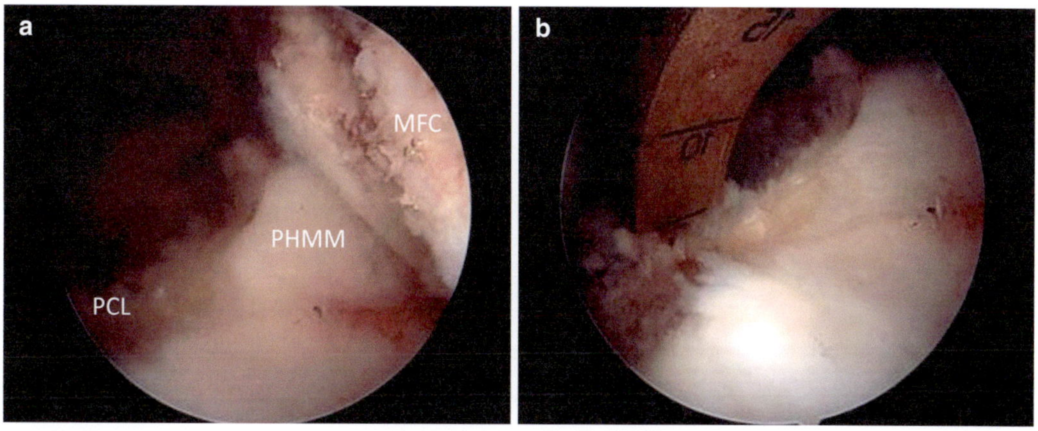

Fig. 8.4 Arthroscopic pictures of a right knee, viewing through the anterolateral portal. (**a**) The PCL remnant is removed and the insertion sites are marked for anatomic tunnel placement. (**b**) The tibial PCL tunnel is drilled first using a drill guide with a guide pin. *PCL* PCL footprint on the tibia, *PHMM* posterior horn medial meniscus, *MFC* medial femoral condyle

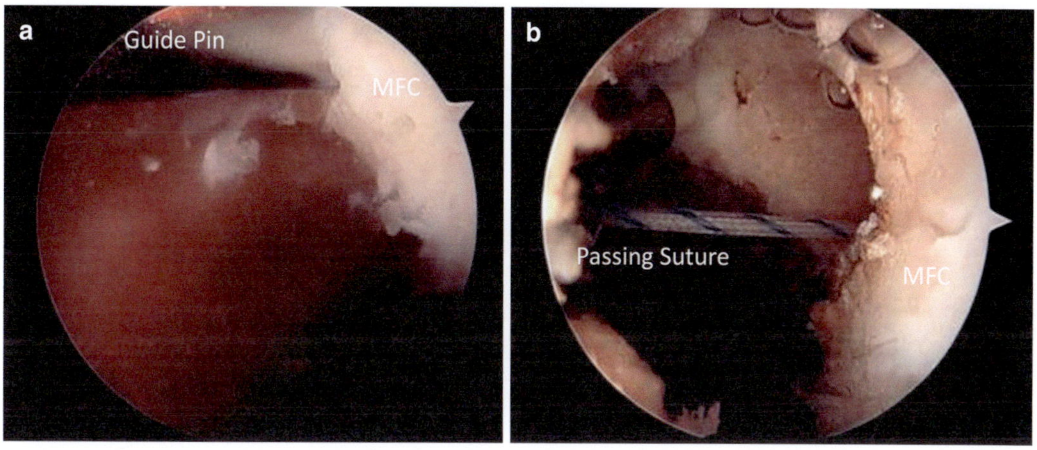

Fig. 8.5 Arthroscopic pictures of a right knee, viewing through the anterolateral portal. (**a**) The femoral PCL tunnel is drilled free hand from the anterolateral portal with a guide pin. (**b**) Next, it is over-reamed to the desired tunnel size. The cortex is broken with a smaller drill to allow passage of the suspensory fixation button and a passing suture is placed. *MFC* medial femoral condyle, *PHMM* posterior horn of medial meniscus

is broken with a smaller drill to allow passage of the suspensory fixation button. A passing suture is placed (Fig. 8.5). A gore smoother is placed up the tibial tunnel and used to facilitate the later graft passage. The gore smoother is then replaced by a passing suture up the tibial tunnel and used to pass the graft up the tibial tunnel (Fig. 8.6). It is then retrieved in the joint and passed up the femoral tunnel using the femoral passing suture (Fig. 8.7). The authors prefer using an all soft tissue allograft with a suspensory fixation button on the femoral side. However, the use of autograft can certainly be considered. The button is flipped and this is confirmed using fluoroscopy. The graft is not fixed on the tibial side until after the PLC is addressed [9].

In the setting of a PLC injury, it can be difficult to contain arthroscopic fluid inside the joint and have adequate visualization. It can help to make the PLC incision early in the case and to place a lap sponge inside the incision to prevent extravasation of the fluid from the joint.

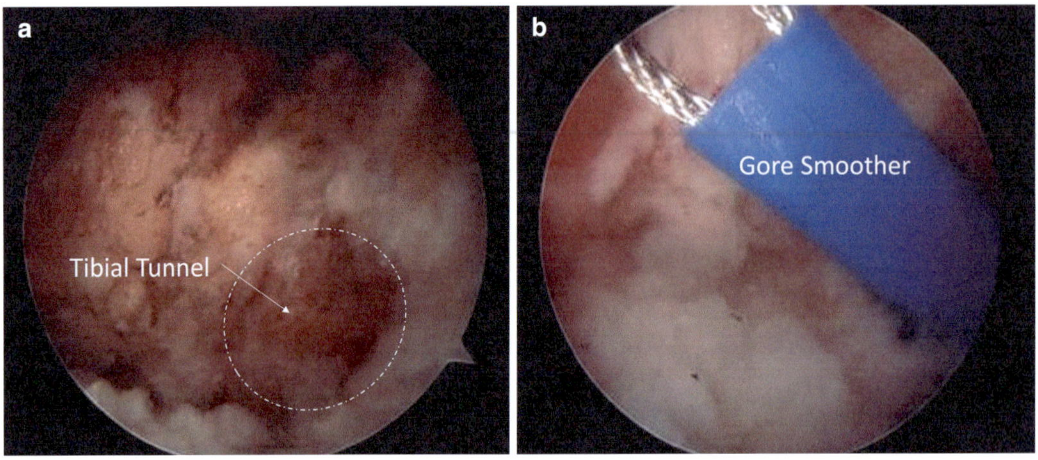

Fig. 8.6 Arthroscopic pictures of a right knee, viewing through the anterolateral portal. (**a**) Demonstrating the location of the tibial tunnel. (**b**) A gore smoother is placed up the tibial tunnel and used to facilitate the later graft passage

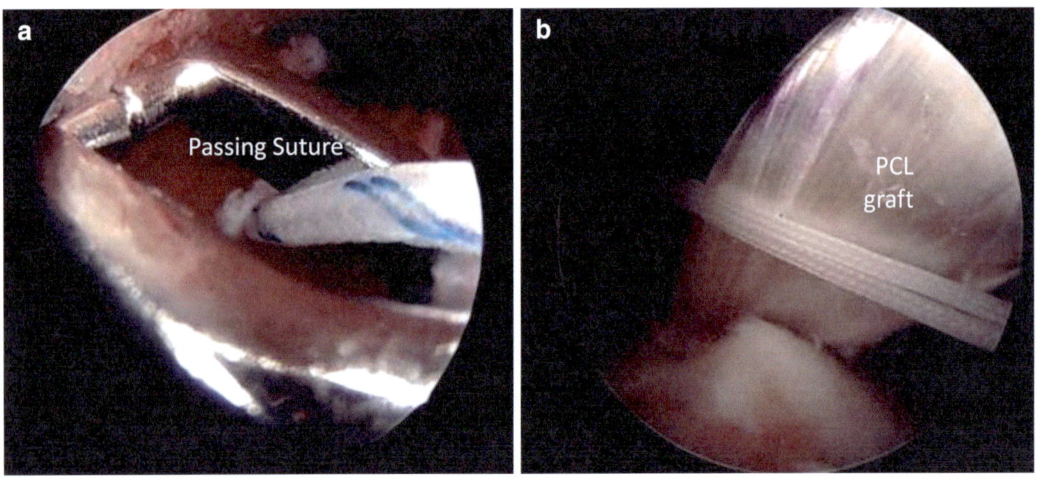

Fig. 8.7 Arthroscopic pictures of a right knee, viewing through the anterolateral portal. (**a**) The gore smoother is replaced by a passing suture up the tibial tunnel and used to pass the graft up the tibial tunnel. (**b**) The graft is then retrieved in the joint and passed up the femoral tunnel using the femoral passing suture

Next, the posterolateral corner repair is performed. A lateral hockey stick incision is placed at the level of the joint line. Skin flaps are mobilized. The fascia is incised between the iliotibial band and biceps femoris (Fig. 8.8). The iliotibial band is retracted anteriorly and the biceps femoris posteriorly. This will expose the PLC structures which are most often avulsed from the tibial/fibular side and can involve a LCL, popliteofibular ligament, popliteus biceps femoral, lateral capsule, and iliotibial band. Care should be taken to identify and protect the peroneal nerve (Fig. 8.9). Next, suture anchors are placed just below the joint line in the proximal tibia and fibular head along the entire lateral aspect of the knee joint. The suture strands are placed through the avulsed posterolateral corner structures, which are generally avulsed circumferential together as a sleeve (Fig. 8.10). All sutures are then tied with the knee in a slight valgus stress, neutral rotation, and at 30° of knee flexion such that the structures are reapproximated to their anatomic origin on the bone. This should reduce the joint and result in equal medial

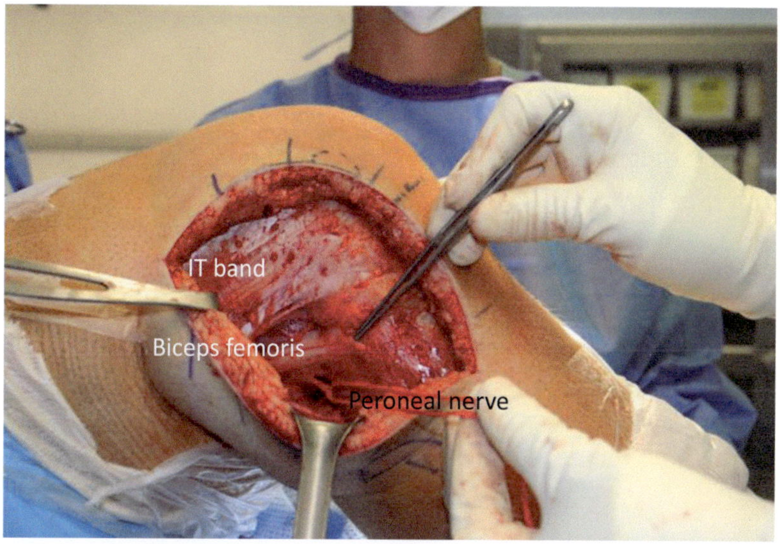

Fig. 8.8 Picture of the lateral aspect of a right knee. A lateral hockey stick incision is placed at the level of the joint line. Skin flaps are mobilized. The fascia is incised between the iliotibial band and biceps femoris. The iliotibial band is retracted anteriorly and the biceps femoris posteriorly

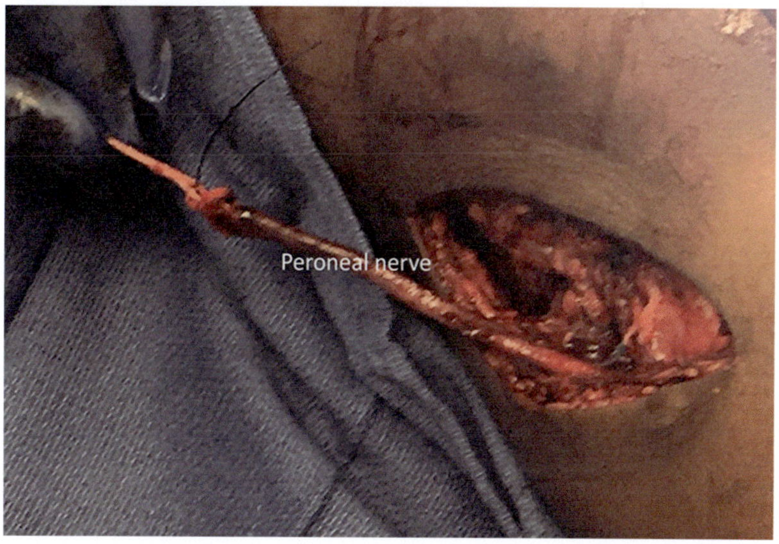

Fig. 8.9 Picture of the lateral aspect of a right knee. This patient had a complete transection of the peroneal nerve as a result of his knee dislocation

and lateral joint space, which can be confirmed using fluoroscopy. In young, healthy patients, repair only is usually sufficient as the tissue quality is excellent. If this is not the case, the repair may be augmented with a soft tissue allograft.

Attention is then turned back to the PCL. The graft is fixed on the tibial side with an interference screw of post and washer with the knee in 90° of flexion [10].

In about 2/3 of cases, repair of the PLC is not possible and reconstruction should be considered. In this case the authors perform reconstruction of the posterolateral corner according to the modified Larson technique, which is less technically demanding and faster than the anatomic technique and produces comparable stability [11]. The surgical approach is the same for the repair. A 6 mm wide all soft tissue allograft is used whipstitched on both ends. A 6 mm oblique tunnel is drilled from anteromedial to posterolateral on the fibula, parallel to the joint line. The graft is pulled through the fibular tunnel (Fig. 8.11). Next, a guide pin is placed at the femoral insertion site of the LCL (Fig. 8.12). A second guide pin is placed at the femoral insertion site of the popliteus tendon. Both guide pins are

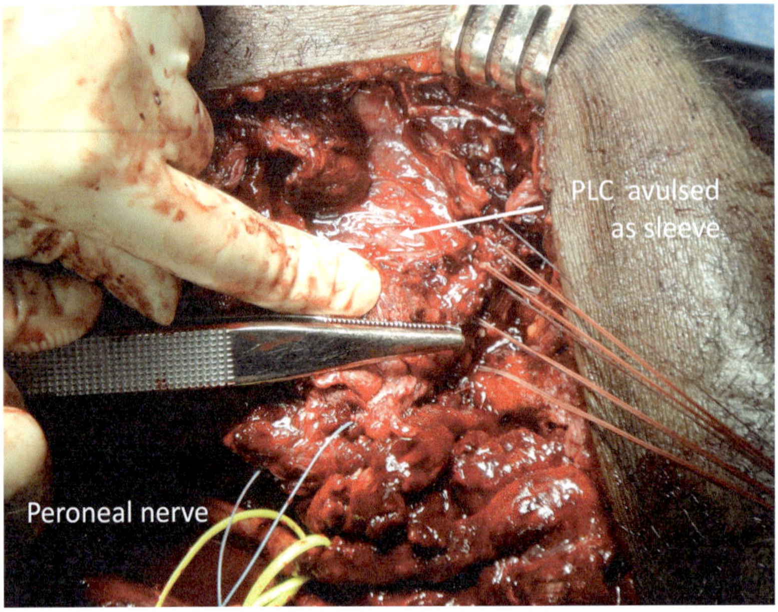

Fig. 8.10 Picture of the lateral aspect of a right knee. Suture anchors are placed in circumferentially around the lateral aspect of the proximal tibial and fibular head, and the corresponding suture strands are placed through the avulsed PLC structures, which are generally avulsed circumferential together as a sleeve. All sutures are then tied with the knee in a slight valgus stress between at 30° of knee flexion such that the structures are reapproximated to their anatomic origin on the bone

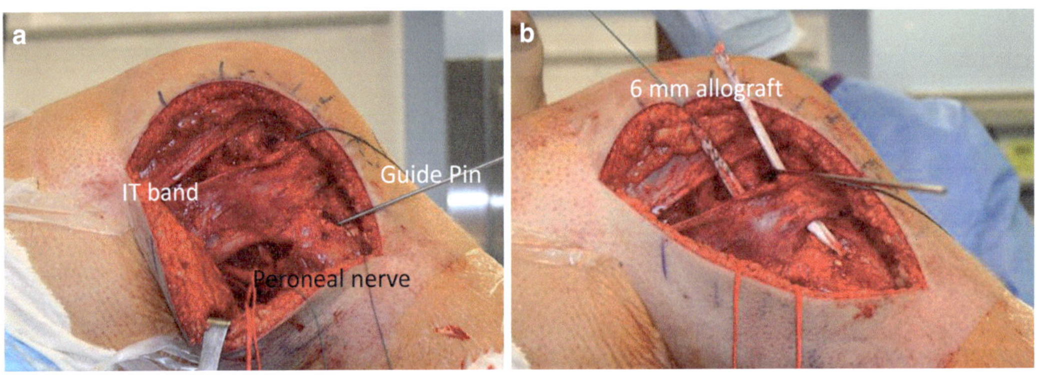

Fig. 8.11 Picture of the lateral aspect of a right knee. (**a**) A guide pin is drilled from anteromedial to posterolateral on the fibula, parallel to the joint line. This is over-reamed to a 6 mm tunnel. (**b**) A 6 mm allograft, whipstitched on both sides, is pulled through the fibular tunnel

over-reamed to a 6 mm tunnel, approximately 20–30 mm in length. The guide pins are replaced by passing sutures, the graft limbs are crossed to create a figure of eight, and each end of the graft is passed into the femoral tunnels to the medial side of the femur. The knee is placed to range of motion with manual tension on the graft to ensure isometry. The graft limbs are then tensioned with the knee flexed at 30°, neutral rotation, and slight valgus and fixed with interference screw fixation. In the setting of PLC reconstruction, the authors perform the PCL reconstruction in a delayed fashion, about 2 months after the PLC surgery.

At the end of the case, all incisions are copiously irrigated and a layered closure is performed. A sterile dressing is placed. Bilateral

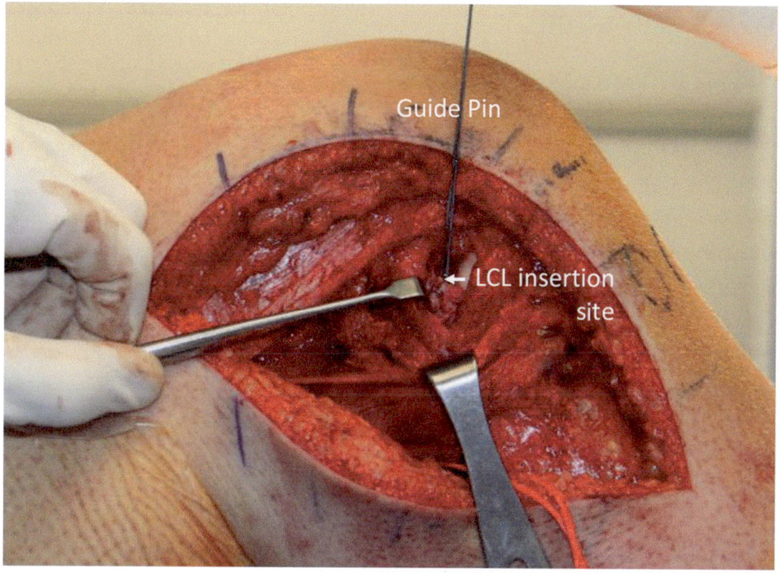

Fig. 8.12 Final view after passing each end of the graft into femoral tunnels. *LCL* lateral collateral ligament

thigh high compression stockings are applied, and the operated knee is placed in a hinged knee brace locked in extension. The most common complications of the surgery are arthrofibrosis and peroneal nerve injury (15–29%).

8.8 Rehabilitation

Postoperative rehabilitation should be conservative for the first 6 weeks. The knee is immobilized in a hinged knee brace in extension for ambulation for 12 weeks. After the second week, it may be unlocked for range of motion exercises. This can start prone to prevent posterior say. At this time, mini squats can then also be started to further strengthen the quad. A stationary bike can be used, but ensure a low resistance, high seat, and no toe clips to prevent hamstring contraction. The authors do not recommend using a continuous passive motion (CPM) machine as this may allow posterior sag. The brace should be locked in extension for straight leg raises for 6 weeks to prevent posterior tibial translation. However, it may remove when quad control is good enough to prevent extension lag. The patient is non-weight-bearing for 6 weeks, then partial weight-bearing for 6 weeks, and then full weight-bearing at 12 weeks. Active hamstring activity should be avoided for 8 weeks, and hamstring strengthening for 16 weeks. Return to manual labor is usually at 3–6 months. Return to sports is between 9 and 12 months. Criteria for return to sports are full painless range of motion, no effusion, quadriceps and hamstring strength ≥90% of the contralateral side, and no apprehension with all sports-specific drills [12].

8.9 Outcome

Across literature, good outcomes are reported for the surgical treatment of multi-ligament injured knees, including those with injuries to the posterolateral corner. However, outcomes are not as good as those for isolated ligament surgery, such as anterior cruciate ligament (ACL) reconstruction. In addition, recovery time, return to work, and sports are slower. Overall, surgical treatment resulted in an International Knee Documentation Committee (IKDC) score of 58%, 72% return to work rate, and 29% return to sports. In comparison for non-operative management, this was only 20% IKDC score, 52% return to work, and 10% return to sports. Those treated with early surgery did better than those treated later. There does not appear to be a difference in outcome between repair and reconstruction [6, 13, 14].

8.10 Conclusion

Combined PCL-PLC injuries are rare and the examination to quantitate these injuries is very challenging. Careful examination comparing the involved and uninvolved knees possibly with the use of stress fluoroscopy can help in grading these injuries. Physical examination should also include a thorough neurovascular exam. Advanced imaging may include (CT) angiography and MRI. Treatment is surgical in the overwhelming majority of cases. This can be acute repair or reconstruction of the posterolateral corner with acute or delayed/staged PCL reconstruction. Rehab, return to work, and sports are slower than isolated ligament reconstruction, such as ACL surgery. Clinical outcomes are also less successful and the patient has to understand this and have realistic expectation. Complications include failure of the repair/reconstruction, peroneal nerve injury, and arthrofibrosis.

Acknowledgement *Declaration of conflicting interests*: Carola F. van Eck, M.D., Ph.D.: no conflicts of interest. Mohsen Hussein, M.D., Ph.D.: no conflicts of interest.

References

1. Fontbote CA, Sell TC, Laudner KG, Haemmerle M, Allen CR, Margheritini F, Lephart SM, Harner CD. Neuromuscular and biomechanical adaptations of patients with isolated deficiency of the posterior cruciate ligament. Am J Sports Med. 2005;33(7):982–9.
2. Ranawat A, Baker CL III, Henry S, Harner CD. Posterolateral corner injury of the knee: evaluation and management. J Am Acad Orthop Surg. 2008;16(9):506–18.
3. Seroyer ST, Musahl V, Harner CD. Management of the acute knee dislocation: the Pittsburgh experience. Injury. 2008;39(7):710–8.
4. Degnan AJ, Maldjian C, Adam RJ, Harner CD. Passive posterior tibial subluxation on routine knee MRI as a secondary sign of PCL tear. Radiol Res Pract. 2014;2014:715439.
5. Harner CD. Treatment of posterolateral knee injuries: complex considerations for complex injuries. J Bone Joint Surg Am. 2011;e108:93–18.
6. Jabara M, Bradley J, Merrick M. Is stability of the proximal tibiofibular joint important in the multiligament-injured knee? Clin Orthop Relat Res. 2014;472(9):2691–7.
7. Harner CD, Waltrip RL, Bennett CH, Francis KA, Cole B, Irrgang JJ. Surgical management of knee dislocations. J Bone Joint Surg Am. 2004;86(A2):262–73.
8. Margheritini F, Mauro CS, Rihn JA, Stabile KJ, Woo SL, Harner CD. Biomechanical comparison of tibial inlay versus transtibial techniques for posterior cruciate ligament reconstruction: analysis of knee kinematics and graft in situ forces. Am J Sports Med. 2004;32(3):587–93.
9. Sekiya JK, West RV, Ong BC, Irrgang JJ, Fu FH, Harner CD. Clinical outcomes after isolated arthroscopic single-bundle posterior cruciate ligament reconstruction. Arthroscopy. 2005;21(9):1042–50.
10. Margheritini F, Rihn JA, Mauro CS, Stabile KJ, Woo SL, Harner CD. Biomechanics of initial tibial fixation in posterior cruciate ligament reconstruction. Arthroscopy. 2005;21(10):1164–71.
11. Apsingi S, Nguyen T, Bull AM, Unwin A, Deehan DJ, Amis AA. A comparison of modified Larson and 'anatomic' posterolateral corner reconstructions in knees with combined PCL and posterolateral corner deficiency. Knee Surg Sports Traumatol Arthrosc. 2009;17(3):305–12.
12. Lynch AD, Chmielewski T, Bailey L, Stuart M, Cooper J, Coady C, Sgroi T, Owens J, Schenck R, Whelan D, Musahl V, Irrgang J, Investigators STT. Current concepts and controversies in rehabilitation after surgery for multiple ligament knee injury. Curr Rev Musculoskelet Med. 2017;10(3):328–45.
13. Levy BA, Dajani KA, Whelan DB, Stannard JP, Fanelli GC, Stuart MJ, Boyd JL, MacDonald PA, Marx RG. Decision making in the multiligament-injured knee: an evidence-based systematic review. Arthroscopy. 2009;25(4):430–8.
14. Fanelli GC, Orcutt DR, Edson CJ. The multiple-ligament injured knee: evaluation, treatment, and results. Arthroscopy. 2005;21(4):471–86.

ACL-PCL Lesions

9

Gaetano Lo Bue and Fabrizio Margheritini

Combinated anterior and posterior cruciate ligament (ACL/PCL) lesions are rare, usually are caused by closed knee dislocations, and often are associated with peripheral injuries. The mechanism of injury can be of two types: high-energy, as a traffic accident, and low-energy mechanism that occurs, for example, during sport contact accidents. The result of bicruciate ligament lesion is a painful and debilitating knee instability. It involves a discomfort for the patient, not only in sports but also in daily activities [1, 2].

The role of the cruciate ligaments is essential in the kinematics of the knee. Respectively, the ACL is the primary restraint to anterior displacement of the tibia on the femur and a secondary stabilizer to tibial rotation; instead the PCL prevents the knee from excessive backward motion of the tibia and secondary restraints to external and internal tibial rotation at flexion angles greater than 90° [3]. Together the cruciate ligaments form a central "pivot" controlling rotational stability to the knee.

Surgical treatment of ACL/PCL lesions is necessary to restore knee kinematics, and although early arthroscopically assisted reconstruction has been recommended by several authors [4, 5], often this is not possible in the polytraumatized patient with severe injuries [6]. In fact surgical timing of acute ACL/PCL repair depends on the vascular status of the extremity, the condition of the skin, the patient's overall health, and the peripheral ligaments tears associated [5].

In the orthopedic literature, surgical treatments of combined ACL/PCL tears are different in timing, techniques, and graft choice [7]. Historically, a two-stage cruciate ligament reconstruction has been advocated because of difficulties in surgical treatment and rehabilitation with one-stage treatment [8, 9]. However since more recently, the single-stage procedure has been popularized due to the possibility of creating a correct central vertical rotation axis, by tensioning and fixing the two grafts at the same time.

Although some authors lean toward delayed surgery because it has been shown to decrease the incidence of arthrofibrosis [10], recent studies have demonstrated that one-stage arthroscopically assisted ACL/PCL reconstruction, when it is possible between 10 days and 3 weeks, is a reliable and safe procedure for ACL/PCL reconstruction [5].

For the reconstruction of cruciate ligaments, a universally accepted graft choice does not exist, and both allografts [11] and autografts [12] have been used. The difficulty in the choice of the grafts depends on advantages and disadvantages of each, like donor-site morbidity, biomechanical

G. L. Bue (✉)
Department of Orthopedics and Traumatology,
University of Rome "Tor Vergata", Rome, Italy

F. Margheritini
Orthopaedics and Traumatology,
University of Rome "Foro Italico", Rome, Italy

F. Margheritini et al. (eds.), *Complex Knee Ligament Injuries*,
https://doi.org/10.1007/978-3-662-58245-9_9

properties of the graft tissue, and weakening of extensor apparatus.

Concerning the surgical techniques, our preferred approach is the full arthroscopic, single-bundle (pro anterolateral (AL) bundle) PCL reconstruction and single-bundle anatomical ACL reconstruction.

9.1 Surgical Technique

9.1.1 Position, Physical Examination, and Imaging

The patient is positioned supine on the operating room table. The legs lie on the fully extended operating table, with a support used to hold the knee at 90 degrees of flexion (Fig. 9.1a, b). This position allows to move the popliteal neurovascular bundle as posterior as possible by simple gravity force. Furthermore, holding the knee at 90° allows an easier access to the posterior area of the joint, in case of emergency, a simple switch to any open peripheral procedure as well as the bleeding reduction. A lateral post is used, while a tourniquet is placed, but in our practice we do not inflate it during all the procedure in order to check the bleeding and in case to control, immediately by using RF system. In our practice a complete X-rays protocol is part of the preoperative assessment including long-standing X-rays films, Rosenberg view, and stress X-rays [13] (Fig. 9.2). MRI is requested in order to confirm the presence of associated both cartilage and meniscal

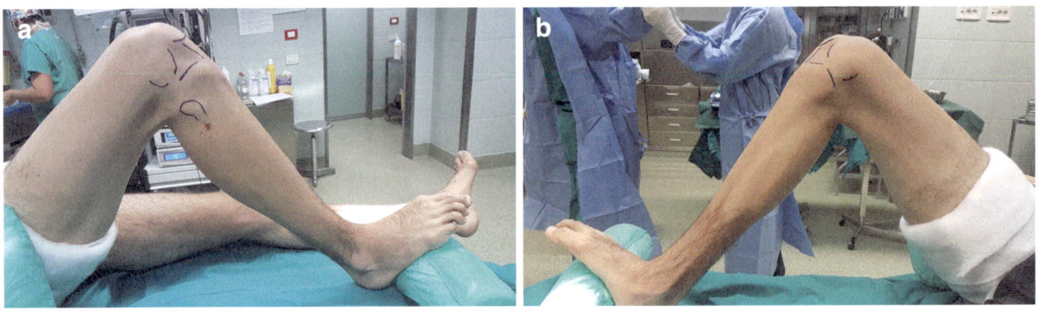

Fig. 9.1 (**a**, **b**) Patient position, the skin is marked to facilitate the placement of arthroscopic portals and the graft harvesting

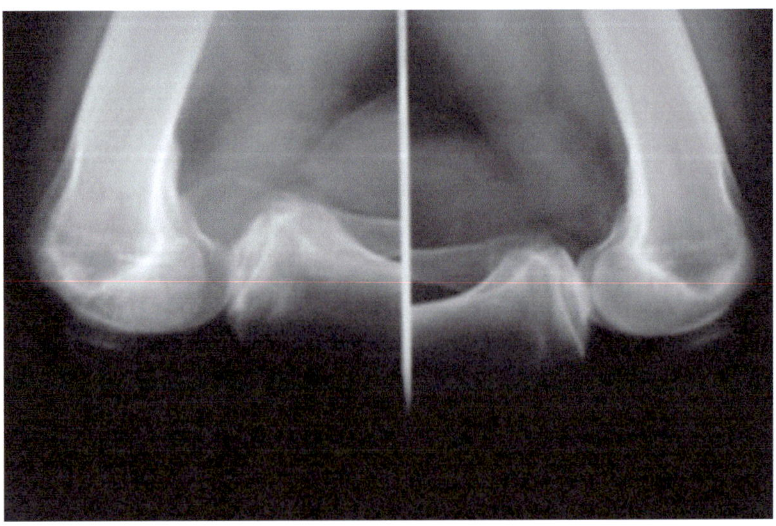

Fig. 9.2 Stress X-ray of right PCL-deficient knee of approximately 13 mm side to side

lesions. An examination under anesthesia (EUA) is always performed in the operating room as it confirms previous physical exam diagnoses.

9.1.2 Graft Selection and Preparation

Our preferred graft choice lies in the autograft hamstring ipsi- and contralateral for both cruciate reconstructions. In case of severe anteroposterior instability, with a posterior tibial subluxation superior than 12 mm, a quadriceps tendon bone is preferred for PCL reconstruction. Graft harvesting is usually accomplished after an initial diagnostic arthroscopy, and in order to save time, an additional surgeon is taking care of the graft preparation in the backtable, locking Krackow whipstitches at each end of the graft with no. 2 FiberWire (Arthrex, Naples, FL).

9.1.3 Arthroscopic Reconstruction

Standard anterolateral and anteromedial portals are used for diagnostic arthroscopy to confirm the bicruciate lesions and to exclude other ligaments and menisci tear. Posteromedial and posterolateral access are established, and a transeptal portal is performed by using alternatively a radiofrequency system (Fig. 9.3) and a motorized shaver inserted through the posteromedial portal, while keeping the camera in the posterolateral access (Fig. 9.4). We found that the use of a transportal access helps in reducing the surgical time, confirming the accuracy of PCL tunnel placement (Fig. 9.5), and controlling unexpected from the middle geniculate artery. In order to control the normal bleeding during the entire procedure (due to the tourniquet unuse), we do use a fluid pump for the entire procedure. By controlling step by step the pressure of the fluid, we reduce the risk of iatrogenic vascular lesion, while drilling the PCL tibial tunnel (by pushing away from the working area the posterior capsule and vessels), while at the same time by keeping the intra-articular pressure of the system as low as possible, we reduce the risk of extravasation.

The tunnels are drilled in the following order: (1) PCL tibial tunnel, (2) PCL femoral tunnel, (3) ACL femoral tunnel, and (4) ACL tibial tunnel. Both tibial tunnels are drilled by meaning different directions and angles in both the coronal and

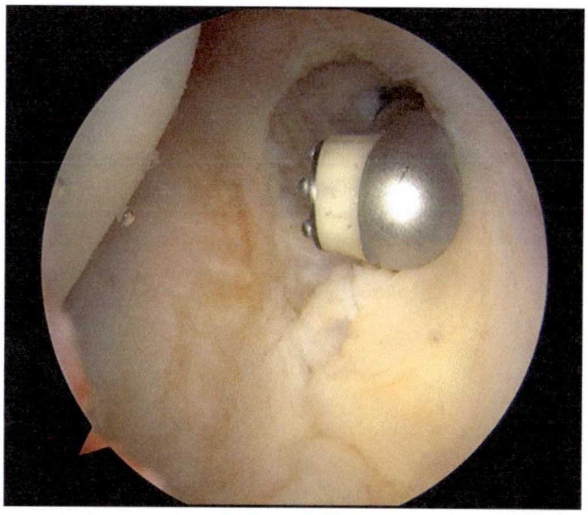

Fig. 9.3 Preparation of the transeptal portal: the camera is on the posterolateral access, while the RF from the posteromedial portal is cleaning the posterior fibrous septum

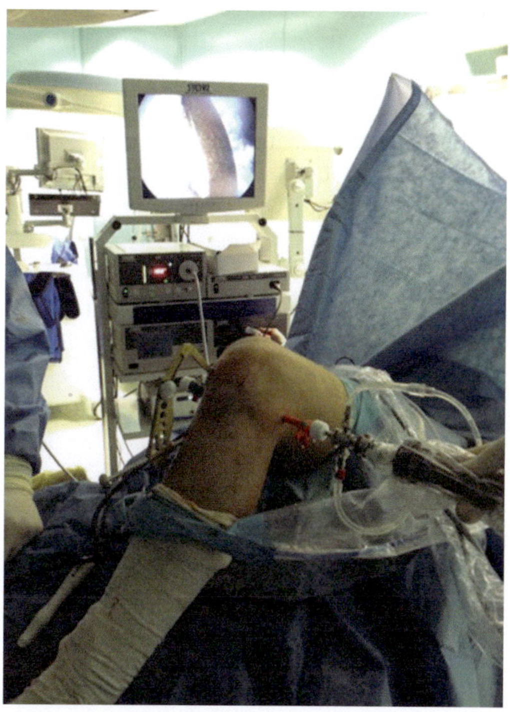

Fig. 9.4 External view of the transeptal portal at the moment of PCL tibial tunnel preparation

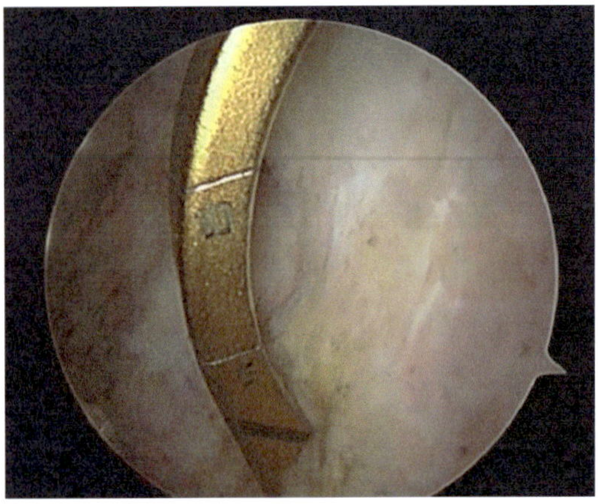

Fig. 9.5 Transeptal view of the tibial PCL guide position

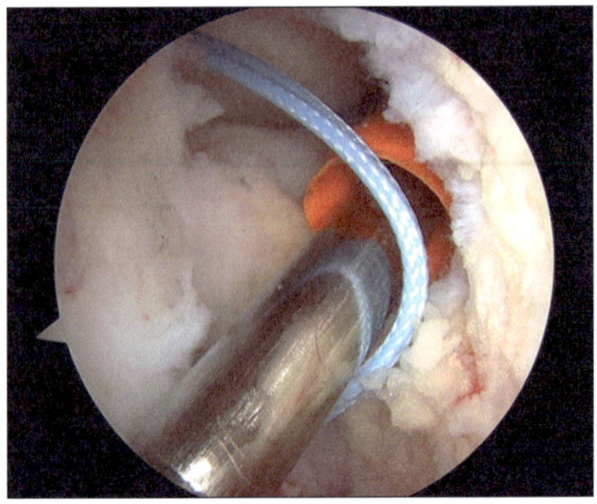

Fig. 9.6 Preparation of the PCL graft passage by using a blunt trocar inserted from the posteromedial access

the sagittal plane, in order to not create crossing tunnels. Ideally we try to drill a PCL tunnel with an angle of 60° or more in the sagittal plane, in order to reduce the killer turn effect. The goal of single-bundle reconstruction is to reproduce the anterolateral component of a PCL. The posterior tibial tunnel opening should exit the posterior tibia within the PCL footprint near the distolateral fibers. The transtibial PCL tunnel is drilled from the anteromedial aspect of the proximal tibia 1 cm below the tibial tubercle and exits posteriorly at approximately 1 cm below the articular surface of the medial tibial plateau slightly lateral to the midline at the PCL insertion site.

A femoral tunnel for the AL bundle of the PCL reconstruction is created with an outside-in technique with the entry point in the joint around 10 mm from the articular cartilage margin and should encompass the AL fibers of the footprint. The ACL is reconstructed by using a single-bundle anatomical technique, after placing an additional low anteromedial portal. After drilling the tunnels, the PCL graft is passed in the joint from distal to proximal. The PCL graft pass around the posterior corner is facilitated by inserting a blunt trocar [14] (Fig. 9.6) from the posterior portal, while the ACL graft is passed in the standard fashion. The proximal graft fixation is accomplished with a bioabsorbable screw for the PCL graft and by using an EndoButton (Smith &Nephew, Andover, MA) for the ACL (Fig. 9.7).

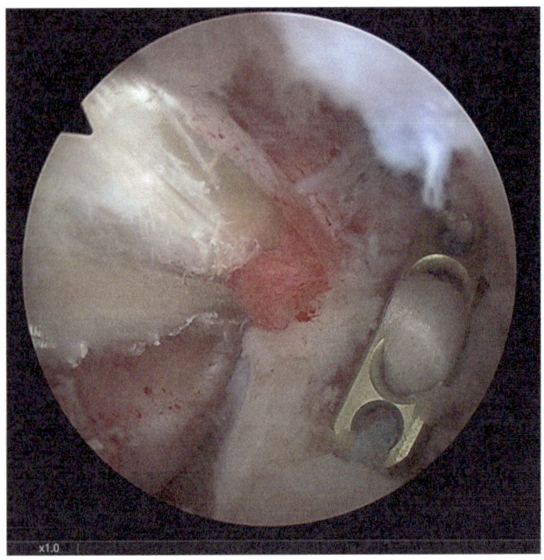

Fig. 9.7 Passage of the ACL graft, on the L side of the picture is visible the PCL graft already in situ

9.1.4 Final Graft Fixation

After cycling the knee 30 times by holding the grafts with a 20 N of tension, the PCL is fixed first. The PCL tibial fixation is placed with the knee in 90° of flexion and under graft suture tension with an anterior drawer placed to establish the normal tibial step-off. A bioabsorbable screw of 1 or 2 mm wider than the tunnel size is used with an anatomical placement closer to the intra-articular tibial tunnel entrance (Fig. 9.8).

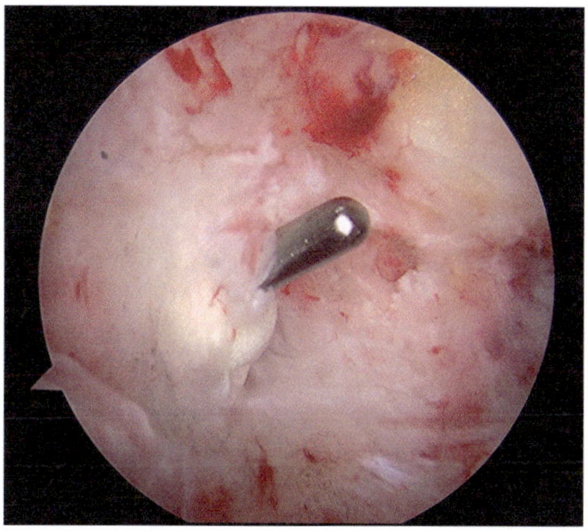

Fig. 9.8 PCL tibial fixation, the camera is in posteromedial position, please note the screw position according to the tibial tunnel entrance in the joint

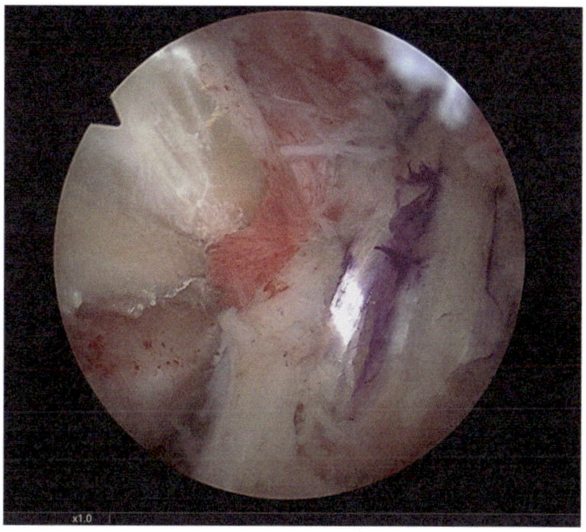

Fig. 9.9 Final arthroscopic view

An additional screw and a washer may be placed at this time in order to produce a better biomechanics [15]. After fixation, a posterior drawer is checked for satisfactory stability. Once confirmed, the ACL tibial fixation is placed. The four limbs of the hamstring graft are splayed apart, and under a manual tensioner, a bioabsorbable screw is placed accommodating the size of the graft. This provides adequate fixation, and an intraoperative Lachman test is performed to ensure stable cruciate fixation (Fig. 9.9).

9.1.5 Postoperative Rehabilitation

The knee is maintained in full extension for 4 weeks non-weight-bearing; then progressive weight-bearing is achieved. Progressive range of motion occurs from weeks 1 through 6, avoiding posterior subluxation by holding the knee with a gentle anterior drawer.

Progressive closed kinetic chain strength training and continued motion exercises are performed from week 4. The brace is discontinued after 10 weeks during the day, while it is kept during the night for some more 4 weeks. Return to sports and heavy labor occurs after 10 months, when sufficient strength and range of motion have returned.

References

1. Kannus P, Bergefeld J, Jarvinen M, Johnson RJ, Pope M, Renstrom P, et al. Injuries to the posterior cruciate ligament of the knee. Sports Med. 1991;12:10–131.
2. Tzurbakis M, Diamantopoulos A, Xenakis T, Georgoulis A. Surgical treatment of multiple knee ligament injuries in 44 patients: 2–8 years follow up results. Knee Surg Sports Traumatol Arthrosc. 2006;14:739–49.
3. Bowman KF Jr, Sekiya JK. Anatomy and biomechanics of the posterior cruciate ligament, medial and lateral sides of the knee. Sports Med Arthrosc. 2010;18:222–9.
4. Clancy WG Jr, Sutherland TB. Combined posterior cruciate ligament injuries. Clin Sports Med. 1994;13:629–47.
5. Fanelli GC, Edson CJ. Arthroscopically assisted combined anterior and posterior cruciate ligament reconstruction in the multiple ligament injured knee: 2- to 10-year follow-up. Arthroscopy. 2002;18:703–14.
6. Stayner LR, Coen MJ. Historic perspectives of treatment algorithms in knee dislocation. Clin Sports Med. 2000;19:399–413.
7. Ohkoshi Y, Nagasaki S, Shibata N, Yamamoto K, Hashimoto T, Yamane S. Two-stage reconstruction with autografts for knee dislocations. Clin Orthop. 2002;398:169–75.
8. Schenck RC Jr, Robert C. Management of posterior cruciate ligament injuries in knee dislocation. Oper Tech Sports Med. 1993;1:143–7.
9. Wen-Lin Y, Yuan-Kun T, Juin-Yih S, Wen-Wei HR. Knee dislocation: treatment of high-velocity knee dislocation. J Trauma. 1999;46:693–701.

10. Wascher DC, Blevins FT, Robinson B. Timing of surgical treatment of the dislocated knee. Arthroscopy. 1999;15:S43.
11. Shapiro MS, Freedman EL. Allograft reconstruction of the anterior and posterior cruciate ligaments after traumatic knee dislocation. Am J Sports Med. 1995;23:580–7.
12. Mariani PP, Margheritini F, Camillieri G. One-stage arthroscopically assisted anterior and posterior cruciate ligament reconstruction. Arthroscopy. 2001;17:700–7.
13. Margheritini F, Mancini L, Mauro CS, Mariani PP. Stress radiography for quantifying posterior cruciate ligament deficiency. Arthroscopy. 2003;19:706–11.
14. Mariani PP, Adriani E, Santori N, Maresca G. Arthroscopic-assisted posterior cruciate ligament reconstruction using patellar tendon autograft: a technique for graft passage. Arthroscopy. 1996;12:510–2.
15. Margheritini F, Rihn JA, Mauro CS, et al. Biomechanics of initial tibial fixation in posterior cruciate ligament reconstruction. Arthroscopy. 2005;21:1164–71.

Management of Combined Anterior Cruciate Ligament and Posterolateral Corner Injury of the Knee

10

Thomas Neri and David Parker

10.1 Introduction

Evaluation of the overall stability of the anterior cruciate ligament (ACL)-deficient knee can be difficult because of the multitude of additional anatomical structures that can be injured. With the improvement of overall knowledge of the knee-stabilizing structures, it is clear that many lesions are not isolated and occur within a potentially complex context of instability. Consequently, the concept of multiligament injury has evolved in recent years due to many anatomical and biomechanical studies which enhance the understanding of injury mechanisms and validate reconstruction techniques. Among those complex ligamentous injuries, the most common association is ACL and posterolateral corner (PLC) [1, 2].

Isolated reconstruction of ACL injury, without treatment of concomitant PLC tear, could lead to altered knee biomechanical behaviour with a high risk of persistent instability, ACL graft failure and early osteoarthritis occurrence [3, 4]. PLC has long been considered as the dark side of the knee, due to the limited understanding of the anatomy, biomechanics function and uncertain surgical outcomes. The objective of this chapter is therefore to offer surgeons help in the management of associated ACL and PLC injuries. After discussing the epidemiology of these injuries, the anatomical and biomechanical aspects of the PLC will be described, highlighting the keys points required to perform an anatomical reconstruction. We will also define the clinical and MRI elements needed to diagnose this combined injury. Finally, we will propose a treatment algorithm based on recent literature.

10.2 Epidemiology

The incidence of multiligament injuries increases each year. With the improvement of diagnosis procedure and awareness, this increase is probably due to the diagnosis of previously unnoticed and underdiagnosed lesions. Subsequently, the true incidence of PLC injury is difficult to estimate. The rate of isolated PLC injury has been reported by clinical studies around 5% of all knee injuries [5], 28% of all PLC injury [6] and around 2% for MRI studies [7]. However, when the PLC injury was associated with a tear of a

T. Neri (✉)
Sydney Orthopaedic Research Institute (SORI), Sydney, Australia

Inter-University Laboratory of Human Movement Biology (LIBM EA 7424), University of Lyon, Jean Monnet, France
e-mail: TNeri@sori.com.au

D. Parker
Inter-University Laboratory of Human Movement Biology (LIBM EA 7424), University of Lyon, Jean Monnet, France

F. Margheritini et al. (eds.), *Complex Knee Ligament Injuries*,
https://doi.org/10.1007/978-3-662-58245-9_10

central cruciate ligament, the incidence is increased: 16% among all knee ligament injuries and 9% among all acute knee injuries with a hemarthrosis [7]. LaPrade et al. [7] reported that 87% of the patients with PLC tear have a multiligament injury and 70% of those PLC patients had a combined ACL injury. Temponi et al. [8] concluded that 20% of the patients with an ACL injury had a concomitant PLC injury. Consequently, two messages are clear: PLC injuries are a common part of a multiligament injury pattern, and the management of a central cruciate ligament tear must include an examination of the lateral side of the knee in order to not miss a PLC injury.

10.3 Anatomy

In order to identify the damaged structures and then reconstruct or repair it, precise knowledge of the anatomy is required. In this paragraph, we will also present the key anatomical points needed to perform an effective reconstruction. The PLC is composed of three primary structures, the fibular collateral ligament (FLC), the popliteus tendon (PLT) and the popliteofibular ligament (PFL), and by many secondary stabilizers, the posterolateral capsule, the biceps femoris tendon, the lateral gastrocnemius tendon, the iliotibial band (ITB), the coronary ligament, the fabellofibular ligament, the arcuate ligament complex and the proximal tibiofibular ligaments. These structures are classified into static and dynamic stabilizers. Their anatomy, their main functions and the main surgery key points are summarized in Table 10.1.

10.3.1 The Fibular Collateral Ligament (FCL)

The femoral insertion is located proximal (1.4 mm) and posterior (3.1 mm) to the lateral epicondyle in a small bony depression [9]. This attachment is posterior and proximal to the PLT insertion. The distance between these two structures, approximately 18.5 mm [9], is a key anatomic relationship that is important to reproduce during the surgical reconstruction, demonstrating the requirement for two femoral tunnels [10]. This proximal insertion can be identified through a longitudinal incision of the ITB. The FCL course is extra-articular underneath the ITB, with an average of 70 mm in length and a maximal length at 30° of knee flexion [9]. The fibres run slightly posterior to terminate on the lateral part of the fibula head. The distal insertion is located 28 mm distal to the tip of the fibula head (fibular styloid) and 8 mm posterior to the anterior margin [9]. During surgery, an incision through the biceps bursa of the biceps femoris tendon is required to identify the distal FCL insertion.

The FCL is the primary restraint to varus of the knee at all flexion angle. In lower degrees of flexion, it also helps to control the external rotation torque [11, 12].

10.3.2 Popliteus Tendon (PLT)

The PLT femoral insertion is located in the proximal fifth of the popliteal sulcus, posterior to the lateral femoral condyle cartilage and anterodistal to the lateral epicondyle [9]. From this attachment the tendons have an intra-articular course (posterior and distal direction), running underneath the FCL, passing lateral to the lateral meniscus (popliteal hiatus) and then becoming extra-articular and curving down to the posterior part of the tibia. It originates from the myotendinous junction of the popliteus muscle, above the soleal line of the tibia posteriorly. The average length is 55 mm [9].

10.3.3 Popliteofibular Ligament (PFL)

The PFL originates from the popliteus musculotendinous junction and inserts on the posteromedial aspect of the fibula head (tip of the styloid process) [9, 12]. It is divided into anterior and posterior sections. The PFL connects the PLT to the styloid process of the fibula head. It consti-

Table 10.1 Anatomic and biomechanics characteristic of main PLC structures

	Origin	Insertion	Main function	Surgery key points
Static stabilizers				
Fibular collateral ligament (FLC)[a]	Lateral femoral epicondyle	Fibula head (lateral part)	Varus control	Distance FLC-PLT = 18.5 mm
Popliteofibular ligament (PFL)[a]	Popliteus musculotendinous junction	Styloid process (fibula head)	External rotation control	
Proximal tibiofibular ligaments	Medial aspect of the fibula head	Lateral aspect of the tibia	Proximal tibiofibular joint stabilizer	Search potential tibiofibular joint instability
Coronary ligament	Lateral meniscus	Posterolateral edge of the tibia	Hyperextension control, posterolateral rotation control	
Fabellofibular ligament	Fabella (or lateral condyle)	Styloid of the fibula head	Hyperextension control	
Arcuate ligament complex	Posterior capsule	Fibula head	Hyperextension control	
Posterolateral capsule	Circumferential with tibial and femoral insertions		Varus stability, hyperextension control	
Dynamic stabilizers				
Popliteus tendon (PLT)[a]	Tibia proximal posterior part	Antero-distal to lateral epicondyle	External rotation control	Femoral attachment is intra-articular
Biceps femoris tendon	Ischial tuberosity	Fibula head	Tibial internal rotation, varus angulation, tibiofemoral anterior translation control	Small longitudinal incision to locate the FLC distal insertion
Lateral gastrocnemius tendon	15 mm posterior to the FLC femoral insertion	Sural triceps	Additional posterolateral stability	Constant anatomic landmark, posteromedial limit do not overstep (neurovascular structure)
Iliotibial band	Iliac crest	Gerdy's tubercle	Internal rotation and varus stress control	Longitudinal incision required to locate the femoral FCL and PLT insertions

[a]Main stabilizers

tutes a pulley for the PLT, allowing it to have a horizontal action.

Both PLT and PFL constitute the popliteal complex which has a dual static and dynamic effect of the knee. Its function is to stabilize external rotation, whilst the knee is hyperflexed (60 to 90° of knee flexion) [11, 13].

10.3.4 Secondary Stabilizers

The long head of the biceps femoris tendon: Before inserting on the fibula head, the long head of the biceps femoris divides into the direct and the anterior arms [11]. Both arms enclosed the FLC insertion on the fibula head. As explained before, to access the distal FCL attachment, a small longitudinal incision through the tendon is required to access the interval (biceps bursa) between the two arms. Moreover, the posterior edge of this tendon, before its attachment on fibula head, is a good anatomic landmark to locate the common peroneal nerve, especially in acute reconstruction. This tendon is a flexor and external rotator of the knee. Its function is to control tibial internal rotation, to provide dynamic stability at varus angulation and to prevent excessive tibiofemoral anterior translation.

The lateral gastrocnemius tendon: The lateral gastrocnemius tendon arises 15 mm posterior to the FLC femoral insertion, courses distally close to the posterior capsule and joins the other head of the sural triceps [1]. Due to its low rate of injury, this tendon is a constant landmark in acute surgery to locate and reconstruct the other structures. Moreover, surgeons do not overstep this posteromedial limit to avoid damaging the posterior neurovascular structure.

The iliotibial band (ITB): The ITB constitutes the superficial layer of the lateral side of the knee and inserts onto the Gerdy's tubercle. During PLC surgery, a longitudinal incision of the ITB has to be performed to locate the femoral FCL and PLT insertions. Its functions are to control excessive internal rotation and varus stresses in extension.

The proximal tibiofibular ligaments: These structures include an anterior and a posterior ligament. By connecting the medial aspect of the fibula head to the lateral aspect of the tibia, these structures are the main stabilizer of the proximal tibiofibular joint. During the surgery, an assessment of the integrity of these ligaments is required in order to treat a potential tibiofibular joint instability.

Posterolateral capsule: The posterolateral capsule is thick and resistant. Its attachments are circumferential with tibial and femoral insertions. The lateral capsular thickening constitutes the mid-third lateral capsular ligament including the meniscofemoral and meniscotibial ligaments. The mid-third lateral capsule is a secondary stabilizer to varus stability [11].

The coronary ligament: The coronary ligament is defined as a meniscotibial structure of the posterolateral capsule. It connects the lateral meniscus and the posterolateral edge of the tibia (under the cartilage). The medial part of this ligament constitutes the medial border of the popliteus hiatus. Arthroscopically, this ligament can be visualized by moving up the free edge of the lateral meniscus with a probe. Its function is to overcome the joint constraint and to stabilize the meniscus when the knee is in hyperextension or tibial posterolateral rotation [14].

The fabellofibular ligament: The fabellofibular ligament is the distal thickening of the capsular arm of the short head of the biceps femoris [11]. It connects the fabella to the styloid of the fibula head. Whilst for some authors these ligaments exist only if the fabella is present [15], for others it is always present [14]. The fabella is an inconstant sesamoid structure (bony or cartilaginous structure) located in the proximal lateral gastrocnemius tendon in 30% of individuals [16]. This structure is tight in extension and relaxed in full flexion. Despite the lack of biomechanical data, the role of this ligament is probably to provide the knee stability close to extension by limiting the hyperextension.

The arcuate ligament complex: The arcuate ligament origin is the posterior part of the capsule, overlying the femoral condyles. After a fibre reunification, this ligament crosses the PLT and inserts into the posterior part of the fibula head [15]. As with other posterior structures, its function is probably largely to limit hyperextension.

10.4 Biomechanics

The PLC structures have two main functions: to resist lateral varus stress and control external tibial rotation. These structures can also be secondary stabilizers of other knee movements, including hyperextension, anteroposterior translation and tibial internal rotation. From biomechanical studies, we have summarized all of these functions in Table 10.2.

10.5 Diagnoses/Evaluation

10.5.1 Injury Mechanism

ACL and PLC injuries occur commonly in high-energy injuries, including sports injuries, falls and motor vehicle accidents. The mechanism is complex, combining hyperextension, varus and external rotation stress and often appearing in knee dislocation [17]. Isolated rupture of PLC is mainly induced by contact on the proximal anteromedial tibia with a postero-

Table 10.2 Biomechanics functions of the PLC structures

Functions	Anatomical structures	Conditions
Primary functions		
Varus	FCL[a]	All degrees of flexion (max: 0–30°)
	Other PLC structures	In FLC-deficient knee
	– Mid-third lateral capsular, ITB	Close extension
	– Popliteus complex	60°
External tibial rotation	Popliteus complex[a]	>30°
	FCL[a]	0–30°
	Other PL structures	
	PCL	In PLC-deficient knee (90°)
Secondary functions		
Internal tibial rotation	ACL, ALL, ITB[a]	
	PLT	
	Biceps femoris	
Anterior tibial translation	ACL[a]	
	PLC	In ACL-deficient knee, close extension
Posterior tibial translation	PCL[a]	
	PLC	In PCL-deficient knee, close extension
Hyperextension	More posterior structures of PLC[a]	
	Posterolateral capsule, coronary ligament, fabellofibular ligament, arcuate ligament complex	

[a]Main stabilizers

lateral directed force and causing hyperextension and varus. However in non-contact injury over a fixed foot with hyperextension, varus stressor external rotation can also damage the PLC [13, 18, 19].

10.5.2 Clinical Evaluation

In acute cases, reported symptoms include pain, ecchymosis, swelling and inability to walk. In chronic cases, the patient may describe side-to-side instability, prominent near extension when weight bearing. Standing examination can reveal abnormal varus malalignment of the lower extremity. PLC injuries can lead to a varus thrust during the initiation of stance phase (loading-response phase), resulting in abnormal gait. Noyes et al. [20] described a "triple varus knee": (1) varus moment on standing due to tibiofemoral geometry, (2) opening of the lateral compartment due to lateral structures injuries and (3) varus recurvatum (hyperextension and external rotation) due to posterolateral structure injury.

For ACL- and PLC-injured knees, a standardized diagnostic approach is required. The physical examination is always important and should include ACL testing (Lachman and pivot shift (PS)) and PLC testing (varus stress, dial test, reverse PS, external rotation recurvatum test and posterolateral drawer test). All of these tests are summarized in Table 10.3.

The varus stress test is performed in both full extension and 30° of flexion. Lateral compartment gapping at 30° of flexion indicates injuries to the FCL and potentially to the posterolateral structures. If this gapping still persists in full extension, a concomitant FLC, PLC and cruciate ligament injury are expected. Conversely, if stability is restored in full extension, an isolated complete tear of the FCL is likely.

The dial test is another helpful test to evaluate tibial external rotation relative to the femur. This test is conducted at 30° and 90° of flexion, with the patient in the prone or supine position. An isolated PCL injury can be presumed if more than 10° of external rotation compared to the contralateral knee is present only at 30° of flexion (not at 90°). A combined PLC and PCL injury is expected, if an increase of more than 10° of external rotation is present at both 30° and 90° of flexion, with an increase at 90° superior than at 30°.

The reverse PS test is also used to assess a PLC instability. This test is performed with the knee flexed to 90° of flexion with valgus and external rotation load. During a slowly extension

Table 10.3 Clinical tests

	Varus stress		Dial test				
	Positive only at 30°	Positive at 0° and 30°	Positive only at 30°	Positive at 0° and 90°	Reverse pivot shift	External rotation recurvatum test	Posterolateral drawer test
Transverse plane	–	–	+ (PLC)	+ (PCL and PCL)	+ (PLC)	+ (PLC) +++ (PCL and PCL)	+ (PLC)
Frontal plane	+ (FCL)	+ (FCL and PLC and cruciate)	–	–	–	–	–
Sagittal plane	–	+ (FCL and PLC and cruciate)	–	+ (PCL and PCL)	–	+++ (PCL and PCL)	–

movement, if the previously subluxated lateral tibial plateau reduces at 40° of flexion (ITB action), with a clicking sound, the test is positive, and a PLC injury is presumed. However, the test has a positive predictive value of 68% and a false-positive rate of 35% under anaesthesia.

The external rotation recurvatum test, first described by Hughston et al. [21], is performed in the supine position, knee in full extension, by grasping the bilateral hallux to lift the leg. Excess hyperextension with the tibia externally rotated and a relative varus angulation suggests a PCL injury. Although the positive predictive value is low (10%) for isolated PLC injury, these positive signs are magnified with a combined PLC and PCL injury.

For the posterolateral drawer test, the knee is flexed to 90° and the foot externally rotated at 15°. A positive test exhibits external rotation associated with posterior displacement of the lateral aspect of the tibia and suggests a PLC injury (PFL and PLT).

10.5.3 Radiological Evaluation

Plain X-ray with standing anteroposterior (AP), lateral and axial views is required to rule out other injuries, including fractures. For acute injuries, bony avulsion fracture, such as fibular head avulsion, or lateral joint widening can be seen on this standard view. For chronic cases, a standing long-leg AP alignment view is necessary to determine whether correction of malalignment by an osteotomy may be necessary prior to or during surgical PCL reconstruction.

Table 10.4 Staging instability evaluation using stress radiography, according to LaPrade [22] and Jackman [23] studies (increased opening compared to contralateral knee)

Stress radiography	Staging variables (mm)	Corresponding instability
Varus stress radiograph	<2.7	Normal-minor sprains
	2.7–4	Isolated FCL injury
	>4	Complete PLC injury
Kneeling PCL radiograph	<4	Normal-minor sprains
	4–12	Isolated PCL injury
	>12	Combined PCL and PLC injury

Stress radiography and varus and kneeling PCL stress X-ray are helpful in the management of PLC injury, with good reliability in the assessment of lateral compartment varus gapping. LaPrade et al. [22] recommend to perform bilateral varus stress radiographs at 20° of flexion. These stress radiographs allow to differentiate isolated FCL from combined FCL and PLC injuries (varus stress) and isolated PCL from combined PCL and PLC injuries (kneeling PCL stress) (Table 10.4).

MRI is another key tool for ACL and PLC injury assessment. It can be useful to determine the full extent of the injury, especially in complex cases, by assessing which structures are injured, and the location of the injury. This allows more precise planning of the surgical procedure. MRI assessment also allows identification of concurrent injuries such as meniscal tears, chondral lesions and occult fractures. Specific T2-weighted coronal oblique imaging sequences (same obliquity as PLT), using 2 mm slices, are recommended in this MRI assessment.

10.5.4 Complications

Neurovascular complications associated with acute injuries must always be detected through careful clinical assessment. Common peroneal nerve injury is frequent (present in 13% of all PLC injuries), and a detailed physical examination must be performed. Popliteal artery injury (up to 32% of knee dislocations) must be suspected in all multiligament knee injuries and should be assessed by careful clinical examination, including serial pulse assessment and ankle-brachial index [24, 25]. If these are normal, then ongoing careful serial neurovascular observations are required, but if there is any clinical suspicion from the examination, then further investigation is mandatory, either through traditional arteriography, CT angiography or MR angiography depending on availability at the treating institution.

10.6 Classification

According to the Schenck classification of knee dislocation, a combined ACL and PLC injury may be classified as a KD I. Concerning the PLC injury, the two following classifications are available and can help for the therapeutic option choice: The Hughston classification [21] is still used for treatment guidance and has three stages depending only on the varus at 30° of flexion (Table 10.5). Stage III corresponds to a complete PLC injury (FCL, PLT, PFL). However, to be optimal a grading system of PLC injury has to include assessment of both varus and rotational stability. Fanelli et al. [26] have subsequently proposed another classification which fulfils this requirement (Table 10.5).

Table 10.5 Clinical grading according to Hughston [21] and Fanelli [26] classification

Hughston classification: varus instability			
Grades	*Varus opening*		
Grade I	0–5 mm		
Grade II	5–10 mm		
Grade III	>10 mm		
Fanelli et al. classification: rotational and varus instability			
Grades	*Instability assessment*		*Damaged structures*
Type A	Isolated rotational instability	10° increase in tibial ER	PFL, PLT
Type B	Rotational instability and mild varus instability	10° increase in tibial ER + 5–10 mm increase in varus load test	PFL, PLT, FCL
Type C	Significant rotational and varus instability	10° increase in tibial ER > 10 mm increase in varus load test	PFL, PLT, FCL, capsule avulsion, cruciate ligament

10.7 Treatment Rationale and Management

The management of a combined ACL and PLC injury is outlined in Fig. 10.1. Three main parameters need to be considered:

- The grade of injury, allowing a decision between nonoperative and operative options.
- The time delay and the location of each injury (bony avulsion or midsubstance injury), in order to decide between repair and reconstruction techniques.

10.7.1 Operative Versus Nonoperative Treatment

Management of lateral side injuries is different to medial side tears. Medial side injuries are more common than lateral, and the majority can have good outcomes with conservative treatment. This finding does not apply for the PLC injury, due to

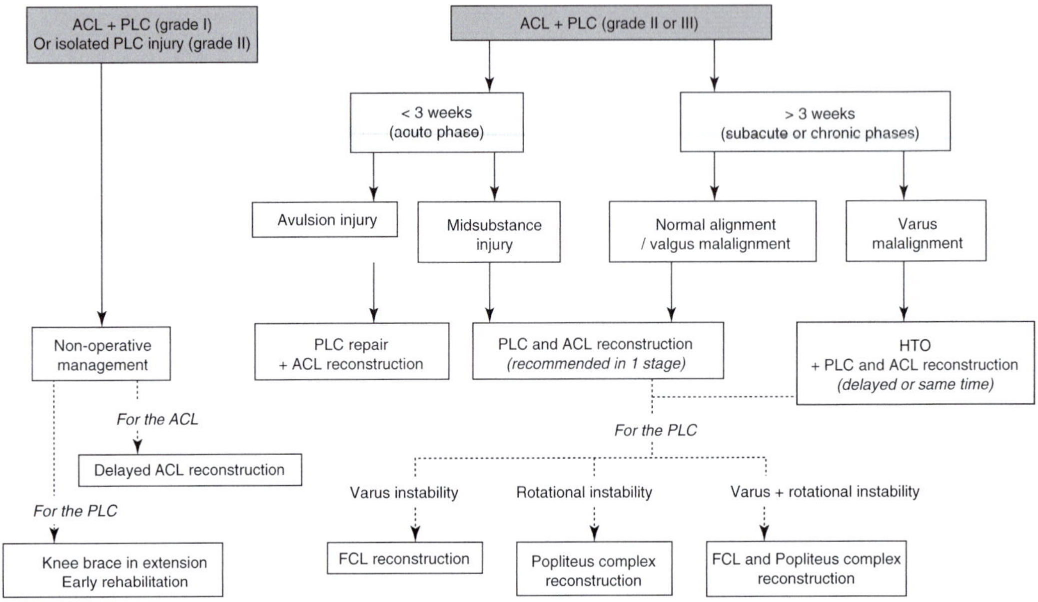

Fig. 10.1 Our algorithm for ACL and PLC management

an inherent anatomic instability of the lateral tibiofemoral compartment. This compartment with a convex lateral tibia plateau articulating with a convex lateral femoral condyle is designed to have more mobility. Consequently, this intrinsic instability does not lead to a spontaneous healing of PLC structures. Moreover, some biomechanical studies have demonstrated the participation of the PLC structures in a better load distribution after an ACL reconstruction. Indeed, increased force on the ACL graft has been reported if the PLC injuries are not addressed [4]. These studies conclude that PLC reconstruction, in addition to being useful for long-term ACL graft stability, is also necessary to restore normal knee kinematic with a good overall stability.

Although definitive guidelines for management of all PLC injuries cannot be derived from the available literature, it would be reasonable to suggest from the available evidence that grade I and II isolated PLC injuries do not usually require surgical treatment, whilst grade II with a combined injury and grade III will be best managed surgically (Fig. 10.1). Regarding a combined ACL and PLC tear, ACL and PLC grade I injuries require only an ACL reconstruction, whilst grade II/III injuries need a reconstruction of all the damaged structures.

Therefore, nonoperative management can only be considered for grade I and II isolated PCL injuries. Regarding combined ACL and PCL injury, only the grade I of PCL injury does not require a surgical procedure. Studies reported good outcomes for nonoperative treatment PCL grades I and II, with minimal radiographic changes at 8-year follow-up [27, 28]. These patients then require careful follow-up and assessment for any residual laxity once recovered, but if the initial assessment was accurate, then a good outcome can usually be obtained. Conversely, nonoperative management for PLC grade III has been shown to result in poor functional outcomes, persistent instability and subsequent development of osteoarthritis. Nonoperative management consists of a hinged knee brace to protect against varus stress and an early mobilization protocol, including gentle and progressive mobilization to avoid stiffness, quadriceps stimulation and gait training. Partial weight bearing is commenced immediately and progressively increased, according to the patient tolerance. Protection with crutches in the first 4 weeks will avoid any falls that may cause varus stress, and the use of a valgising unloader brace may have additional benefits in protecting the injured lateral structures if available.

For operative management, there are many things to consider. In addition to questions concerning the technique used, the question around the surgical sequence used, in one stage or multi-stage, remains an important discussion. The advantages of ACL and PLC reconstruction in one stage are to address all of the pathology at once, decreasing the risk of graft failure and allowing an earlier rehabilitation to avoid stiffness. Disadvantages of this one-stage surgery are a longer surgery time and a more technical and complex surgery and the need to source graft at short notice. Conversely, multistage techniques are easier, and require fewer grafts, but have an increased recovery time and a higher risk of graft failure between the two stages. Therefore, we recommend one-stage surgery in the majority of cases, when possible, for ACL and PLC reconstruction. The only exception is varus malalignment in the chronic cases, which require correction of alignment through high tibial osteotomy (HTO). In these cases, one study [29] reported that in 38% of cases, the PLC laxity is satisfactorily addressed by the HTO alone, supporting isolated HTO without PLC reconstruction as the initial and possibly definitive procedure for these patients. In this chapter, discussion of the operative treatments will be divided into two parts: repair and reconstruction technique.

10.7.2 Repair Versus Reconstruction Techniques

Regarding the timing of surgery, acute treatment (<3 weeks after the injury) is reported to have better outcomes than treatment in subacute (3–12 weeks) or chronic phases (>3 months) [30, 31]. Acute PLC injuries may be treated by direct repair, augmentation or reconstruction. Primary repairs of bony avulsions of FCL and PLT, without midsubstance injury, can be done only during the acute phase. After this endpoint, the fibrosis associated with tissue healing makes anatomic reduction and reattachment of injured structures difficult to achieve. Therefore, injuries older than 3 weeks are difficult to achieve primary repair and will usually require a reconstruction [32]. Stannard and Levy et al. reported 37–40% failure rate with repair compared to 6–9% with reconstruction [26, 33]. However, there can be difficulties in making definitive recommendations from these studies due to the heterogenous nature of patient groups, but as a general guideline, reconstruction, or augmentation with a reconstruction, is usually required when a satisfactory repair cannot be achieved. This is mostly in the case of midsubstance injuries, which in the acute setting are best dealt with by primary repair augmented by a reconstruction. Bony avulsions which can be reduced and secured will usually do well without reconstruction, and indeed in these cases, the usual reconstruction is not technically possible due to the fibular head avulsion.

In the surgical management of acute injuries, the position of the common peroneal nerve is usually altered by the surrounding avulsion injury. Therefore, careful exploration and identification of this nerve and a neurolysis are recommended, to allow careful retraction of the nerve to avoid injury. This should be the first step of the surgical procedure prior to commencing the repair and reconstruction components.

For chronic PLC injuries, reconstruction is always recommended, regardless of the location of the injury [32]. Alignment of the lower limb is of course an important prognostic factor to consider (Fig. 10.1). Malalignment of more than 3° of varus, associated with a varus thrust when walking, can lead to increased stress on the graft and increase the failure rate. This should therefore not be ignored as it will most likely lead to failure of the reconstruction. For these cases, a HTO, either as an initial procedure alone or combined with reconstruction, is recommended.

In patients with concomitant ACL injuries, reconstruction is usually advised at the same time as the lateral-sided procedure.

10.8 Surgical Repair

Regarding acute management of PLC injuries, bony avulsions should be fixed. This is most commonly an avulsion of the fibular head but may also involve avulsions from the lateral tibial plateau. As with any internal fracture fixation, the size of the fragment will determine which fixation device, and which size, is most appropriate. For larger fragments, screws with soft tissue washers can be used, whereas smaller, more comminute fragments may require suture anchors, with the sutures passed through the bony fragments and attached soft tissues. Suture imbrication is possible when the PLT musculotendinous tendon region is injured. Sutures are passed through the remaining tendon and anchors in the posterior part of the tibia. The PFL can be repaired in the same way. Moreover, it is necessary to diagnose and treat all of the additional lateral side injuries. Initial surgical dissection should identify the zone of injury and all structures within that zone that are injured and need to be repaired. Capsular structures, such as the coronary ligament, the proximal tibiofibular ligaments, the mid-third lateral capsular ligament and the ITB, all need to be repaired, usually by anchoring into their bone attachments.

For midsubstance injuries, a good quality isolated repair is not usually able to be achieved and hence usually requires augmentation with a reconstruction to reduce the risk of recurrent laxity. Some authors recommend a repair with an augmentation using synthetic ligament, whereas most commonly the augmentation reconstruction would use a soft tissue graft [34].

Apart from these specific injuries in the acute phase, the preference would generally be towards reconstruction for PLC injuries. Regarding associated ACL injuries, with the exception of bony avulsions, the recommendation would clearly be for reconstruction.

10.9 Reconstruction Treatments

Several reconstruction techniques are available. However, there is not one specific reconstruction that has proven superiority or would be agreed upon by all experts. Not surprisingly, there are no randomized controlled studies to rationalize this choice. Given that these injuries are uncommon, it is important that the surgeon chooses a familiar and mastered technique. For the ACL reconstruction, all available techniques recommended for isolated ACL reconstruction can be used, the choice coming down to surgeon preference. This chapter will therefore only present two techniques of PLC reconstruction, which seem to be currently the most commonly used in current practice: a modified Larson technique (Fig. 10.2) and LaPrade technique (Fig. 10.3).

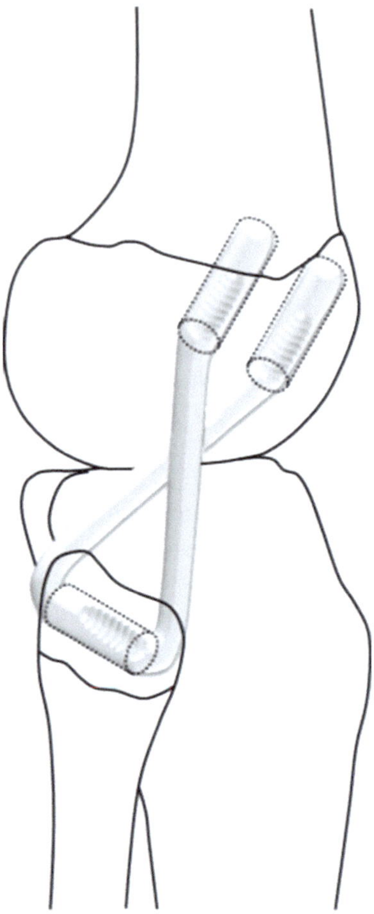

Fig. 10.2 Our modified Larson technique

In our experience, we prefer to use the modified Larson technique, the "modification" being the use of two tunnels on the femur to allow a more anatomical reconstruction and independent tensioning of the two grafts. When compared to the LaPrade technique, it is faster, requires less extensive dissection and requires only one graft. Nevertheless, it is not perfectly anatomical in that it does not allow accurate reconstruction of the popliteal complex. LaPrade technique was created to anatomically reconstruct the popliteal complex but is still not an accurate reproduction of anatomy. As explained, the PLT has one dynamic muscular action which is impossible to reconstruct with a graft, and the PFL has a pulley function. In

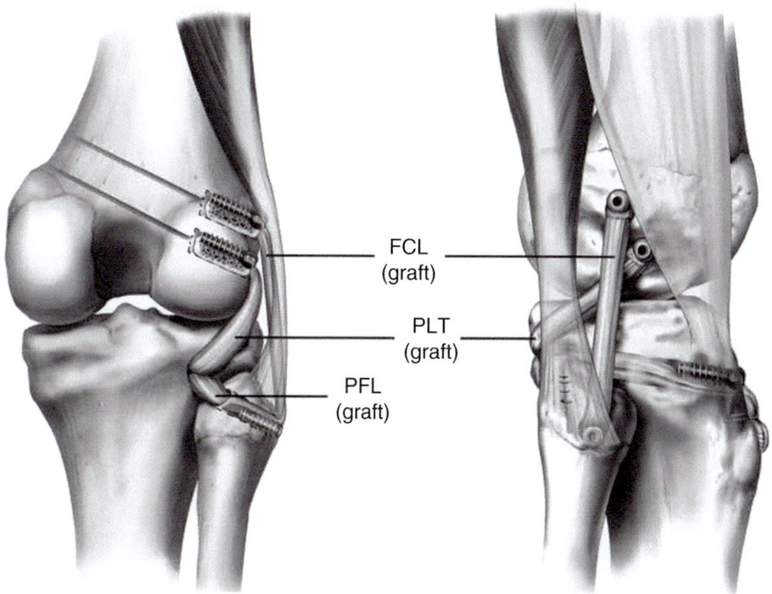

Fig. 10.3 LaPrade technique. (Reprinted with permission from Am J SportsMed. 2010;38:1674–80)

the LaPrade technique, the "PFL graft" is not dynamic as it would be in the native knee, because the graft goes directly between the fibula head and the tibia without clear dynamic action with the PLT, even if the two grafts are sutured to one another. For us, the main advantage of this technique is to stabilize the fibula head. It is possible also that the attachment to the posterolateral tibia is advantageous in controlling hyperextension.

Therefore, we used the modified Larson technique in all cases, except when a proximal tibiofibular joint instability is observed. In these specific cases, we use the LaPrade technique, after separately stabilizing the tibiofibular joint. We would also recommend the LaPrade technique in cases of abnormal hyperextension and in certain revision cases in which the modified Larson technique is not possible.

Below we will provide a more detailed description for our preferred modified Larson technique, followed by a description of the LaPrade technique.

10.9.1 Modified Larson Technique

Patient positioning: After an examination under anaesthesia, the patient is placed in supine position, knee flexed at 90° of flexion, with a tourniquet. The main anatomic landmarks are marked: fibula head, biceps femoris, peroneal nerve and lateral femoral epicondyle (Fig. 10.4).

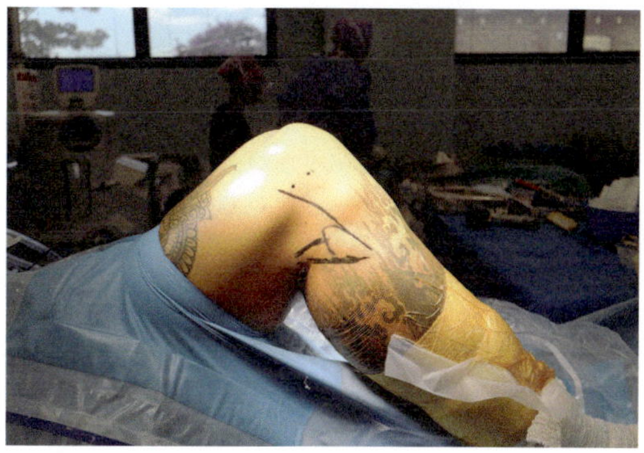

Fig. 10.4 Patient positioning and anatomic landmarks

Graft preparation: Usually, for the ACL the ipsilateral semitendinosus (ST) is harvested and prepared as a four-strand graft by quadrupling the tendon over two tightrope loops. Contralateral ST, or anon-irradiated allograft, is used for the PLC reconstruction. We prefer to use a tibialis anterior allograft due to its robust size and strength. A whipstitch is placed in either end of the tendon, and it is sized to pass through 5 mm tunnel, and both grafts are stored in a moist vancomycin-soaked gauze (Fig. 10.5).

Approach and soft tissue dissection: A lateral longitudinal incision is made from the lateral epi-

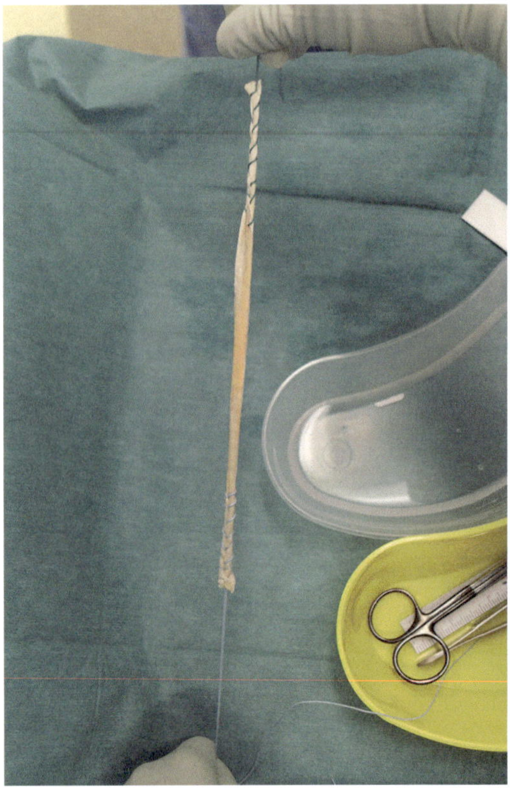

Fig. 10.5 Allograft preparation for the PLC reconstruction

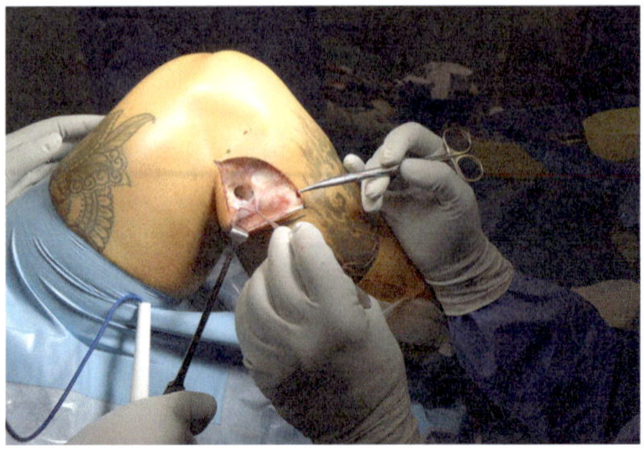

Fig. 10.6 Identification of the interval between ITB and short head of biceps

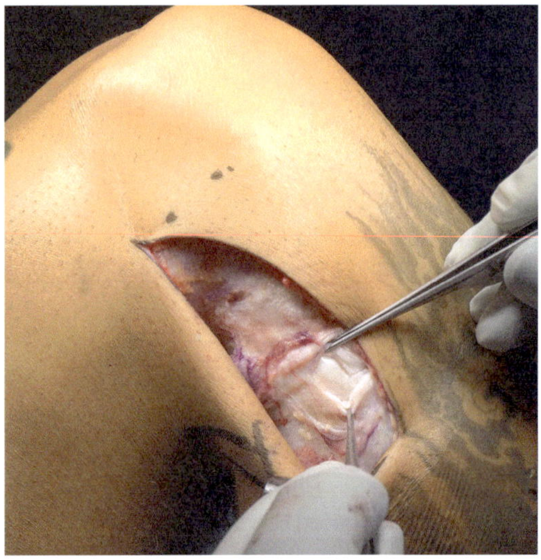

Fig. 10.7 Distal FLC footprint identification through a biceps bursa incision

condyle down to the neck of the fibula. Dissection proceeded to expose the deep fascia. The common peroneal nerve is visualized through the fascia posterior to biceps tendon. During the acute phase, a peroneal nerve neurolysis is recommended to eliminate a potential injury and to protect it during the gesture due to anatomic changes. In chronic phase, peroneal nerve neurolysis is not obligatory. If the nerve is visualized and palpated in the typical location posterior to the biceps tendon, it is not mobilized, but it is protected throughout the procedure. The interval between the short head of biceps and the ITB is developed and dissection undertaken to expose the posterolateral corner anterior to the lateral head of gastrocnemius (Fig. 10.6). A small incision longitudinally is made into the anterior arm of the long head of the biceps and its bursa to expose the insertion of the FCL on the fibula (Fig. 10.7). Putting tension on the tag stich allows to identify the FCL proximal insertion.

Fibula tunnel: A guidewire is then passed from the FCL distal footprint (anteromedial aspect of the fibula head) in a posterior, medial and proximal direction to exit the posterior aspect of the fibula head just distal to the styloid and overdrilled with a 5 mm drill taking care to protect the soft tissues. For this step, the surgeon can use a pin alignment guide or target his finger insert into the interval previously created. A stay suture is placed in this tunnel (Fig. 10.8).

Femoral tunnels: The ITB is split allowing the exposure of the lateral femoral condyle. The popliteus tendon insertion is identified on the condyle after a short arthrotomy (Fig. 10.9). A guidewire is passed from this point approxi-

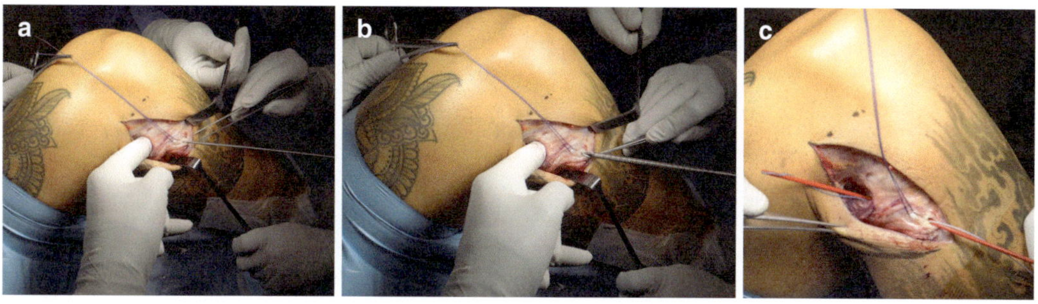

Fig. 10.8 Fibula tunnel preparation: (**a**) guidewire passing; (**b**) drilling; (**c**) stay suture placement

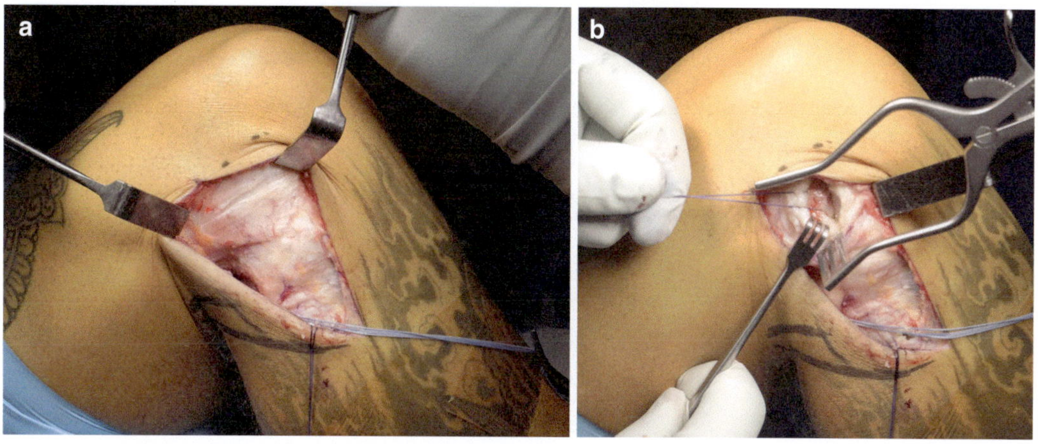

Fig. 10.9 (**a**) ITB incision, (**b**) PLT insertion identification after a small arthrotomy

mately 30° anteriorly and proximally to exit the medial skin of the thigh (Fig. 10.10). A temporary guidewire is placed at the attachment point for the FCL reconstruction just proximal and posterior to the lateral epicondyle. According to the anatomic studies, the length between the two femoral insertions should be approximately 18.5 mm. The graft is then passed into the fibular tunnel and secured with a 6 mm interference screw, keeping equal lengths of graft on either side of the fibula. The anterior limb of the graft, for the FCL, is then passed deep to the ITB and passed around the previously placed temporary guidewire, and the isometry is checked by moving the knee from flexion to extension and guidewire position adjusted if necessary to achieve isometry. The definitive guidewire is then passed from this point parallel to the popliteus guidewire and out through the medial skin of the thigh. The two femoral guidewires are then overdrilled with a 6 mm drill up to but not through the lateral cortex and a 4.5 mm drill through the medial cortex.

The popliteus limb of the graft is then passed through the joint, through the popliteal hiatus to the site of attachment on the femur (Fig. 10.11). Both grafts are then passed into the femoral tunnels. With the knee at 90° and the foot in neutral rotation with an anterolateral drawer, the popliteus limb of the graft is fixed on the femoral side using a 7 mm interference screw (Fig. 10.12). The knee is then brought out to 20–30° of flexion, with the foot still in neutral rotation. After applying tension on the fibular collateral graft and some slight valgus force, this graft is then fixed to the femur using a 7 mm interference screw (Fig. 10.12).

In the setting of combined reconstruction with ACL, we would usually do the arthroscopic ACL reconstruction first, followed by the open proce-

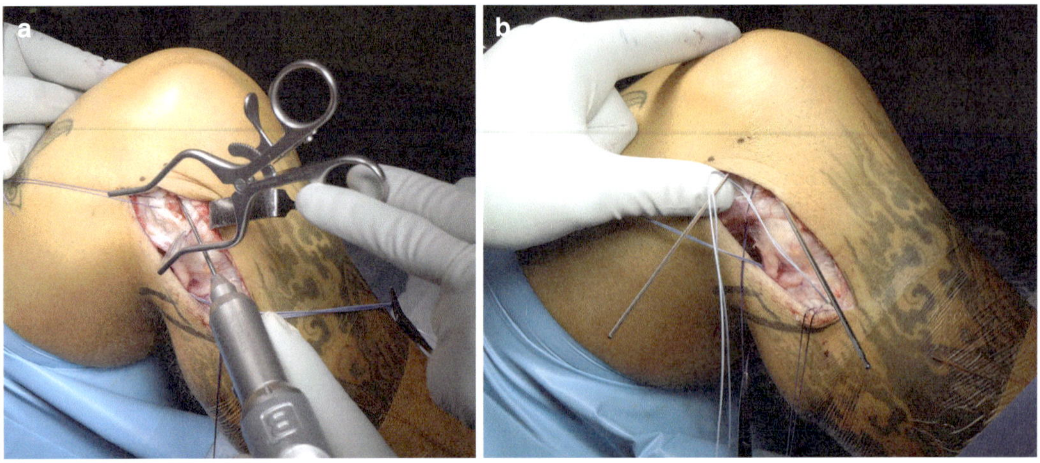

Fig. 10.10 (**a**) Positioning of the first guidewire in the PLT footprint, (**b**) positioning of a second guidewire, at 18.5 mm to the first one, in the FCL footprint, and isometry testing

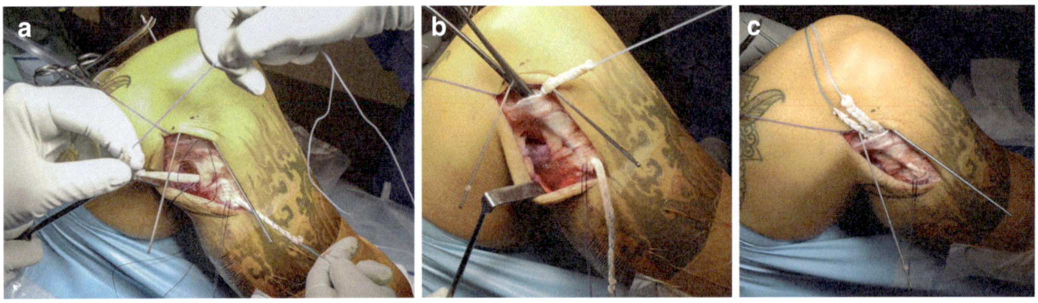

Fig. 10.11 (**a**) Passing of the graft into the fibular tunnel, (**b**) passing of posterior strand through the joint to reconstruct the popliteus complex, (**c**) passing of anterior strand under the ITB to reconstruct the FCL

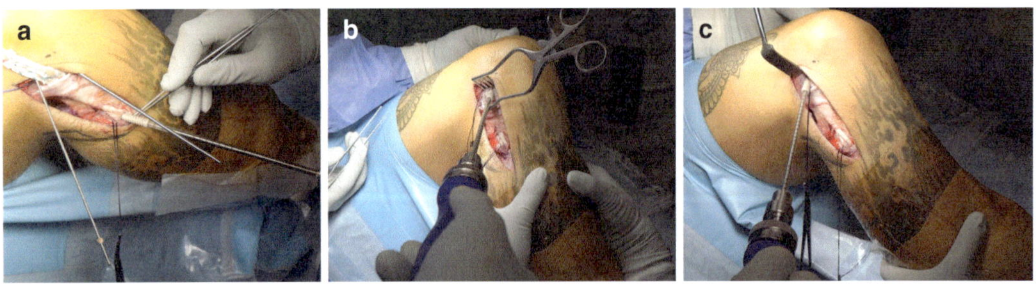

Fig. 10.12 (**a**) Firstly, the graft is fixed into the fibular tunnel. (**b**) Secondly, the popliteus graft is fixed with the knee at 90° of flexion, the foot in neutral rotation after applying an anterior drawer. (**c**) Finally, the FCL graft is fixed with the knee at 30° of flexion, the foot in neutral rotation after applying tension on the fibular collateral graft and some slight valgus force

dure. In the acute setting, care should be taken to monitor possible extravasation of arthroscopic fluid into the leg compartments, and if any concern then the lateral exposure can be done first to avoid this. Typically, the sequence of surgery would be (a) ACL reconstruction with graft fixed on femoral but not tibial side; (b) lateral dissection and preparation of all structures for repair and reconstruction, including fixation of graft to fibula but not to femur; (c) fixation of ACL graft on tibia with knee

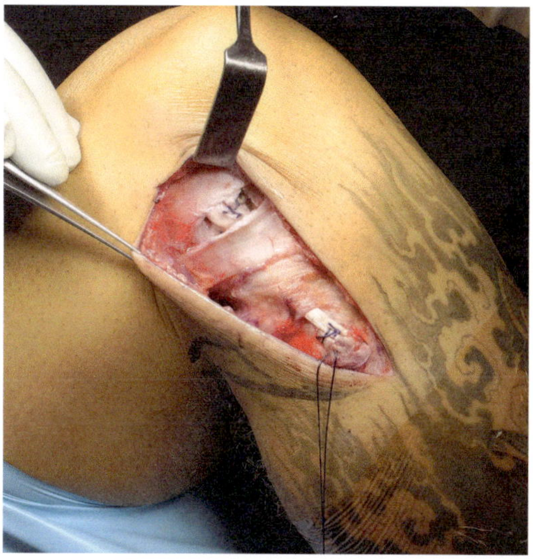

Fig. 10.13 Final view before closure

at full extension; (d) tensioning and fixation of popliteus and FCL grafts as described above.

Final testing: Before closure, the knee has to retain a full range of motion with a normal testing for PLC and ACL. Figure 10.13 represents the final view.

Closure: The incisions of the anterior capsule, the biceps bursa and the ITB are closed. The interval between the short head of biceps and the ITB is left open.

10.9.2 LaPrade Technique [35, 36]

Patient positioning: After an examination under anaesthesia, the patient is placed in supine position, knee flexed at 70–90° of flexion, with a tourniquet.

Graft harvest and preparation: For the ACL an ipsilateral patellar tendon or ST is harvested and prepared. A nonirradiated allograft is used for the PLC reconstruction. For the PLC reconstruction, a split Achilles allograft is used to have two different grafts. The two calcaneal blocks are shaped to be 9 × 25 mm. The non-osseous aspects of each graft are tubulized for an easy passing into 7-mm-diameter tunnel sizer.

Approach and soft tissue dissection: A lateral hockey stick is made from the distal femoral shaft along the ITB and extending distally between fibula head and Gerdy's tubercle. In addition to the steps previously described, a careful dissection is performed between the soleus and the lateral gastrocnemius to identify the musculotendinous junction of the popliteus.

Fibula tunnel: A 7 mm fibula tunnel is drilled from the distal FCL footprint to the posteromedial aspect of the fibula head.

Tibia tunnel: A 9 mm tibia tunnel anteroposterior is drilled from the flat area distal and medial to the GT to the musculotendinous junction spot of the popliteus. This targeted point is about 1 cm proximal and 1 cm medial to the fibular tunnel posterior exit point.

Femoral tunnels: After the same approach and preparation as previously described, two femoral tunnels, 18.5 mm spaced, are performed with a 9 mm reamer.

Graft passing and fixation: Both grafts are fixed in the femur with 7 mm interference screws. The FCL graft is passed under the ITB and then through the fibular tunnel and fixed with a 7 mm interference screw, with the knee at 20–30° of flexion, the foot in neutral rotation and applying a slight valgus stress. The popliteus graft is passed through the joint. Both grafts (popliteus and PFL) are passed into the tibial tunnel and fixed with a 9 mm interference screw with the knee flexed at 60° of flexion in neutral rotation.

Final fixation sequence: LaPrade et al. recommend the following order for the combined ACL and PLC reconstruction: (1) femoral ACL fixation, (2) femoral PLC fixation, (3) fibula fixation, (4) tibial fixation and (5) tibial ACL fixation.

10.10 Postoperative Rehabilitation

Currently, there is no consensual protocol of rehabilitation. Based on our clinical experience and gait studies, we prefer to have some minor residual laxity than stiffness. Therefore, we encourage an earlier active rehabilitation protocol. Typically, the patient will remain in the hospital for one to two nights until comfortable. Whilst in hospital he has antibiotic and deep vein thrombosis prophylaxis. We recommend the use of a hinged knee brace allowing 10–90° for the first 4 weeks and then full range for the next

4 weeks. An unloader brace could also be used if available. Regarding weight bearing, whilst LaPrade [35] recommends non-weight bearing for 6 weeks, we usually allow the patient to have partial weight bearing to 50% for 4 weeks and then weight bearing as tolerated in the brace for the next 4 weeks.

10.11 Conclusion

Whilst ACL injuries are common and management protocols well defined, PLC injuries are less common and more varied in their nature and therefore require the treating surgeon to have a good understanding of the pathology and the ideal treatment algorithm for each case. In this chapter we have outlined the anatomy, epidemiology and clinical assessment of these injuries and provided a treatment algorithm to ensure ideal management for each scenario. If the treating surgeon has a good understanding of the injury and is able to provide the appropriate treatment individualized for each case, good outcomes can usually be achieved.

References

1. Chahla J, Moatshe G, Dean CS, LaPrade RF. Posterolateral corner of the knee: current concepts. Arch Bone Joint Surg. 2016;4(2):97–103.
2. Kennedy NI, LaPrade CM, LaPrade RF. Surgical management and treatment of the anterior cruciate ligament/posterolateral corner injured knee. Clin Sports Med. 2017;36(1):105–17.
3. Harner CD, Vogrin TM, Höher J, Ma CB, Woo SL. Biomechanical analysis of a posterior cruciate ligament reconstruction. Deficiency of the posterolateral structures as a cause of graft failure. Am J Sports Med. 2000;28(1):32–9.
4. LaPrade RF, Resig S, Wentorf F, Lewis JL. The effects of grade III posterolateral knee complex injuries on anterior cruciate ligament graft force. A biomechanical analysis. Am J Sports Med. 1999;27(4):469–75.
5. LaPrade RF, Gilbert TJ, Bollom TS, Wentorf F, Chaljub G. The magnetic resonance imaging appearance of individual structures of the posterolateral knee. A prospective study of normal knees and knees with surgically verified grade III injuries. Am J Sports Med. 2000;28(2):191–9.
6. Geeslin AG, LaPrade RF. Location of bone bruises and other osseous injuries associated with acute grade III isolated and combined posterolateral knee injuries. Am J Sports Med. 2010;38(12):2502–8.
7. LaPrade RF, Wentorf FA, Fritts H, Gundry C, Hightower CD. A prospective magnetic resonance imaging study of the incidence of posterolateral and multiple ligament injuries in acute knee injuries presenting with a hemarthrosis. Arthroscopy. 2007;23(12):1341–7.
8. Temponi EF, de Carvalho Júnior LH, Saithna A, Thaunat M, Sonnery-Cottet B. Incidence and MRI characterization of the spectrum of posterolateral corner injuries occurring in association with ACL rupture. Skelet Radiol. 2017;46(8):1063–70.
9. LaPrade RF, Ly TV, Wentorf FA, Engebretsen L. The posterolateral attachments of the knee: a qualitative and quantitative morphologic analysis of the fibular collateral ligament, popliteus tendon, popliteofibular ligament, and lateral gastrocnemius tendon. Am J Sports Med. 2003;31(6):854–60.
10. LaPrade RF. Anatomic reconstruction of the posterolateral aspect of the knee. J Knee Surg. 2005;18(2):167–71.
11. Sanchez AR, Sugalski MT, LaPrade RF. Anatomy and biomechanics of the lateral side of the knee. Sports Med Arthrosc Rev. 2006;14(1):2–11.
12. Sugita T, Amis AA. Anatomic and biomechanical study of the lateral collateral and popliteofibular ligaments. Am J Sports Med. 2001;29(4):466–72.
13. Amis AA, Bull AMJ, Gupte CM, Hijazi I, Race A, Robinson JR. Biomechanics of the PCL and related structures: posterolateral, posteromedial and meniscofemoral ligaments. Knee Surg Sports Traumatol Arthrosc. 2003;11(5):271–81.
14. Terry GC, LaPrade RF. The posterolateral aspect of the knee. Anatomy and surgical approach. Am J Sports Med. 1996;24(6):732–9.
15. Seebacher JR, Inglis AE, Marshall JL, Warren RF. The structure of the posterolateral aspect of the knee. J Bone Joint Surg Am. 1982;64(4):536–41.
16. Kawashima T, Takeishi H, Yoshitomi S, Ito M, Sasaki H. Anatomical study of the fabella, fabellar complex and its clinical implications. Surg Radiol Anat. 2007;29(8):611–6.
17. Fanelli GC, Orcutt DR, Edson CJ. The multiple-ligament injured knee: evaluation, treatment, and results. Arthroscopy. 2005;21(4):471–86.
18. Baker CL, Norwood LA, Hughston JC. Acute posterolateral rotatory instability of the knee. J Bone Joint Surg Am. 1983;65(5):614–8.
19. LaPrade RF, Terry GC. Injuries to the posterolateral aspect of the knee. Association of anatomic injury patterns with clinical instability. Am J Sports Med. 1997;25(4):433–8.
20. Noyes FR, Barber-Westin SD, Hewett TE. High tibial osteotomy and ligament reconstruction for varus angulated anterior cruciate ligament-deficient knees. Am J Sports Med. 2000;28(3):282–96.

21. Hughston JC, Andrews JR, Cross MJ, Moschi A. Classification of knee ligament instabilities. Part II. The lateral compartment. J Bone Joint Surg Am. 1976;58(2):173–9.
22. Laprade RF, Heikes C, Bakker AJ, Jakobsen RB. The reproducibility and repeatability of varus stress radiographs in the assessment of isolated fibular collateral ligament and grade-III posterolateral knee injuries: an in vitro biomechanical study. J Bone Joint Surg Am. 2008;90(10):2069–76.
23. Jackman T, LaPrade RF, Pontinen T, Lender PA. Intraobserver and interobserver reliability of the kneeling technique of stress radiography for the evaluation of posterior knee laxity. Am J Sports Med. 2008;36(8):1571–6.
24. McDonough EB, Wojtys EM. Multiligamentous injuries of the knee and associated vascular injuries. Am J Sports Med. 2009;37(1):156–9.
25. Sanders TL, Johnson NR, Levy NM, et al. Effect of vascular injury on functional outcome in knees with multi-ligament injury: a matched-cohort analysis. J Bone Joint Surg Am. 2017;99(18):1565–71.
26. Fanelli GC, Stannard JP, Stuart MJ, et al. Management of complex knee ligament injuries. Instr Course Lect. 2010;92(12):2235.
27. Kannus P. Nonoperative treatment of grade II and III sprains of the lateral ligament compartment of the knee. Am J Sports Med. 1989;17(1):83–8.
28. Krukhaug Y, Mølster A, Rodt A, Strand T. Lateral ligament injuries of the knee. Knee Surg Sports Traumatol Arthrosc. 1998;6(1):21–5.
29. Arthur A, LaPrade RF, Agel J. Proximal tibial opening wedge osteotomy as the initial treatment for chronic posterolateral corner deficiency in the varus knee: a prospective clinical study. Am J Sports Med. 2007;35(11):1844–50.
30. Clancy JW, Sutherland TB. Combined posterior cruciate ligament injuries. Clin Sports Med. 1994;13(3):629–47.
31. Geeslin AG, LaPrade RF. Outcomes of treatment of acute grade-III isolated and combined posterolateral knee injuries: a prospective case series and surgical technique. J Bone Joint Surg Am. 2011;93(18):1672–83.
32. Levy BA, Stuart MJ. Treatment of PCL, ACL, and lateral-side knee injuries: acute and chronic. J Knee Surg. 2012;25(4):295–305. https://doi.org/10.1055/s-0032-1324813.
33. Levy BA, Dajani KA, Morgan JA, Shah JP, Dahm DL, Stuart MJ. Repair versus reconstruction of the fibular collateral ligament and posterolateral corner in the multiligament-injured knee. Am J Sports Med. 2010;38(4):804–9.
34. Geeslin AG, Moulton SG, LaPrade RF. A systematic review of the outcomes of posterolateral corner knee injuries, Part 1: Surgical treatment of acute injuries. Am J Sports Med. 2016;44(5):1336–42.
35. LaPrade RF, Johansen S, Agel J, Risberg MA, Moksnes H, Engebretsen L. Outcomes of an anatomic posterolateral knee reconstruction. J Bone Joint Surg Am. 2010;92(1):16–22.
36. McCarthy M, Camarda L, Wijdicks CA, Johansen S, Engebretsen L, Laprade RF. Anatomic posterolateral knee reconstructions require a popliteofibular ligament reconstruction through a tibial tunnel. Am J Sports Med. 2010;38(8):1674–81.

Acute Knee Dislocations

11

Conor I. Murphy, Philip P. Roessler, Tracye J. Lawyer, and Volker Musahl

11.1 Epidemiology and Injury Mechanism

Acute knee dislocations are regarded to be very rare. It is estimated that they account for less than 0.02% of all musculoskeletal injuries, although this number may be underestimated due to spontaneous reduction and missed diagnosis [1, 2]. Frequency is higher in male patients with a peak age around 35 years [3] with about 44% of cases presenting as polytrauma [4]. Most frequent mechanisms are either high-velocity injuries (e.g., motorcycle accidents) or low-velocity injuries (e.g., pivoting or cutting movements during sports activities), although recent studies also indicate a rising amount of ultralow-velocity injuries (around 10%), especially with regard to obese patients [5]. Incidences are 0.06% patients for closed and 0.012% for open dislocations [3]. Femorotibial joint dislocation may take the following directions: anterior, posterior, medial, lateral, and rotary combined. Proximal tibiofibular dislocations are very rare but may occur isolated as well as alongside femorotibial dislocations [6].

Depending on the injury mechanism, a certain trauma pattern can be noted in most cases. Anterior dislocations (40%) usually involve hyperextension above 30° and thus rupture of the posterior capsule and at least the anterior cruciate ligament [7] (ACL). In contrast, posterior dislocations (30%) are commonly "dashboard injuries" to the flexed knee involving rupture of the posterior cruciate ligament (PCL). Lateral (18%) and medial (4%) dislocations damage the opposite collateral and posterior corner of the knee occasionally leading to concomitant tibial plateau fractures. Rotatory combined injuries usually manifest a mixed soft tissue injury pattern.

11.2 Classification

Different systematics have been used over the past years to classify the extent of injury and concomitant damages to the periphery of the knee joint. As surgical strategies may vary between fractured and non-fractured states, it appears to be appropriate to use both, the Schenck/Wascher and Moore classification systems [8, 9] (Tables 11.1 and 11.2).

11.3 Concomitant Injuries

Despite the occurrence of fractures and associated soft tissue trauma, the most common concomitant injuries affect the neurovascular structures around the knee.

The original version of this chapter was revised. A correction to this chapter can be found at https://doi.org/10.1007/978-3-662-58245-9_19

C. I. Murphy · P. P. Roessler · T. J. Lawyer
V. Musahl (✉)
Department of Orthopaedic Surgery, University of Pittsburgh, Pittsburgh, PA, USA
e-mail: murphyci@upmc.edu; musahlv@upmc.edu

F. Margheritini et al. (eds.), *Complex Knee Ligament Injuries*,
https://doi.org/10.1007/978-3-662-58245-9_11

Table 11.1 Schenck/Wascher classification of knee dislocation

Class[a]	Injury
KD I	ACL or PCL torn, MCL/LCL variable pattern
KD II	ACL/PCL torn, MCL/LCL intact
KD III	ACL/PCL torn, either MCL (subtype M) or LCL (subtype L) torn
KD IV	ACL/PCL and MCL/LCL torn
KD V	Knee fracture dislocation (see Moore classification)

[a]Subtype C refers to a presence of arterial injuries, while subtype N refers to nerve injuries

Table 11.2 Moore classification of knee fracture dislocation

Class	Injury
I	Split fractures through medial or lateral plateau
II	Complete fractures separating entire medial or lateral plateau
III	Rim avulsion fractures
IV	Rim compression fractures
V	Four-part fracture

11.3.1 Vascular Injuries

Vascular injuries in acute knee dislocation most commonly are a result of shear forces or rapid deceleration, possibly leading to major bleeding or decreased distal perfusion. In those cases, urgent surgical intervention after joint reduction may be required, often resulting in a two-staged procedure to manage both the ligamentous and soft tissue trauma.

Injuries of the popliteal artery show the highest incidence (76%) and mostly occur in dislocations KD III and above. Further vessels at risk with lower injury incidences include the medial genicular artery, anterior tibial artery, posterior tibial artery, superficial femoral artery, as well as common femoral artery [10]. As the popliteal artery is anatomically suspended to the adductor canal proximally and to the soleus arch distally, it is most likely to be injured than all other vessels. Corresponding injuries to the popliteal vein are less morbid but may subsequently result in thrombosis [11]. In case of any suspicion of ischemia or potentially life-threatening bleeding, immediate vascular surgical intervention is advised. Treatment strategies include watchful waiting with pharmacologic anticoagulation, thrombectomy or thrombolysis, as well as vascular surgical repair or bypass. In 12% of cases, severe ischemia may necessitate distal amputation [10]. Continuous clinical assessment for the first few days in the immediate postoperative or post-injury period is necessary to rule out compartment syndrome or reperfusion injury.

11.3.2 Nerve Injuries

Common peroneal nerve palsy has been reported in up to 40% of multi-ligamentous knee injuries, largely during varus stress, due to tethering of the nerve to the fibular head and the boundaries of the popliteal fossa [12]. In contrast, tibial nerve palsy is a rare condition as the structure is not tethered like the peroneal nerve. Most incomplete palsies recover over time. Complete palsies also exhibit a high rate of spontaneous recovery if they are painless and without any further signs of deep denervation upon presentation. Positive predictors of recovery are young patient age [13] and incomplete palsies upon first clinical presentation [14]. Complete palsy recovery is rarely noted in cases accompanied by severe pain and positive Tinel sign [15].

Besides true continuity lesions, extrinsic pressure due to distortion, fracture, or posttraumatic hematoma is the most common cause for neurologic symptoms after knee dislocations. Treatment strategies are dependent on the extent of neurological symptoms. Surgical exploration with decompression or neurolysis should be considered in all clinically apparent palsies with open injuries. Closed injuries should be explored no later than 2 weeks following onset of symptoms. Following this, watchful waiting is an option for anatomically intact nerves. Timely referral to a specialist for nerve grafting is advised for continuity lesions with a gap below 6 cm, while gaping over 6 cm usually demands nerve transfer or grafting with the ipsilateral sural [16]. Recurrent neurophysiology and electromyography (EMG) assessment helps quantify nerve injury and prognosis for recovery.

11.4 Assessment

Assessment begins with primary survey according to Advanced Trauma Life Support (ATLS) protocols. Clinical suspicion based on mechanism and patient history is vital. The examiner needs to be able to rapidly recognize and manage knee dislocations in a systematic fashion (Fig. 11.1).

11.4.1 Reduction

Immediate reduction of the knee joint to prevent further damage to surrounding soft tissues and neurovascular structures is imperative. Prior to reduction, document the vascular examination with palpation and Doppler ultrasound when available. With the patient adequately sedated, reduce the knee with manual axial traction. In certain circumstances, if the injury is witnessed and the patient can be examined immediately, reduction can be performed in the field. Postreduction radiographs are necessary to confirm reduction and stabilization.

The knee may exhibit a "dimple sign" in the skin along the medial joint line signifying a buttonholing of the medial femoral condyle through the medial capsule. In this case, closed reduction is not possible and should not be attempted due to the risk of skin necrosis.

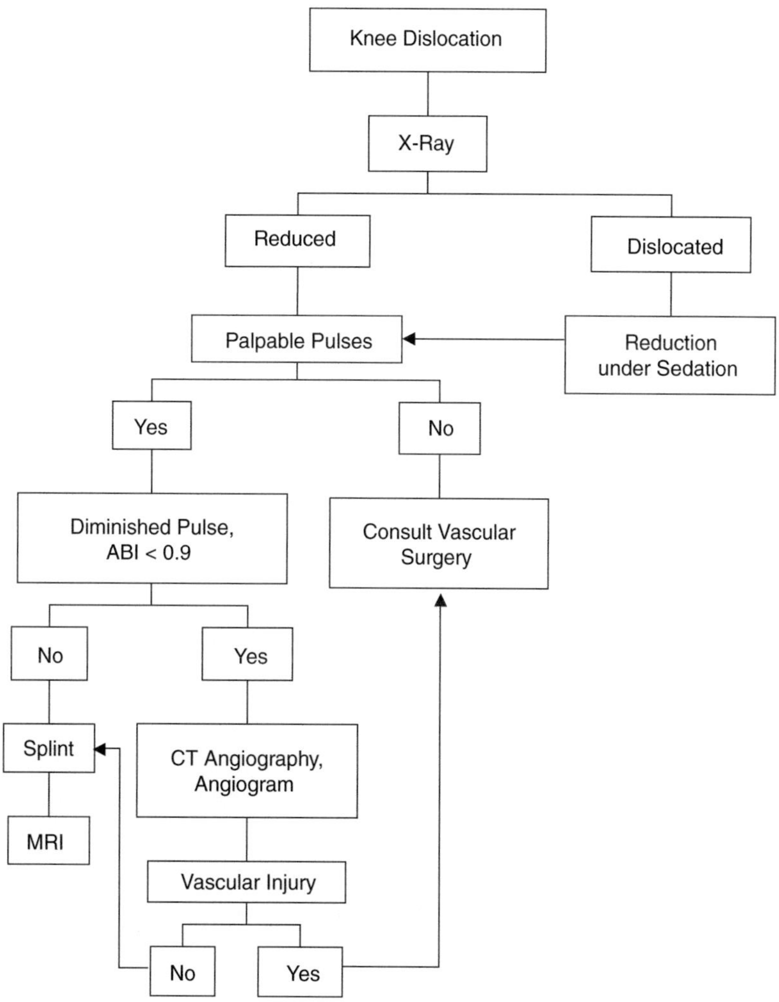

Fig. 11.1 Decision tree directing acute management of a knee dislocation upon initial presentation

11.4.2 Clinical Exam

Secondary survey should then shift to a focused assessment of the knee. Pre- and post-reduction vascular status must be examined and documented. Vascular assessment includes palpation of distal pulses, Doppler ultrasound of distal arteries, and measurement of the ankle-brachial pressure index (ABI). Absent postreduction distal pulses on palpation or Doppler ultrasound demands immediate vascular surgery consultation and surgical exploration. If the pulses are palpable but diminished compared to the contralateral limb or the ABI is less than 0.9, advanced imaging and vascular surgery consultation should be ordered [17].

Neurological assessment includes peripheral sensory and motor strength exam as well as pain scale and reflexes. In subacute and elective cases, neurophysiology and EMG are the diagnostic tools of choice to localize nerve lesions topographically. Conventional clinical examination using varus/valgus stress and Lachman test to check for instabilities is largely unreliable in the alert and painful patient. If sedation is required for reduction, these tests should be performed while the patient is sedated for improved diagnostic accuracy.

11.4.3 Radiographic Assessment (Immediate)

Plain radiographs of the knee are the primary initial imaging studies. Diagnosing the direction of dislocation, associated fractures, osteochondral defects, and overall joint congruency is paramount to establishing subsequent intervention (Fig. 11.2a, b). Subtle joint incongruences or subluxations may be the sole evidence of pathology in instances where spontaneous reduction occurred.

If there is evidence of vascular compromise manifested by diminished distal pulses or abnormal ABI then the patient should be sent for CT angiography or formal angiogram to identify the location of the vascular injury. An injured limb with absent pulses after reduction does not require vascular imaging.

Injuries to the cruciate ligaments, collateral ligaments, meniscus, chondral surfaces, and structures comprising the posterolateral and posteromedial corners are clarified with magnetic resonance imaging (MRI) (Fig. 11.3a–c).

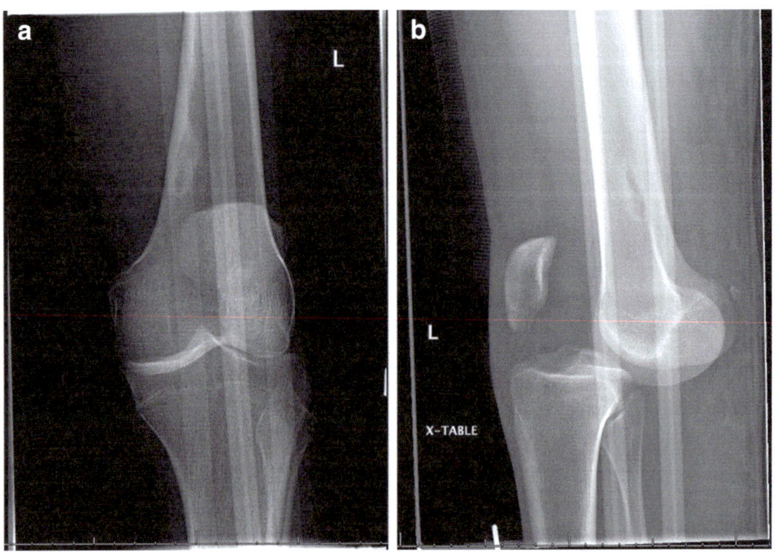

Fig. 11.2 (**a**) AP radiograph left knee dislocation, (**b**) Lateral radiograph left knee anterior dislocation

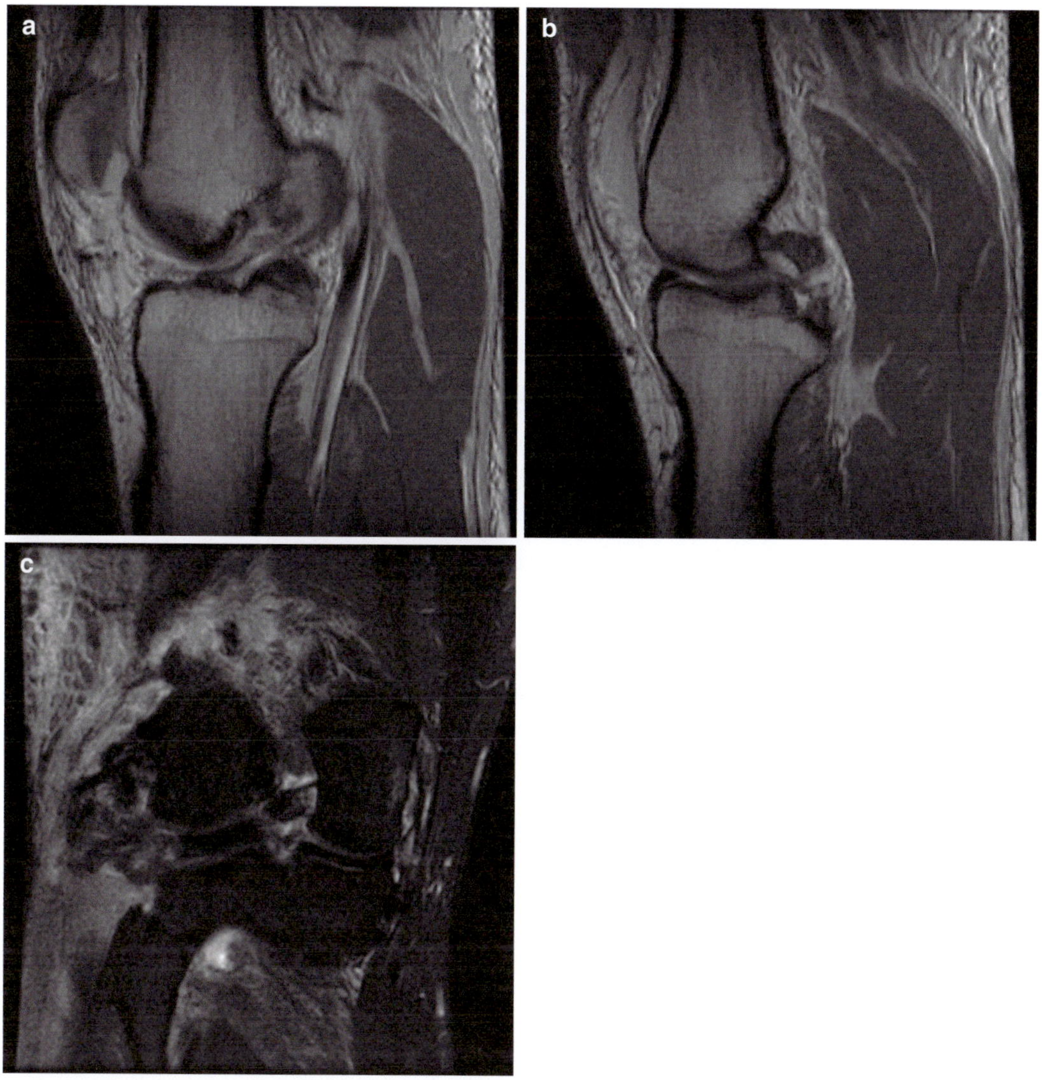

Fig. 11.3 (**a**) MRI sagittal view left knee demonstrating complete disruption ACL, (**b**) MRI sagittal view left knee demonstrating PCL injury, (**c**) MRI coronal view left knee demonstrating posterolateral corner disruption

This study should be delayed until reduction and stabilization of the dislocated knee and confirmation that there is no vascular injury or other associated limb- or life-threatening injuries.

Computed tomography (CT) provides utility in the context of a tibial plateau fracture with intra-articular extension. Open reduction and internal fixation of the tibial plateau will be necessary prior to any ligamentous reconstruction. Often, CT is necessary in these cases to identify the fracture pattern and formulate a preoperative plan for the fixation construct.

11.5 Initial Stabilization (Operative Versus Non-operative)

After reduction and confirmation with X-ray, the knee must be initially immobilized with a posterior splint in 20° to 30° of flexion to stabilize the

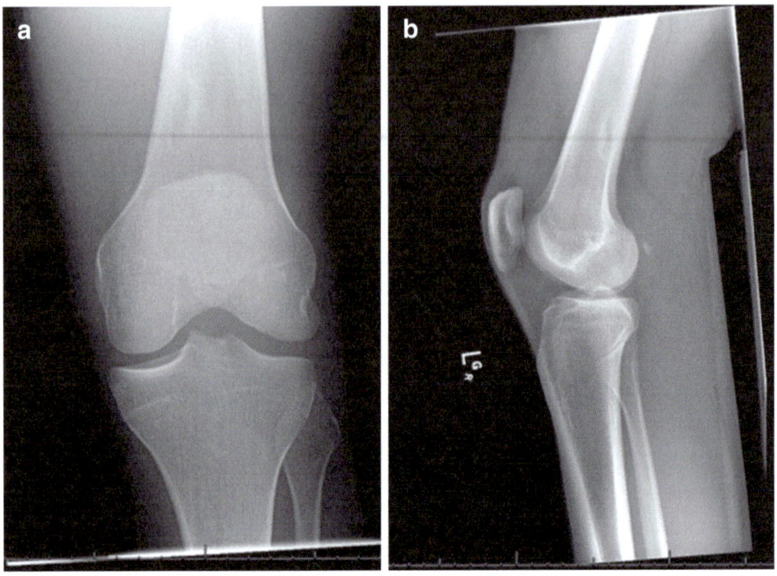

Fig. 11.4 (**a**) AP radiograph reduction left knee dislocation, (**b**) Lateral radiograph reduction left knee dislocation

joint (Fig. 11.4a, b). If the postreduction and splinting X-rays demonstrate adequate alignment and congruency of the joint, then the splint can be maintained or the patient can transition to a knee brace, such as a hinged knee brace or knee immobilizer, until discharge from the hospital and follow-up as an outpatient for surgical planning.

If there is persistent malreduction or subluxation of the knee joint then temporary surgical stabilization with knee-spanning external fixation is necessary to protect the joint from further soft tissue, vascular, and nervous injury. External fixation may also be necessary after vascular repair depending on the extent of injury and confidence in the repair integrity by the vascular surgeon.

11.6 Surgical Management and Technique

The PCL is reconstructed first followed by the ACL, followed by the posterolateral complex and/or medial side. Reconstruction of the medial or lateral collateral ligaments requires a functional central pivot for accurate determination of isometry.

11.6.1 Graft Selection

Allograft is preferred for these complex surgical procedures. Preferred graft for the PCL is Achilles tendon allograft for single-bundle PCL reconstructions and Achilles tendon and tibialis anterior allografts for double-bundle PCL reconstructions. Achilles tendon allograft is preferred for the ACL reconstruction. The preferred graft material for the posterolateral corner is allograft tissue combined with a primary repair or a posterolateral capsular shift procedure. Preferred method for medial collateral ligament (MCL) and posteromedial reconstructions is a primary repair and/or posteromedial capsular advancement with allograft supplementation as needed [18].

11.6.2 PCL Reconstruction

PCL reconstruction technique can be performed transtibial, open, or arthroscopic tibial inlay. The preferred technique by the senior author is arthroscopic transtibial PCL reconstruction. An examination under anesthesia is performed to assess posterior drawer, posterior sag, dynamic stress tests for collateral ligaments, and posterolateral and

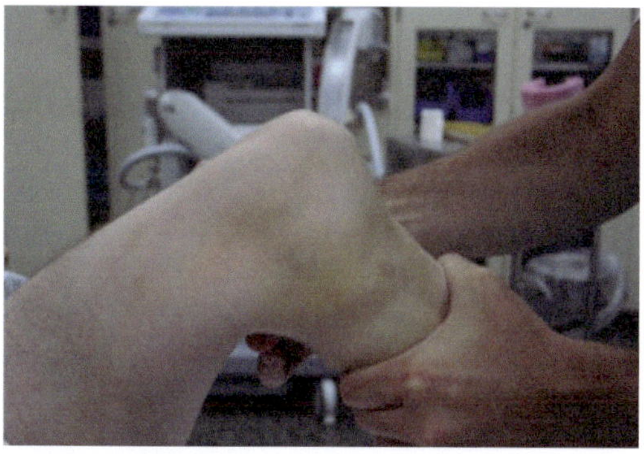

Fig. 11.5 Intraoperative dynamic posterior drawer stress test with positive posterior translation of tibia

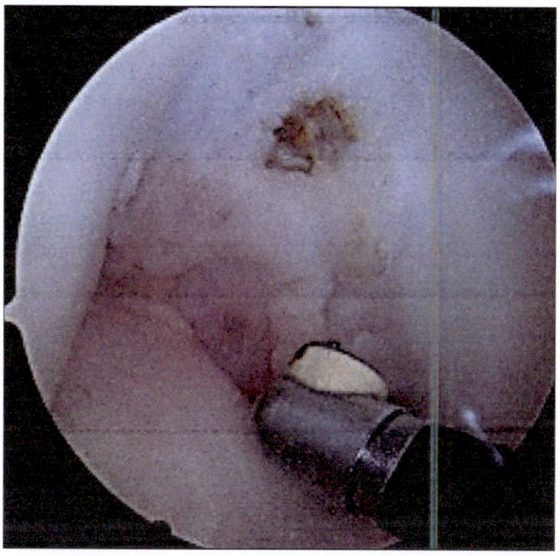

Fig. 11.6 Arthroscopic view from anterolateral portal of PCL debridement

posteromedial corner (Fig. 11.5). Diagnostic arthroscopy is performed through standard anterolateral portal with 30°arthroscope. The PCL is examined and debrided (Fig. 11.6). Preserve footprint for tunnel placement. Establish posteromedial portal under spinal needle guidance. A posteromedial arthroscopic portal is helpful to create the tibial tunnel for the PCL reconstruction arthroscopically. With a posteromedial portal, using a 30° or 70° scope either from the posteromedial position or through the notch can help expose the posterior tibial ledge. Preparation of the area can then be easily accomplished by working through either an anterior portal or the posteromedial portal. Dissect

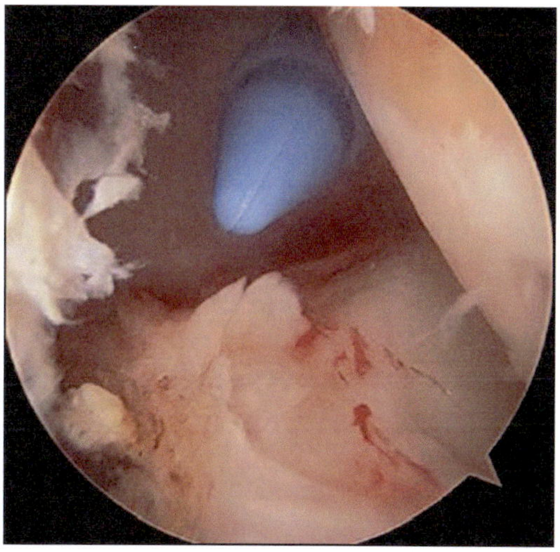

Fig. 11.7 Establishment of posteromedial working portal

behind ACL, 10–12 mm below joint line to cephalad border of popliteus (Fig. 11.7).

Place tibial guide on inferior aspect of PCL facet, lateral to posterior root of medial meniscus (Fig. 11.8a, b). Use fluoroscopy for tibial tunnel creation which aids in accurate and safe placement of a guidewire into the appropriate site on the posterior tibia. The anterior entry site for the tibial tunnel is well distal to the usual ACL tunnel site. The exit site of the tunnel, at the back of the tibia, is critical. The guidewire should exit in the middle of the posterior facet of the natural PCL origin. This ensures that the reconstructed ligament will be anchored far enough posteriorly to function properly. A properly placed guidewire, when seen on fluoroscopy on the lateral view, parallels the angle made by the joint of the proximal tibia with the fibula and runs just superior and parallel to the posterior curve of the proximal tibia cortex just underneath the posterior ledge.

Set the initial length of the guidewire from tip to drill chuck, such that when the guidewire has been advanced to the point at which the drill chuck hits the drill guide, the guidewire has just reached the inner table for the posterior tibial cortex.

Advance the guidewire under radiologic control from the beginning of the procedure.

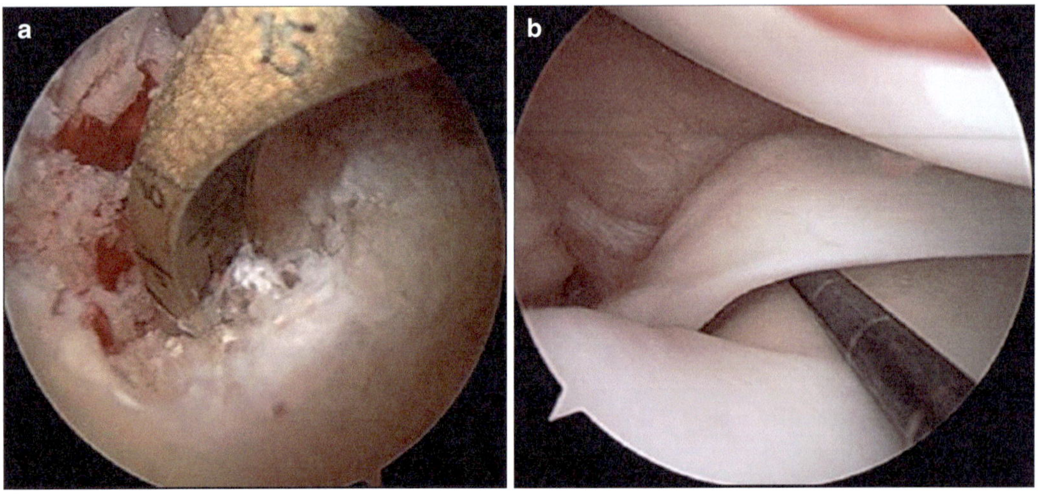

Fig. 11.8 (**a**) Tibial guide in place at the PCL facet, (**b**) Visualization of posterior root of medial meniscus

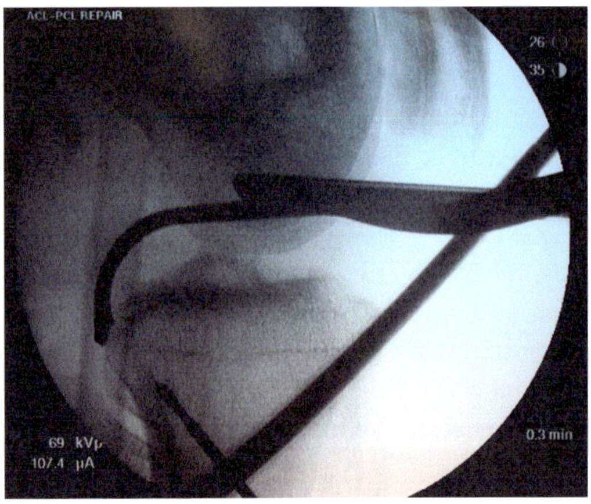

Fig. 11.9 Intraoperative lateral fluoroscopic images demonstrating the proper entry point, trajectory, and exit point for the tibial drill and guide pin for PCL reconstruction

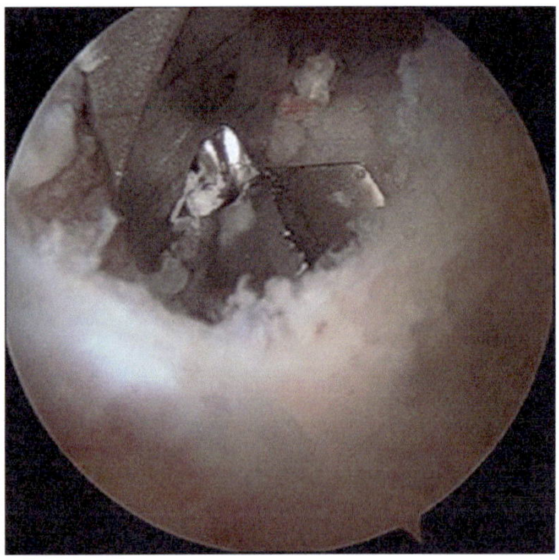

Fig. 11.10 Overreaming tibial tunnel by hand viewed from posteromedial portal

Stop advancement of the wire under power when the posterior cortex is reached (Fig. 11.9).

Penetrate the posterior cortex slowly, viewing it directly from the posterior medial portal with 70°arthroscope. Grasp the guidewire with an arthroscopic grasper to ensure that it is not advertently driven further posteriorly during reaming over the wire. Set the length of the reamer, from tip to drill chuck, to prevent inadvertent penetration of the reamer past the posterior tibial cortex. Drill over the guidewire while viewing the advancing reamer with frequent fluoroscopic radiographic spot pictures. Complete reaming by hand to protect neurovascular structures (Fig. 11.10).

The site for the femoral tunnel in PCL reconstruction is chosen at a point anterior and superior on the medial wall of the intercondylar notch. Center guide primarily within anterolateral bundle with anterior tunnel margin 2 mm off chondral junction at roof of the notch. When the notch is viewed with the knee flexed at 70–90° and is at the axilla of the medial wall and the roof of the notch, the point of guidewire placement is optimal. A low

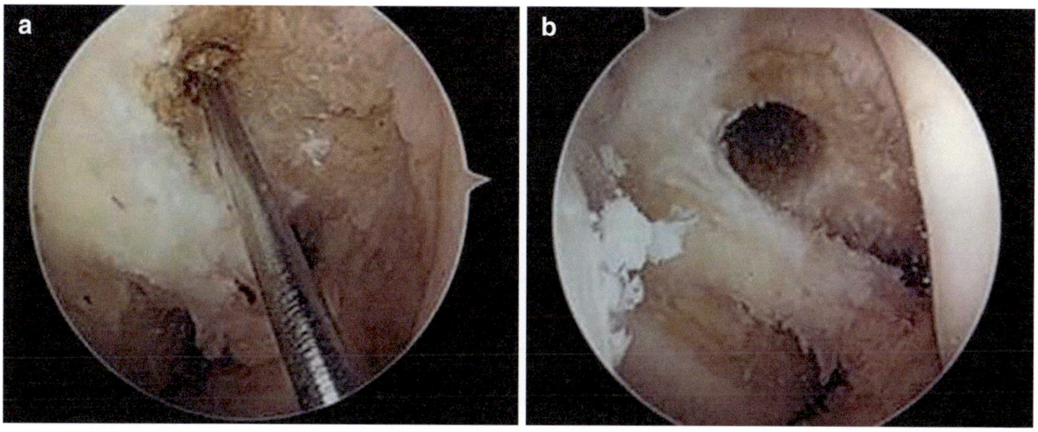

Fig. 11.11 (**a**) Guidewire position at femoral insertion of PCL, (**b**) Femoral tunnel socket at PCL insertion site viewing from low anterolateral portal

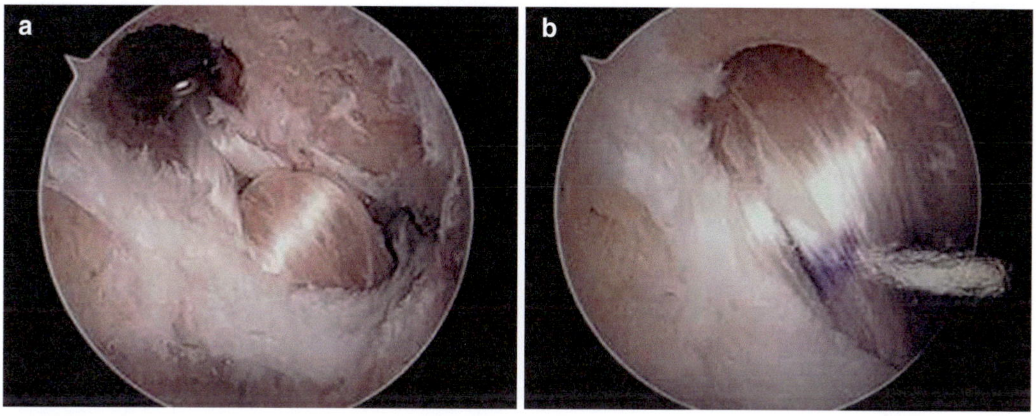

Fig. 11.12 (**a**) Passage of PCL graft into femoral tunnel, (**b**) Final position of PCL graft at femoral tunnel

anterolateral portal helps to view the PCL femoral insertion site. The guidewire is placed from the anteromedial cortex of the distal femur into the chosen position in the intercondylar notch using a standard drill guide, and the tunnel is made by reaming over the guidewire with the appropriate-sized reamer (Fig. 11.11a, b).

PCL graft is passed through anteromedial portal and retrograde in tibia. Fixation occurs at 90° flexion with anterior drawer. Suspensory fixation is used for femoral tunnel and double fixation is used for tibia. The senior author's preferred fixation method is Endobutton for femoral tunnel and interference screw with suture post screw for tibial fixation (Fig. 11.12a, b).

11.6.3 ACL Reconstruction

The tibial tunnel for the ACL is made in typical fashion using a standard drill guide and reamer system. A femoral tunnel for the ACL is also made in standard endoscopic fashion on the wall of the lateral femoral condyle (Fig. 11.13).

When all required tunnels have been constructed, the PCL graft is positioned first followed by the ACL graft. When both grafts are in place, the PCL graft is tensioned and fixed in place first, followed by tensioning and fixation of the ACL graft. The knee must be properly reduced during fixation of the PCL graft to recreate the normal step-off. Proper tensioning of the PCL is best achieved with knee at 70° of flexion.

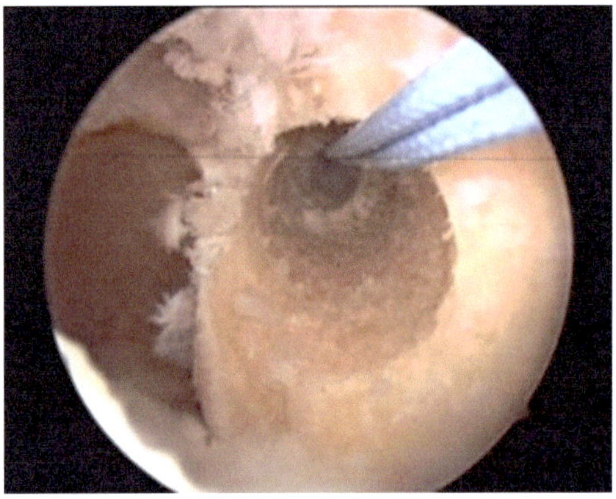

Fig. 11.13 Femoral tunnel ACL reconstruction

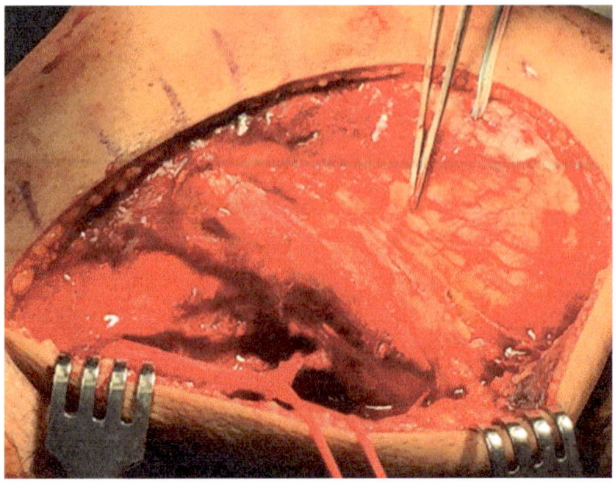

Fig. 11.14 Exposure of lateral knee and identification of peroneal nerve with vessel loop

Additional fixation can be used with fastening the draw sutures with either a ligament button or staples. The ACL graft is tensioned and fixed with interference screws with the knee in full extension and properly reduced [19, 20].

11.6.4 Posterolateral Reconstruction (Fibular-Based)

A curvilinear incision is made in the lateral aspect of the knee extending from the lateral femoral epicondyle to the interval between Gerdy's tubercle and the fibular head. The peroneal nerve is dissected free and protected through the procedure. A neurolysis of the common peroneal nerve can be performed as necessary. The nerve is typically located posteromedially to the long head of the biceps femoris (Fig. 11.14).

The fibular head is exposed and a tunnel is created in an anterior-posterior direction at the area of maximal fibular diameter. The tunnel is created by passing a guide pin followed by a cannulated drill usually 6–7 mm in diameter. The free tendon graft is then passed through the fibular head drill hole (Fig. 11.15).

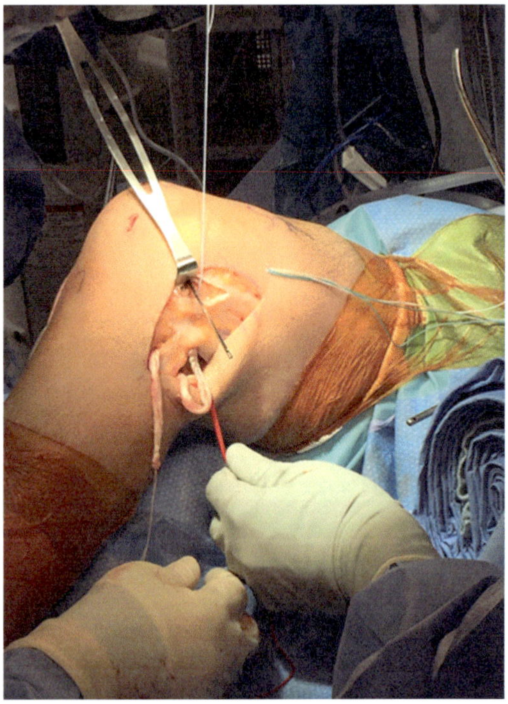

Fig. 11.15 Graft passed through the fibular tunnel with guidewire in femoral tunnel

Next step is to identify the proximal insertions of the lateral collateral ligament (LCL) and the popliteus tendon. An incision is then made in the iliotibial band in line with fibers directly overlying the lateral femoral epicondyle. The LCL insertions can be located approximately 1.5 mm proximal and 3 mm posterior to the lateral epicondyle. The femoral attachment of the popliteus tendon is located approximately 18.5 mm anterior to the LCL insertion. The femoral aiming guide is placed between the LCL and popliteus tendon over the proximal LCL attachment. The guide pin should exit the medial aspect of the distal thigh, anterior and proximal relative to the entry point. A longitudinal incision is made in the

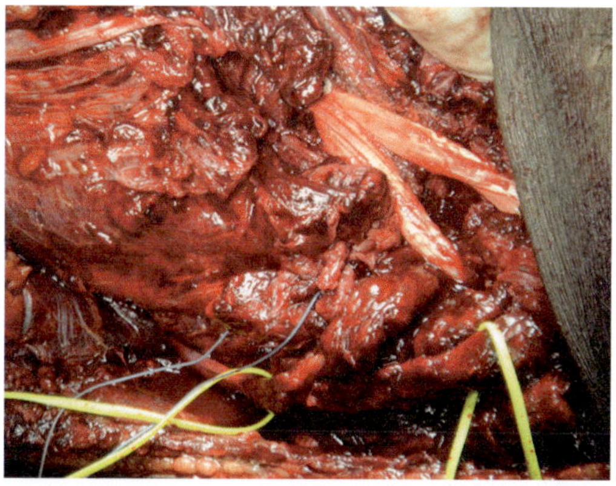

Fig. 11.16 Final position LCL graft into interference screw (yellow vessel loop around peroneal nerve and blue sutures tied to biceps femoris)

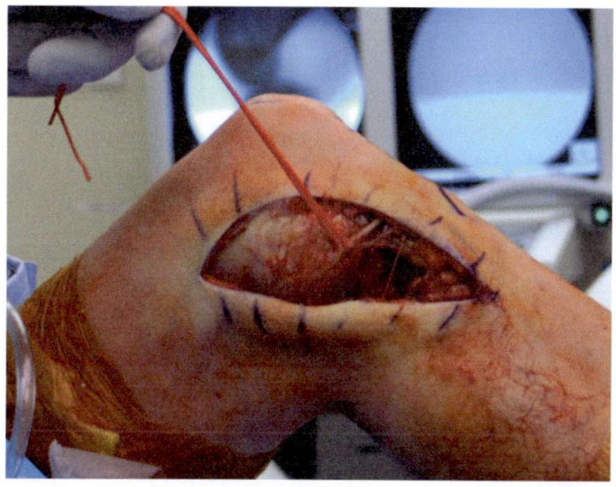

Fig. 11.17 Medial knee incision with identification of saphenous nerve

lateral capsule just posterior to the LCL. The graft material is passed medial to the iliotibial band and secured to the lateral femoral epicondylar region, either with a screw and spiked ligament washer or with interference screw (Fig. 11.16).

The final graft tensioning position is approximately 20° of knee flexion and neutral rotation while applying a gentle valgus force to reduce any lateral compartment laxity [21].

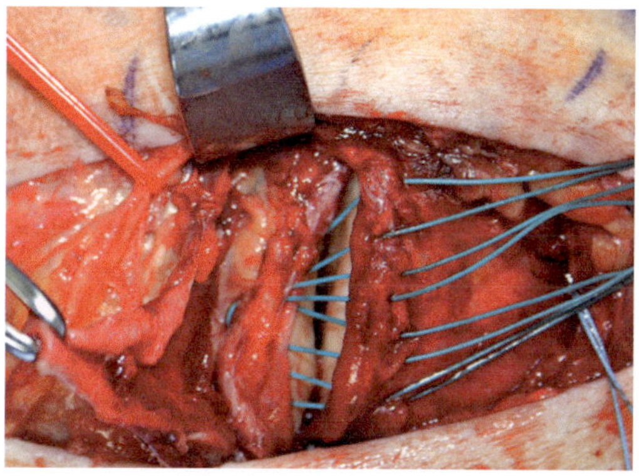

Fig. 11.18 Repair of medial meniscus. MCL has been pulled out from within the joint held by instrument

11.6.5 Posteromedial Reconstruction (MCL and PMC)

Posteromedial and medial reconstructions are performed through a medial hockey stick incision. Saphenous nerve is identified (Fig. 11.17). The superficial medial collateral ligament is exposed, and a longitudinal incision is made just posterior to the posterior border of the superficial MCL. The interval between the posteromedial capsule and medial meniscus is developed. The posteromedial capsule is shifted anterosuperiorly. The medial meniscus is repaired to the new capsular position, and shifted capsule is sewn into the MCL using permanent braided suture for posteromedial instability (Fig. 11.18).

Fluoroscopy is used to obtain a perfect lateral of the distal femur. The femoral attachment of the superficial MCL is found where Blumensaat's line intersects a line extended along the anterior aspect of the posterior cortex of the femoral shaft. A guide pin is inserted and a cannulated reamer is used to drill a socket for the screw (Fig. 11.19).

Either allograft or autograft may be used when reconstructing the posteromedial corner (PMC). When multiple ligaments are to be addressed, it is often beneficial to use allograft to limit morbidity to the patient. An incision is made longitudinally following the posteromedial border of the tibia. The anterior graft will recreate the MCL, and the posterior graft reconstructs the posterior oblique ligament (POL) providing stability to the PMC.

Just proximal to the insertion of the semitendinosus tendon, a bicortical drill hole is created. The anterior limb of the graft is taken directly inferior from its femoral insertion in line with the MCL. The posterior graft tunnels under the

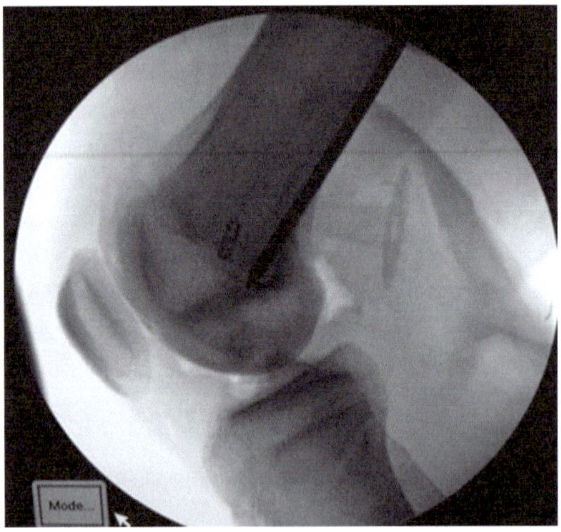

Fig. 11.19 Lateral radiographic knee with guidewire located at femoral attachment of superficial MCL

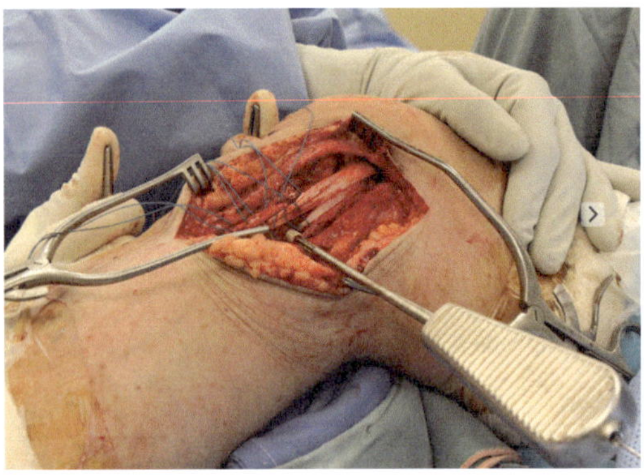

Fig. 11.20 Completed posteromedial corner reconstruction tension at 30° with varus stress

semimembranosus in a posterior to anterior direction toward the tibia. This graft recreates the POL as well as the direct insertion of the semimembranosus. The graft is tensioned at 30° knee flexion with gentle varus stress (Fig. 11.20). The posteromedial capsular advancement is performed in conjunction with a strut graft to enhance the reconstruction and sewn into the newly reconstructed MCL (Figs. 11.21 and 11.22).

11.6.5.1 Summary: Order of Surgical Steps [19]

1. Examination under anesthesia and finalizing surgical plan.

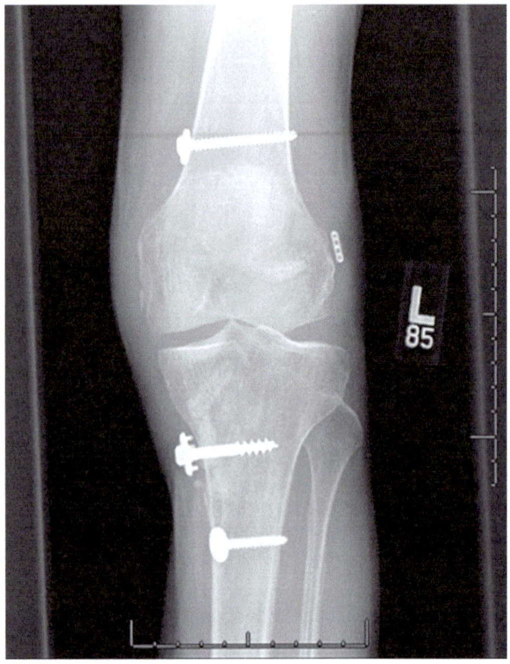

Fig. 11.21 Final AP radiograph of a right knee after ACL, PCL, posterolateral corner, and posteromedial corner reconstruction

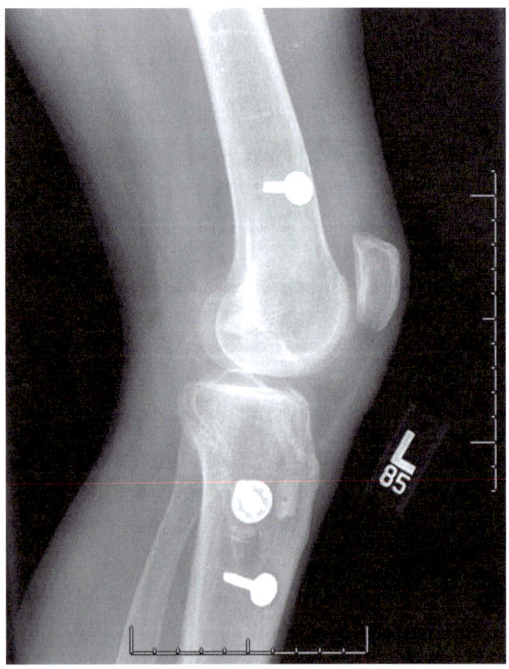

Fig. 11.22 Final lateral radiograph of a right knee after ACL, PCL, posterolateral corner, and posteromedial corner reconstruction

2. Graft harvesting/preparation.
3. Diagnostic scope.
4. Meniscus repair.
5. Debride torn ACL and PCL.
6. Place ACL/PCL pins and confirm positions by C-arm fluoroscopy.
7. PCL femoral tunnel drilled.
8. ACL femoral tunnel drilled.
9. PCL tibial tunnel drilled.
10. ACL tibial tunnel drilled.
11. Pass PCL graft and fix femoral side.
12. Pass ACL graft and fix femoral side.
13. Pass PLC grafts.
14. Place pins medial side and confirm positions by C-arm fluoroscopy.
15. Tension PCL and fix femoral tibial side at 90° of knee flexion.
16. Tension ACL and fix tibial side at full extension.
17. Tension and fix PLC on femoral side at 30° of knee flexion with slight valgus.
18. Tension and fix superficial MCL on tibial and femoral side at 30° of knee flexion with slight varus.

11.6.5.2 Postoperative Rehabilitation [18]

While protection after multiligament knee injuries surgery is important to allow the surgically repaired or reconstructed tissues to heal, massive injuries and complicated surgeries are more likely to develop knee joint stiffness, loss of motion, and arthrofibrosis. Rehabilitation after surgery for multiligament knee injuries depends on the condition of the host, including comorbidities, the anatomic structures that were injured, the quality of the repaired/reconstructed tissues, the strength of the fixation method, and any associated injuries. Careful progression should reduce the risk for postoperative complications and maximize clinical outcomes for patients.

11.6.5.3 Criterion-Based Rehabilitation Progression.

Goals: Return individuals to (1) normal activities of daily living and (2) work, military duty, and sports activities at the same level or participation.

Three phases:

1. Tissue Protection.
   (a) Restoration of knee motion.
   (b) Prevention of muscle atrophy.
   (c) Re-establishment of gait patterns with assistive devices.
   - Initially, weight-bearing should be performed in a locked, double upright knee brace to prevent sagittal or frontal plane motion.
   - Gait activities are progressed based on knee inflammation and ROM, quadriceps strength, and neuromuscular control.
2. Restoration of motor control.
   (a) Goals include full ROM compared to the opposite limb, symmetrical muscle strength, normal gait, and return to activities of daily living.
3. Optimization of function.
   (a) Most tissue-specific considerations are not relevant, and the rehabilitation specialist is able to advance function without restrictions of tissue protection.

References

1. Peskun CJ, Levy BA, Fanelli GC, et al. Diagnosis and management of knee dislocations. Phys Sportsmed. 2015;38:101–11.
2. Hegyes MS, Richardson MW, Miller MD. Knee dislocation. Complications of nonoperative and operative management. Clin Sports Med. 2000;19:519–43.
3. Arom GA, Yeranosian MG, Petrigliano FA, et al. The changing demographics of knee dislocation: a retrospective database review. Clin Orthop Relat Res. 2014;472:2609–14.
4. Almekinders LC, Dedmond BT. Outcomes of the operatively treated knee dislocation. Clin Sports Med. 2000;19:503–18.
5. Sillanpää PJ, Kannus P, Niemi ST, et al. Incidence of knee dislocation and concomitant vascular injury requiring surgery: a nationwide study. J Trauma Acute Care Surg. 2014;76:715–9.
6. Ogden JA. Subluxation and dislocation of the proximal tibiofibular joint. J Bone Joint Surg Am. 1974;56:145–54.
7. Kennedy JC. Complete dislocation of the knee joint. J Bone Joint Surg Am. 1963;45:889–904.
8. Schenck RC, Richter DL, Wascher DC. Knee dislocations: lessons learned from 20-year follow-up. Orthop J Sports Med. 2014;2:2325967114534387.

9. Moore TM. Fracture-dislocation of the knee. Clin Orthop Relat Res. 1981:128–40.
10. Medina O, Arom GA, Yeranosian MG, et al. Vascular and nerve injury after knee dislocation: a systematic review. Clin Orthop Relat Res. 2014;472:2621–9.
11. Lachman JR, Rehman S, Pipitone PS. Traumatic knee dislocations: evaluation, management, and surgical treatment. Orthop Clin North Am. 2015;46:479–93.
12. Seroyer ST, Musahl V, Harner CD. Management of the acute knee dislocation: the Pittsburgh experience. Injury. 2008;39:710–8.
13. Peskun CJ, Chahal J, Steinfeld ZY, Whelan DB. Risk factors for peroneal nerve injury and recovery in knee dislocation. Clin Orthop Relat Res. 2012;470:774–8.
14. Krych AJ, Giuseffi SA, Kuzma SA, et al. Is peroneal nerve injury associated with worse function after knee dislocation? Clin Orthop Relat Res. 2014;472:2630–6.
15. Woodmass JM, Romatowski NPJ, Esposito JG, et al. A systematic review of peroneal nerve palsy and recovery following traumatic knee dislocation. Knee Surg Sports Traumatol Arthrosc. 2015;23:2992–3002.
16. Wascher DC, Dvirnak PC, DeCoster TA. Knee dislocation: initial assessment and implications for treatment. J Orthop Trauma. 1997;11:525–9.
17. Mills WJ, Barei DP, McNair P. The value of the ankle-brachial index for diagnosing arterial injury after knee dislocation: a prospective study. J Trauma. 2004;56:1261–5.
18. Lynch AD, Musahl V, Irrgang J. Current concepts and controversies in rehabilitation after surgery for multiple ligament knee injury. Curr Rev Musculoskelet Med. 2017;10(3):328–45.
19. Sgaglione NA, Lubowitz JH, Provencher MT. The knee: AANA advanced arthroscopic surgical techniques. Slack Incorporated and AANA. 2016.
20. Reider B, Terry MA, Provencher MT. Operative Techniques: sports medicine surgery: operative techniques. 2009.
21. Cruz RS, LaPrade RF. Anatomic posterolateral corner reconstruction. Arthrosc Tech. 2016;5:e1–9.

12 Chronic Knee Dislocations

John M. Pinski, Matthew Salzler, and Christopher D. Harner

12.1 Introduction

Knee dislocations involve a complex and heterogeneous set of injuries with various clinical presentations [1, 2]. A multi-ligament knee injury is typically defined as a tear of at least two of the four major knee ligament structures: the anterior cruciate ligament (ACL), the posterior cruciate ligament (PCL), the lateral collateral ligament (LCL), and the medial collateral ligament (MCL) [3, 4]. Multi-ligament knee injuries have a high association with knee dislocations, and these terms are sometimes used interchangeably. Because over 50% of knee dislocations reduce spontaneously, clinicians must maintain a high degree of suspicion for dislocation-associated neurovascular injury [5]. The most commonly used classification to describe multi-ligamentous knee injuries was described in 1994 by Schenck to characterize knee dislocations based on the number of ruptured ligaments (Table 12.1) [6]. In addition to the KD classification, one must also know the timing of the injury, location (proximal, mid, distal), grade (1–3), any associated injuries to the menisci and articular cartilage and their grade, and any injuries to tendons about the knee (patella, biceps, etc.)

Table 12.1 Anatomic classification of knee dislocations described by Schenck. Roman numerals are used to designate the severity of the dislocations

Anatomic classification of knee dislocations (KD)	
Class	Injury
KD I	PCL or ACL intact knee dislocation, variable collateral involvement
KD II	Both cruciates torn, collaterals intact
KD III	Both cruciates torn, one collateral torn, subset M (medial) or L (lateral)
KD IV	All four ligaments torn
KD V	Knee fracture dislocation

Subtypes include medial sided (M), lateral sided (L), arterial injury (C), and neurologic injury (N) [6]

Surgical treatment of all multi-ligamentous knee injuries requires thoughtful preoperative planning, a detailed understanding of the technical aspects of surgery, and careful attention to the patient in the postoperative rehabilitation phase. In chronic cases, there is potential for the development of a progressive malalignment that may need to be corrected with a uniplanar or biplanar osteotomy. With regard to the surgical technique, we will discuss surgical tips and tricks including our recommendations for graft choice, the sequence of reconstruction, tunnel position and orientation, and the order of graft tensioning.

J. M. Pinski · M. Salzler (✉)
Department of Orthopaedics, Tufts Medical Center, Boston, MA, USA
e-mail: jpinski@tuftsmedicalcenter.org; Msalzler@tuftsmedicalcenter.org

C. D. Harner
Department of Orthopaedic Surgery, University of Texas at Houston, Houston, TX, USA

F. Margheritini et al. (eds.), *Complex Knee Ligament Injuries*,
https://doi.org/10.1007/978-3-662-58245-9_12

12.2 Case Presentation

A 19-year-old male collegiate wrestler sustained a knee dislocation after a twisting injury. His knee was reduced and splinted at an outside hospital, and he underwent a CT angiogram which was negative for vascular pathology. He was initially treated with a brace and crutches. He was referred to the office 8 weeks after the injury neurovascularly intact with a reduced knee. His preoperative range of motion was 3–100 versus 0–130 on his contralateral knee. He was sent to physical therapy to improve his range of movement (ROM) and strength. His preoperative exam and imaging demonstrated a complete ACL tear, a proximal MCL tear, and a high-grade partial PCL tear which based on the knee dislocation classification system is a KD III-M. Though this classification system is helpful in understanding the knee injury in broad terms, a more specific diagnosis is required and is necessary to determine an operative plan. Specifically, the diagnosis should refer to the timing of the injury, location and grade of injury of all ligaments, as well as injuries to the menisci and cartilage, and any underlying neurovascular injuries and deformities. We would specifically classify this particular injury as a chronic grade 3 mid-substance ACL tear, grade 3 PCL mid-substance tear, and grade 3 MCL mid-substance tear with intact menisci and articular cartilage.

12.3 Preoperative Evaluation

A thorough history and physical exam are necessary when evaluating a patient with a potential multi-ligamentous knee. A history of previous knee surgeries or vascular surgeries should be noted as it may affect surgical planning. Signs and symptoms of a deep venous thrombosis (DVT) should be routinely assessed with physical exam and a preoperative lower extremity duplex ultrasound [7]. The preoperative exam is of critical importance when assessing for multiligamentous knee injuries as concurrent ligamentous injuries can often be missed in the acute presentation of a knee injury. Clinical examination should include assessment of active and passive knee range of motion, anterior and posterior drawer tests, Lachman test, McMurray test, dial testing, and stability with varus and valgus stress at 0 and 30° of knee flexion. These tests should be compared to the non-injured knee for symmetry and firmness of endpoints. Preoperative knee range of motion and lower extremity strength are important to evaluate when determining timing of reconstructions [8–10]. Once in the chronic setting, assuming the knee is concentrically reduced, we recommend preoperative physical therapy to regain a near full range of motion and strength.

In addition to magnetic resonance imagining (MRI) of the knee and standard weight-bearing knee radiographs, stress view and/or kneeling knee radiographs are essential for identifying and quantifying posterior tibial translation. With chronic multi-ligamentous knee injuries, long leg weight-bearing radiographs are required to assess for potential limb malalignment. A corrective osteotomy should be considered for any deviation greater than 5° from the contralateral side and for chronic posterolateral corner instability in patients with varus alignment as varus limb alignment can lead to stretching and subsequent failure of reconstructive grafts [11].

Reconstructive graft choices should be discussed with the patient prior to surgery and they include autografts and allografts. Allograft choices include bone-patellar tendon-bone, anterior tibialis tendon, posterior tibialis tendon, or Achilles tendon, while autograft choices include quadriceps tendon, hamstring tendon, or bone-patellar tendon-bone. Fanelli et al. [12] found no significant difference in functional improvement or knee stability between autograft or allograft multi-ligament knee PCL reconstructions. When possible, we prefer autograft for ACL and PCL reconstruction in young patients. If autograft is chosen for PCL reconstruction, our preference is quadricep autograft with bone block as it has a length of 10–12 cm which is necessary for the reconstruction. Otherwise, we often favor allografts for the collateral reconstructions with consideration to patient factors and concomitant injuries in determining the graft choice for the

ACL reconstruction. Allografts eliminate donor site morbidity while simultaneously reducing the number of surgical incisions which could potentially reduce the postoperative pain and stiffness associated with autograft harvest. Possible disadvantages for allograft include greater cost, potential for disease transmission, and a slower rate of incorporation [13]. When allografts are not available or not considered the best choice, autografts are a viable option as there have been good results of reconstructions of multi-ligamentous knee injuries with hamstring or bone-patellar tendon-bone (BPTB) grafts [14]. Avoid ipsilateral hamstring graft with concomitant MCL injuries as the hamstrings may also be injured and are a secondary medial stabilizer and avoiding ipsilateral BPTB or quadriceps tendon autografts these grafts choices in the setting of PCL injuries as the extensor mechanism is a stabilizing force in these injuries.

12.4 Operating Room Setup

The patient is placed supine on a radiolucent operating room table with a knee post and bar which allows for knee flexion to 90°. The arthroscopic tower should be located on the non-injured side with fluoroscopy or flat plate radiographs if fluoroscopy is not available and located on the operative side of the patient. It is the senior surgeon's preference not to use a tourniquet, but it is acceptable to place a well-padded non-sterile thigh tourniquet. Though it may be placed, it should rarely be inflated. It should be known that these cases often last 3–6 h, and the maximum time length for a tourniquet is 2 h, and, once it is let down, there is often a venous tourniquet. A sequential compression device boot is applied to the non-operative leg for mechanical DVT prophylaxis, and chemical DVT prophylaxis should be considered taking into account patient risk factors. We typically recommend aspirin 325 mg daily for 4–6 weeks at a minimum and consider a prophylactic dose of Lovenox for 4 weeks if the patient is a smoker, is on oral contraceptives, or has a personal or family history of DVT.

Overview of surgical technique: chronic multi-ligamentous knee injury
1. Exam under anesthesia.
2. Diagnostic arthroscopy.
3. Preparation of the ACL and PCL tunnels with associated grafts.
4. Pass the PCL graft and secure it on the femoral side.
5. Pass the ACL graft and secure it on the femoral side.
6. Open MCL reconstruction (and/or posterolateral corner).
7. Tibial fixation of both the ACL and PCL grafts.
8. Post-reconstruction exam under anesthesia.

12.5 Surgical Technique

A fluoroscopic examination under anesthesia (EUA) is done using the same preoperative exam physical exam tests of both the injured knee and the uninjured knee prior to starting the reconstruction (Fig. 12.1).

After EUA, administration of preoperative antibiotics, and an appropriate surgical time-out, the operative knee joint is injected with 20 ml of local anesthetic with epinephrine through the superior lateral approach. A curvilinear incision centered over the medial joint line is drawn out along with standard anterolateral and anteromedial arthroscopic portal sites (Fig. 12.2).

These sites are also infiltrated with local anesthetic with epinephrine. Though we place a tourniquet, we prefer to use epinephrine and meticulous hemostasis over tourniquet inflation. A #11 blade is used to create an anterolateral portal, and an anteromedial portal is created under spinal needle localization with arthroscopic visualization to prevent injury to the medial meniscus. A diagnostic arthroscopy is performed examining for loose bodies, meniscal injuries, cartilage injuries, and injuries to the ACL, PCL, and intra-articular popliteus tendon.

The PCL graft is fashioned from an Achilles tendon allograft bone block, the ACL graft is fashioned from a bone-tendon-bone allograft, and the MCL graft is fashioned from a posterior tibialis tendon allograft. Each graft is soaked in warm saline until they reach room temperature.

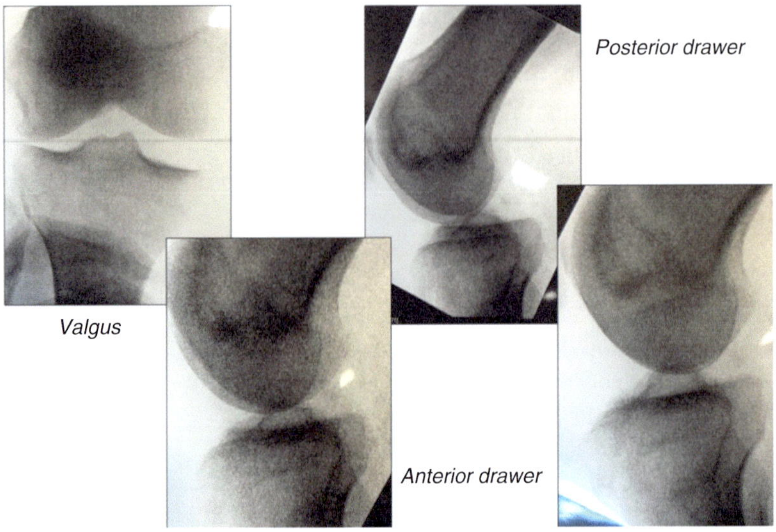

Fig. 12.1 Intraoperative radiographs of an exam under anesthesia demonstrating an AP fluoroscopic image with valgus stress, lateral images in neutral and with an anterior drawer and posterior drawer force applied

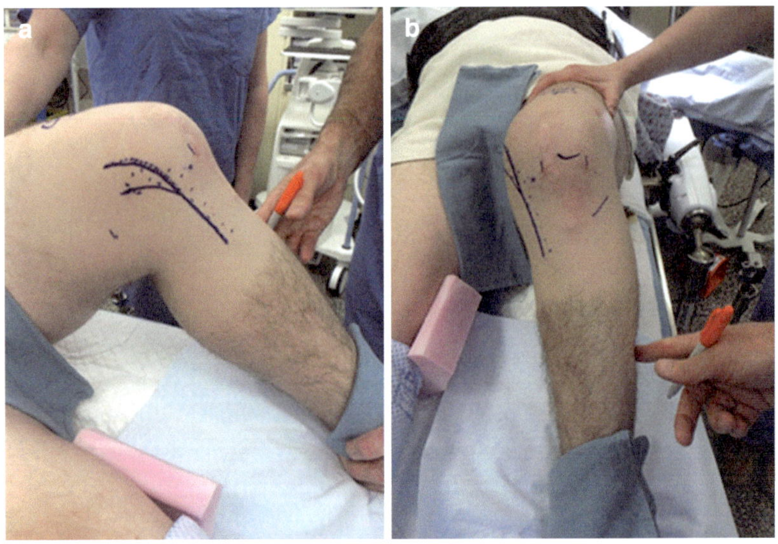

Fig. 12.2 (**a**) Lateral and (**b**) AP of planned surgical incisions for an MCL reconstruction with concurrent arthroscopic ACL and PCL reconstructions

Bone blocks are fashioned to the appropriate size; we typically use a size 10. Two #2 heavy nonabsorbable sutures are placed through drill holes in each of the bone blocks, and the soft tissues ends of all grafts are whipstitched with #5 sutures. Of note, if a posterior oblique ligament (POL) reconstruction is to be performed, the Achilles allograft can be used, and the soft tissue portion of the graft is separated into two limbs such that one limb can function as the MCL and the other can function as the POL. Each graft is placed on 15–20 pounds of tension for 15 min overwrapped in saline-soaked gauze.

The ACL and PCL stump sites are prepared with an oscillating shaver. It is important to preserve the meniscofemoral ligaments and the posteromedial portion of the PCL whenever possible, but we prepare the anterolateral portion. A PCL reconstruction guide is placed on the tibial PCL facet, and a guidewire is passed starting on the anteromedial tibia up to the origin of the PCL through a single transtibial technique. A mini C-arm is used to confirm the placement of the tip-aiming guide (Fig. 12.3). On an anteroposterior (AP) radiograph, it is located at the center of the tibial spines and on a lateral radiograph; it is

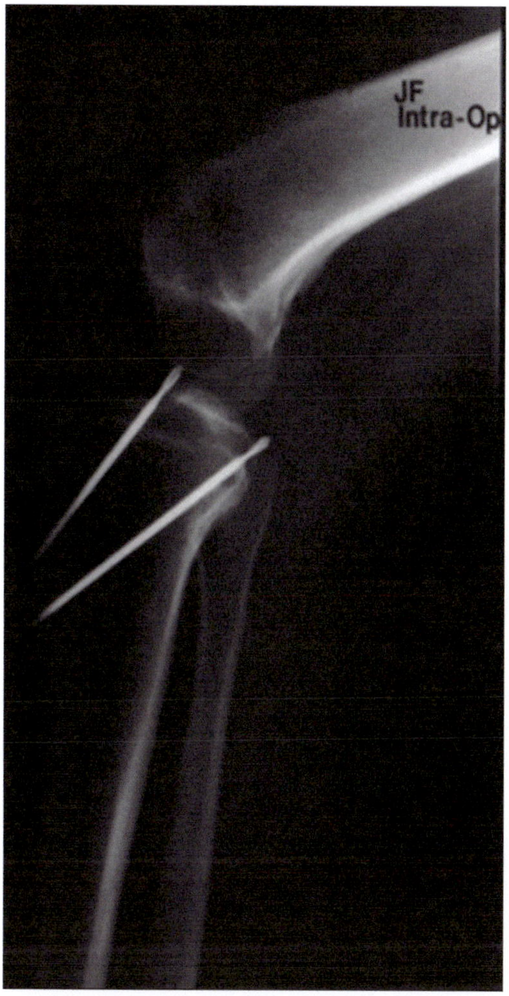

Fig. 12.3 Intraoperative radiograph showing the trajectory of the tibial tunnels for the PCL and ACL reconstruction. The divergent tunnel trajectory is crucial to a successful reconstruction

70% on the way from proximal and anterior to posterior and distal along the PCL facet on lateral imaging [15].

A microfracture awl mark or an outside-in femoral tip-aiming guide is placed as anterior as possible on the medial femoral condyle; the tunnel is then drilled after confirmation of the pin placement. We recommend under drilling the tunnels by a half to full size and hand dilating up to the desired size. A flexible rasp is passed and used to smooth the edges of the PCL tunnel to aid in passage and final incorporation of the graft (Fig. 12.4).

The origin of the ACL on the lateral femoral condyle is identified, marked with a microfracture awl, and confirmed by viewing the tunnel location through the anteromedial portal. The knee is then hyperflexed and the femoral tunnel is drilled out the lateral cortex of the femur. Drilling instruments are passed with caution as to avoid damage to the medial femoral condyle. The femoral tunnel is then hand-dilated to the appropriate size based on the size of the graft. The stump of the tibial ACL, if present, is identified. A tip-aiming guide is centered between the tibial spines at the level of the posterior border of the anterior horn of the lateral meniscus. A Steinmann pin is drilled up to the tip-aiming guide, and the location of the pin is confirmed with fluoroscopy on AP (40% of the way from the medial to lateral tibial spine) and lateral (40% of the way from the anterior to posterior tibial plateau) views (Fig. 12.5).

After drilling with an undersized half acorn reamer, the tibial tunnel is hand-dilated to the appropriate size based on the size of the graft. The PCL graft is then passed with the soft tissue side first retrograde up the tibia then passed through the medial side of the knee. The PCL graft is then anchored to the femur using screw fixation. The appropriate lengths on the ACL graft from the adjustable cortical suture button and graft are marked. The sutures from the suture button are brought retrograde through the tibial tunnel using the previously passed PDS suture. After visualizing that the cortical button flip outside the lateral cortex, it is confirmed with fluoroscopy, and the graft is then seated in the femoral tunnel (Fig. 12.6).

The previously described medial incision is created using a #15 blade. Electrocautery is used to coagulate any bleeding vessels, and the dissection is continued down to the level of the fascia using Metzenbaum scissors. Care is taken to identify and preserve the branches of the saphenous nerve. Though the medial layers of the knee are often still torn in the acute setting, in a chronic injury, they are often scarred together and may be healed with excess laxity. Because of this, careful attention is paid to dissecting and tagging each layer individually. Tagging sutures

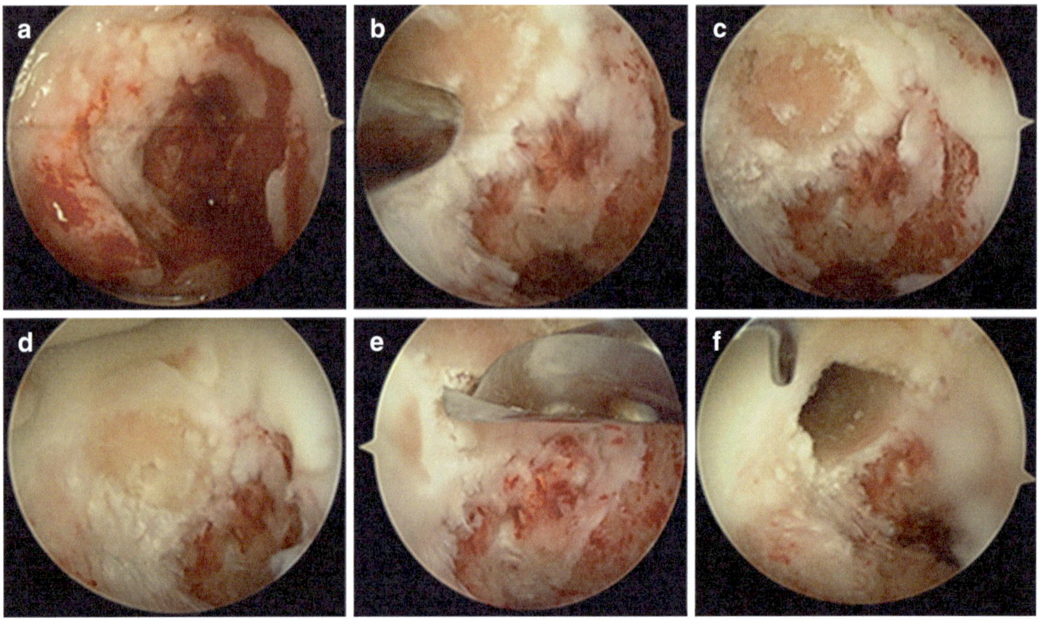

Fig. 12.4 Intraoperative arthroscopic images of the wall preparation and drilling of the PCL femoral tunnel. (**a**) Identification of the PCL insertion site on medial femoral condyle. (**b, c**) PCL femoral insertion site debrided. (**d**) PCL tunnel site marked with a microfracture awl. (**e**) Drilling of the femoral PCL tunnel. (**f**) Completed femoral PCL tunnel. Note preservation of the meniscofemoral ligaments and PM component to the PCL in the bottom right of the image

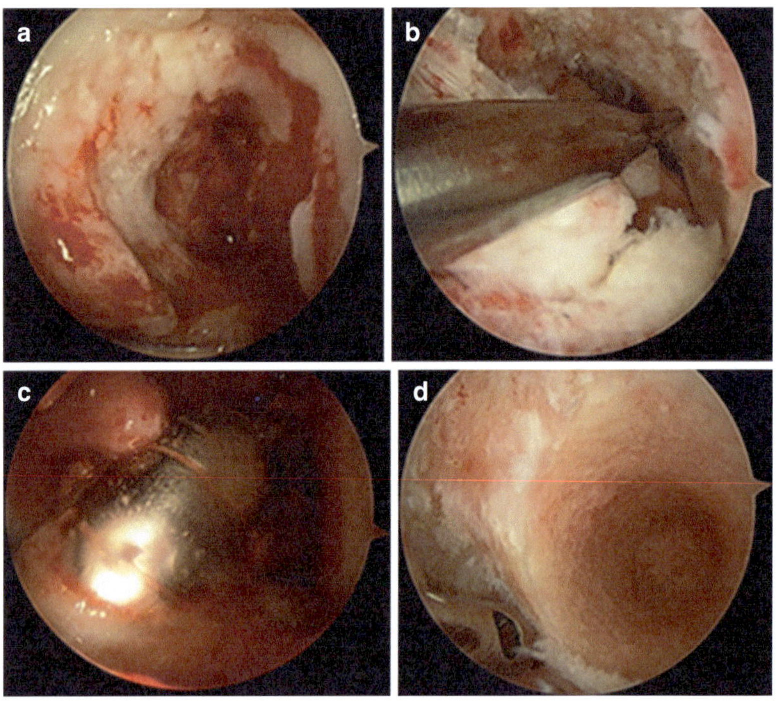

Fig. 12.5 Intraoperative arthroscopic images detailing the preparation and drilling of the tibial and femoral tunnels for the ACL graft. (**a**) ACL insertion site on the tibia identified with the tip-aiming guide. (**b**) Drilling of the ACL tibial tunnel. (**c**) Identification of the insertion of the ACL on the femur using the lateral intercondylar ridge is with a microfracture awl for placement of the femoral sided tunnel. (**d**) Completed ACL femoral tunnel

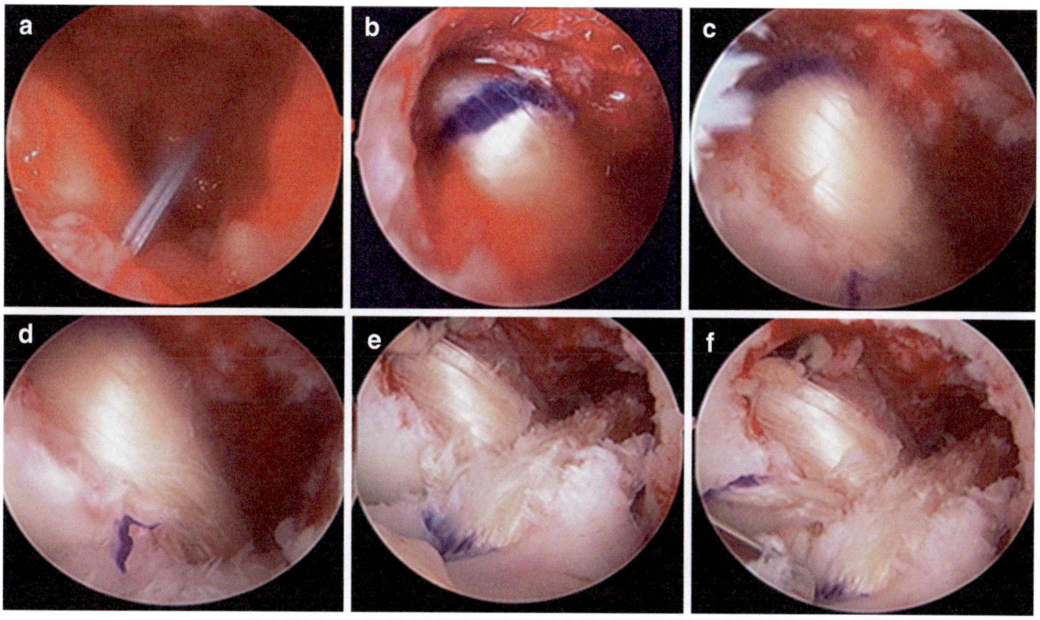

Fig. 12.6 Intraoperative arthroscopic images depicting the passage of the PCL and ACL reconstructive grafts. The PCL graft is anchored to the femur prior to passage and fixation of the ACL graft. (**a**) Graft suture passing through the femoral ACL tunnel. (**b**, **c**) Passing of the PLC graft into the femoral tunnel. (**d**) PCL graft in place. (**e**, **f**) Both the PCL and ACL grafts have been passed into their respective tunnels

can both facilitate closure as well as allow for retensioning in conjunction with a reconstruction. The anterior border of the POL is identified, and a vertical incision is made exposing the deep MCL and POL below the level of the sartorius fascia.

Next, the medial epicondyle of the knee as well as the origin of the MCL on the femoral condyle are identified. A Beath pin is placed in the origin of the MCL and passed across the lateral side of the knee ensuring that the pin is extra-articular. Pin placement is confirmed with fluoroscopy to ensure that the patellofemoral joint and prior tunnels are avoided. The MCL tunnel is drilled to 30 mm over the Beath pin, and the allograft is passed into the tunnel and secured with an interference screw. If there is rotatory instability, the POL can be both retensioned using a pants-over-vest technique and reconstructed with a separate limb of graft to the proximal tibia. The MCL soft tissue limb is brought down and slightly proximal to the MCL insertion to avoid the semitendinosus and gracilis tendons. With the knee in approximately 15° of flexion with a maximum valgus force, the graft is then secured in place with a screw and a spiked washer (Fig. 12.7).

After reconstruction of the MCL, the PCL and the ACL grafts will be anchored on the tibia. The knee is cycled a minimum of 10 times under maximal tension to remove any creep from the grafts. An anterior drawer force is then placed on the knee with the knee in 90° of flexion, and the PCL graft bone block is secured in place under maximal hand tension. The knee is then brought into 20° of flexion with a posterior drawer force applied to the tibia, and the ACL graft is secured under maximal hand tension. If tunnel fixation is utilized, backing up the fixation with a post and washer may be considered. The arthroscope is placed back into the knee to evaluate the tension of the ACL and PCL as well to inspect the joint for any protruding hardware. The knee is then reexamined for translation with anterior and posterior draw and for laxity at 0 or 30°. Local anesthetic is injected into the knee joint, the sartorius fascia is repaired and retensioned with 0-Vicryl, and all other incisions are closed. The incisions

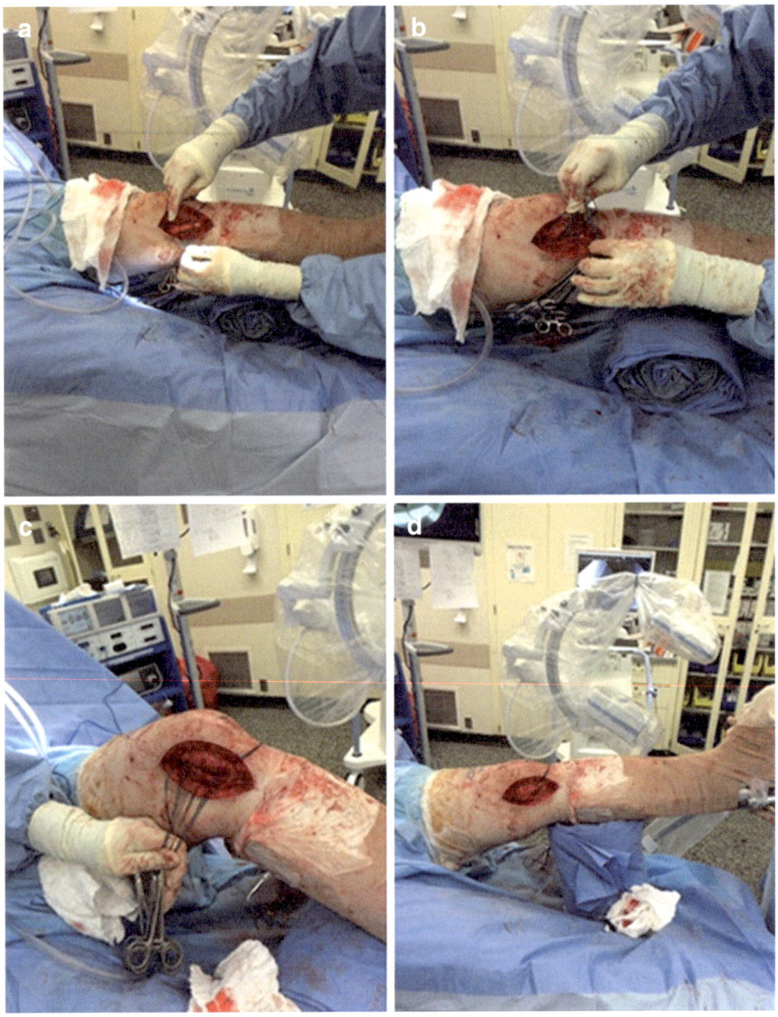

Fig. 12.7 Open MCL reconstruction with a tibialis anterior allograft. (**a**, **b**) Placement of the allograft to reconstruct an anatomic MCL. (**c**, **d**) Closure of the MCL and POL reconstruction using tagging sutures placed during the initial dissection

are dressed with sterile dressings, wrapped in an ACE wrap, and placed in a hinged knee brace locked in extension.

12.6 Postoperative Rehabilitation Protocol

Appropriate rehabilitation with close follow-up is necessary to ensure a good outcome from a multi-ligament reconstruction. We typically keep a patient locked in extension for 4 weeks and consider casting if there are concerns about patient compliance. We recommend seeing patients every week for the first 2–3 weeks, every other week for weeks 3–7, and then every 6 weeks after to ensure that the patient is progressing well. In addition to reminding the patients of their rehabilitation instructions, we recommend a low threshold to return to the operating room for either a dropout cast for extension problems or a manipulation under anesthesia for flexion problems. If a patient is still having problems with flexion at 8 weeks, we would recommend a weekly follow-up and a manipulation under anesthesia at 12 weeks if they are not making significant progress.

Every multi-ligamentous knee injury and reconstruction is different, and their rehabilitation protocols need to be individualized. However, general considerations include weight-bearing as tolerated for PCL and ACL reconstructions. With collateral reconstructions, the patient is made non-weight-bearing for 3 weeks followed by partial weight-bearing for 3 weeks with full weight-bearing at 6 weeks post-op in a hinged knee brace. The brace is kept locked in extension for 4 weeks. The first 2 weeks of rehabilitation are focused on pain control and achieving full extension. Straight leg raises in all planes, calf pumps, quadriceps sets, and electrical stimulation can be performed. Phase 2 is from weeks 2 to 6 and includes prone passive knee flexion to 90° with care to avoid posterior tibial sag. Wall slides can be progressed to mini squats (0–45°) when the patient exhibits good quadriceps control. Phase 3 is from week 6 to 12, and the goals are to achieve full flexion, establish normal gain, and progress to strengthening and endurance. The patient is full weight-bearing with the brace unlocked and may discontinue the brace when the gait has normalized. Phase 4 is from 3 months to 6 months, and goals include maintaining full range of motion with improved strength and proprioception. During this phase improvement on flexibility and closed chain strengthening exercises are initiated. Jogging can be initiated around 4–5 months when quadriceps strength is 90% of the contralateral side. Phase 5 is 6–9 months postoperative and goals with the goal of return to all recreational and sporting activities by 9 months. Agility drills and plyometric exercises are used to meet the criteria for return to sport which include full painless range of motion, quadriceps and hamstring strength that is 90% of the contralateral side, and no apprehension with all sport-specific drills.

Surgical tips and tricks: chronic multi-ligamentous knee injuries

1. Ensure the ACL and PCL tibial pins, the ACL and PLC femoral pins, and the PCL and MCL femoral pins are divergent using fluoroscopy prior to tunnel drilling.
2. Avoid intra-articular placement of the MCL guide pin.
3. Tensioning tips:
   (a) ACL: 20° of flexion with a posterior drawer force applied to the tibia.
   (b) PCL: 90° of flexion with an anterior drawer force applied to tibia.
   (c) MCL: 15° of flexion with a maximum valgus force.
   (d) LCL: 15° of flexion, maximum varus force, neutral tibia.
4. Do not forget about rotational instability; the POL and posteromedial corner or posterolateral corner may need to be reconstructed.
5. Postoperative rehabilitation: be conservative in the initial 6 weeks while grafts are healing. Immediate ROM exercises should be done with caution, and all exercises should be closed chain.

References

1. Levy BA, Dajani KA, Whelan DB, et al. Decision making in the multiligament-injured knee: an evidence-based systematic review. Arthroscopy. 2009;25:430–8.
2. Moatshe G, Chahla J, LaPrade RF, et al. Diagnosis and treatment of multiligament knee injury: state of the art. J ISAKOS. 2017;2:152–61.
3. Eastlack RK, Schenck RC Jr, Guarducci C. The dislocated knee: classification, treatment, and outcome. US Army Med Dep J. 1997;11(12):2–9.
4. Schenck R. Classification of knee dislocations. Oper Tech Sports Med. 2003;11:193–8.
5. Wascher DC, Dvirnak PC, DeCoster TA. Knee dislocation: initial assessment and implications for treatment. J Orthop Trauma. 1997;11:525–9.
6. Schenck R, Richter D, Wascher D. Knee dislocations lessons learned from 20-year follow-up. Orthop J Sports Med. 2014;2(5):2325967114534387.
7. Sems SA, Levy BA, Dajani K, Herrera DA, Templeman DC. Incidence of deep venous thrombosis after temporary joint spanning external fixation for complex lower extremity injuries. J Trauma. 2009;66:1164–6.
8. Mariani PP, Santoriello P, Iannone S, et al. Comparison of surgical treatments for knee dislocation. Am J Knee Surg. 1999;12:214–21.
9. Fanelli GC, Giannotti BF, Edson CJ. Arthroscopically assisted combined posterior cruciate ligament/posterior lateral complex reconstruction. Arthroscopy. 1996;12:521–30.
10. Harner CD, Waltrip RL, Bennett CH, et al. Surgical management of knee dislocations. J Bone Joint Surg Am. 2004;86-A:262–73.
11. Arthur A, LaPrade RF, Agel J. Proximal tibial opening wedge osteotomy as the initial treatment for chronic posterolateral corner deficiency in the varus knee: a prospective clinical study. Am J Sports Med. 2007;35:1844–50.
12. Fanelli GC, Giannotti BF, Edson CJ. Arthroscopically assisted combined anterior and posterior cruciate ligament reconstruction. Arthroscopy. 1996; 12(1):5–14.

13. Cox C, Spindler K. Multiligamentous knee injuries—surgical treatment algorithm. N Am J Sports Phys Ther. 2008;3(4):198–203.
14. Fanelli GC, Orcutt DR, Edson CJ. The multiple-ligament injured knee: evaluation, treatment, and results. Arthroscopy. 2005;21(4):471–86.
15. Salim R, Salzler MJ, Bergin MA, Zheng L, Carey RE, Kfuri M Jr, Zhang X, Harner CD. Fluoroscopic determination of the tibial insertion of the posterior cruciate ligament in the sagittal plane. Am J Sports Med. 2015;43(5):1142–6.

Part III

Specific Scenario

Fractures Associated with Knee Ligamentous Injury

13

Ciaran Thrush, Timorthy S. Whitehead, Jérôme Murgier, and Brian M. Devitt

13.1 Introduction

Injuries to the knee are often complex with significant involvement of both soft tissue and bony structures. Fractures are related to the position of the knee at the time of impact and the mechanism of injury involved. As such, a number of common fracture patterns have been described. In the treatment of these complex injuries, particular attention should be paid to the timing of operative intervention, surgical rationale, and order of treatment. Three broad categories of fractures are discussed in relation to these complex knee injuries: avulsion and impaction fractures commonly related to knee injury, articular or periarticular fractures with resultant soft tissue injuries, and fractures remote to knee injury.

13.2 Epidemiology

Becker et al. [1] published a report investigating multiligamentous knee injury patterns presenting to a level 1 trauma centre. Of the 106 knee ligament injuries examined over an 8-year period, 25% had associated ipsilateral tibial plateau fractures, and 19% had associated ipsilateral femoral fractures. A further study by Shepherd et al. [2], investigating the prevalence of soft tissue injuries in nonoperative tibial plateau fractures, determined that 40% had complete ligament disruption and 80% had meniscal tears. Considering tibial plateau fractures requiring operative intervention, Gardner et al. [3], in their study of 103 consecutive patients, revealed that 77% sustained a complete tear or avulsion of one or more cruciate or collateral ligaments and 68% had tears of one or more of the posterolateral corner structures of the knee; the most frequent fracture pattern was a lateral plateau split-depression (Schatzker II), sustained in 60% of patients. Stannard et al. [4], in a similar study, determined that 71% of patients with tibial plateau fractures tore at least one major ligament, while 55% of patients tore multiple ligaments. Therefore combinations of soft tissue injury and bony injury are common and should be considered in conjunction with one another.

13.3 Soft Tissue Knee Injury and Associated Fractures

In general, multiligamentous knee injuries, rather than isolated soft tissue knee injuries, are often associated with avulsion or impaction fractures [5]. Many of these fractures are visible on plain radiographs and are indicative of ligamentous disruption and possible reduced knee dislocation. Schenck described the anatomical classification

C. Thrush · T. S. Whitehead · J. Murgier
B. M. Devitt (✉)
OrthoSport Victoria, Epworth Healthcare, Richmond, VIC, Australia
e-mail: tswhitehead@osv.com.au; bdevitt@osv.com.au

F. Margheritini et al. (eds.), *Complex Knee Ligament Injuries*,
https://doi.org/10.1007/978-3-662-58245-9_13

of knee dislocation based on the ligaments and structures that were injured [6], including four combinations of ligament injury (KD I to KD IV). An additional category, KD V, was added by Wascher et al. [7] to encompass fracture dislocations. KD V is specific to periarticular fractures and does not include avulsion fractures or fractures remote to the knee. The other fracture patterns encountered include Segond fractures, 'reverse-Segond' fractures, tibial spine avulsions, tibial plateau compression fractures, fractures of the fibular head, avulsions of the popliteus, osteochondral fractures, and marginal tibial plateau fractures. It is imperative to identify these fractures, as they should raise suspicion for associated neurovascular pathology that should not be overlooked when assessing a multiligamentous injured knee. It is the experience of the authors that isolated repair of avulsion injuries may give rise to residual laxity due to the plastic deformity to the ligament or capsular structure prior to the bony avulsion and that reconstruction may be more appropriate.

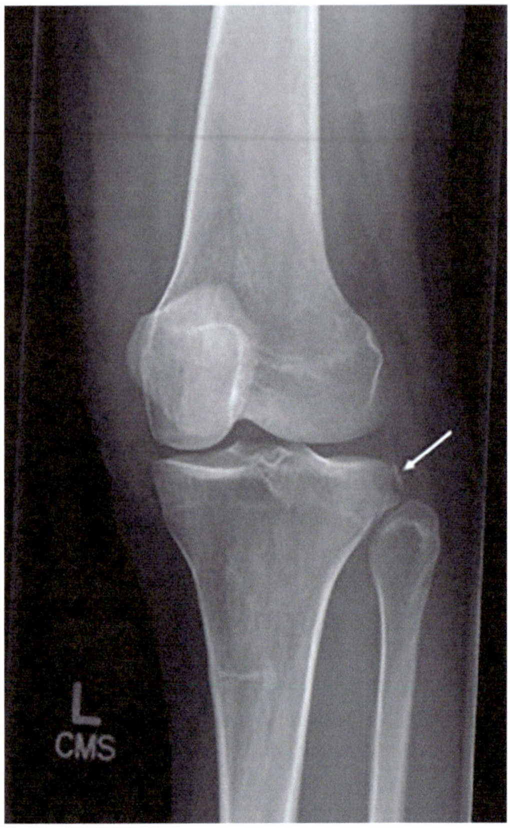

Fig. 13.1 Anteroposterior radiograph of the left knee depicting a Segond fracture (white arrow). This fracture is an avulsion of the anterolateral aspect of the tibial plateau and is associated with rupture of the anterior cruciate ligament. (Image courtesy of Dr. Ryan Martin, Calgary, Canada)

13.3.1 Segond Fracture

Segond fractures, first described in 1879, occur as a result of excessive varus and internal rotation and involve a bony avulsion from the tibia just distal to the lateral tibial plateau [8] (Fig. 13.1). The Segond fracture is caused by an avulsion of the anterolateral complex [9]. In a recent study, a magnetic ressonance imaging (MRI) analysis revealed that soft tissue attachments to the Segond fracture are the posterior fibres of the iliotibial band (ITB) and the lateral capsule in most of the cases [10]. These structures are involved in the control of the rotational stability of the knee. A Segond fracture, therefore, can be associated with significant knee damages, including anterior cruciate ligament (ACL) tears, meniscal tears, and injury to the posterolateral corner in addition to other ligamentous injuries [5, 11, 12]. Traditionally they are regarded as pathognomonic for ACL rupture, but any patient with a Segond fracture in the trauma setting should be evaluated for a concomitant multiligamentous injury, including a detailed vascular examination. It is possible to sustain a Segond fracture without ACL injury [13]; therefore a high index of suspicion should be maintained for other injuries.

Typically the Segond fracture is not treated directly, but as it indicates a high likelihood of other significant knee pathologies, investigation and treatment are directed at that underlying pathology.

13.3.2 Reverse Segond Fracture

'Reverse Segond' fracture is the term attributed to avulsion fractures from the medial tibial

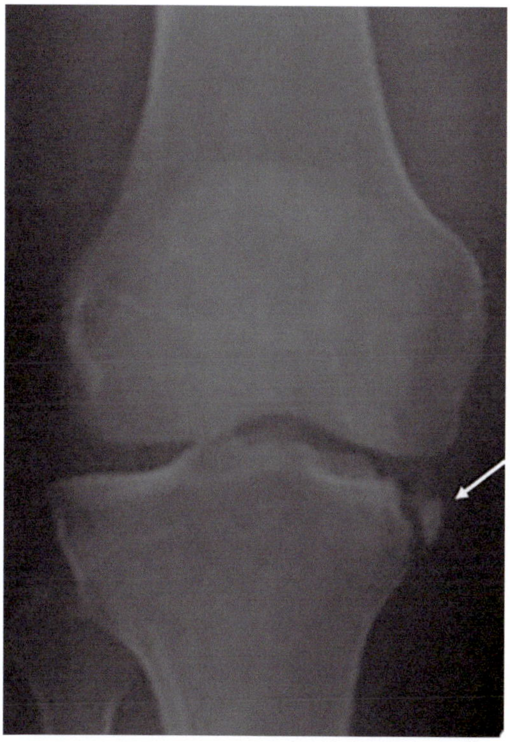

Fig. 13.2 Anteroposterior radiograph of the right knee demonstrating a 'reverse Segond' fracture. This is an avulsion fracture of the anteromedial aspect of the tibial plateau which is associated with medial collateral ligament and posterior cruciate ligament injuries

plateau (Fig. 13.2). This fracture is brought about by the opposite mechanism to that which creates a Segond fracture, valgus, and internal rotation of a flexed knee and typically requires a higher energy mechanism than a Segond fracture [14]. It has been associated with combined posterior cruciate ligament (PCL) and medial collateral ligament (MCL) injuries [14, 15]. Merrit et al. [16] have described a spectrum of pathology associated with the 'reverse-Segond' fracture, including intra-substance tears of the superficial, deep, and/or posterior oblique fibres of the MCL, in addition to extensive stripping of the soft tissue attachments off the proximal tibia on the medial side.

Treatment of these fractures is best performed in the acute setting. The avulsed bony fragment is identified and repaired with the adjacent soft tissue. A variety of techniques, including bone anchors and AO fracture reduction principles, can be employed. After 6 weeks, capsular structures, left unrepaired, tend to shorten, and anatomic reduction is difficult to achieve.

13.3.3 Anterior Cruciate Ligament Avulsion

Avulsion fractures of the tibial insertion of the ACL (Fig. 13.3) are common and are also frequently associated with a multiligamentous knee injury pattern [17]. Tibial eminence fractures are normally indicative of injury to the ACL and/or PCL as well as almost certain disruption to some or all of the meniscal root [16]. Traditionally, avulsion fractures of the tibial eminence have been described in the paediatric population using the Meyers and McKeever classification [18]. However, this classification can be applied to the adult population and may help to guide treatment.

Fixation of ACL avulsions allows early range of motion to avoid undue arthrofibrosis and assurance that the tibial footprint of the ACL is

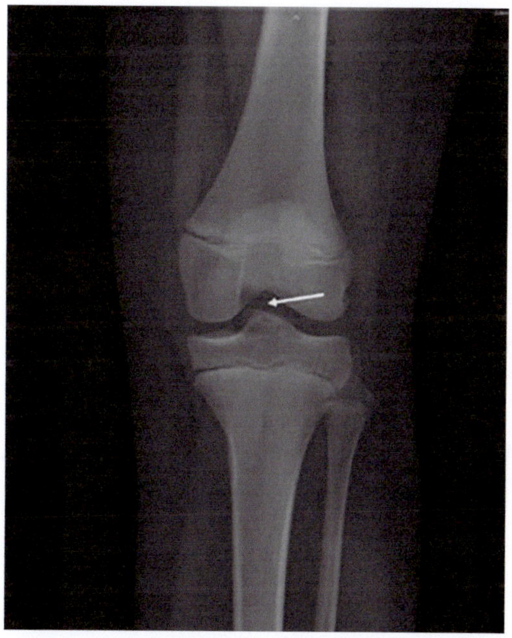

Fig. 13.3 Anteroposterior radiograph depicting (white arrow) an avulsion of the tibial spine in a paediatric patient

restored. Arthroscopic repair of tibial eminence fractures is possible and allows concurrent assessment and treatment of any meniscal pathology. An arthrotomy may be required to assist reduction, and fixation may take the form of screws or trans-osseous sutures or a button device [19]. Krakow sutures through the ligament are often necessary to supplement screw fixation.

13.3.4 Posterior Cruciate Ligament Avulsion

Much like a tibial avulsion of the ACL, the PCL may be avulsed, typically in combination with injury to the posterolateral corner (PLC) (Fig. 13.4). Unlike midsubstance tears of the PCL, bony avulsions should be primarily repaired to restore function to the PCL. Fixation of a bony avulsion of the PCL can be achieved using an open approach, either directly posteriorly or posteromedially, which avoids direct dissection of the popliteal neurovascular structures [20]. Similar to an ACL avulsion, fixation may be achieved with screws or suture and button devices. Arthroscopic or arthroscopic-assisted techniques may also be used [21], which avoid the morbidity associated with open approaches.

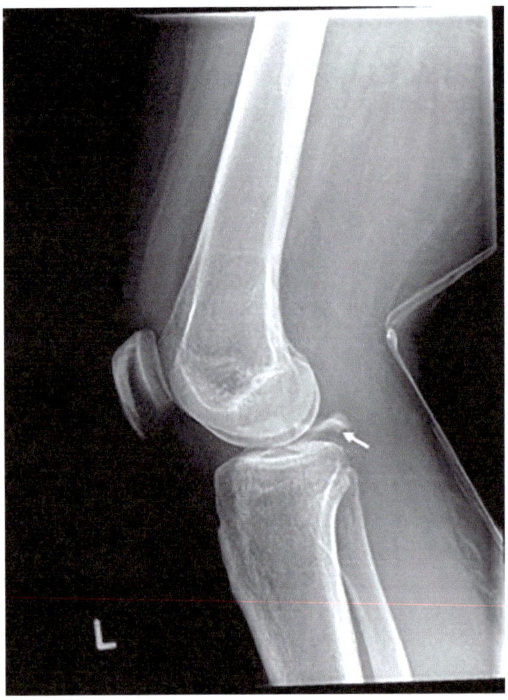

Fig. 13.4 Lateral radiograph of the left knee depicting a displaced avulsion fracture of the tibial attachment of the posterior cruciate ligament (white arrow) (Image courtesy of Dr. Ryan Martin, Calgary, Canada)

13.3.5 Impaction Fractures

The force imparted on the knee during injury may also give rise to impaction fractures (Fig. 13.5a, b). The mechanism of injury is typically a compression force with hyperextension and differs to that of avulsion fractures, which commonly involve a tensile force with or without a rotational element [5, 22, 23]. These fractures are often seen on the anteromedial aspect of the tibia and anterior medial femoral condyle and are associated with PCL and PLC/lateral collateral ligament (LCL) injuries [24].

Bony compression fractures may also occur on the distal femoral articular surface as a result of its impact on the tibial plateau [25]. This force is most commonly found with an ACL tear and joint subluxation in the classic pivot shift pattern.

The treatment of impaction fractures can be difficult. If dealt with acutely, anatomical reduction of the depressed subchondral fragment may be possible and held with a small buttress or 'washer' plate. 'Retrograde disimpaction' has been described to elevate the subchondral depression on the femoral side [26].

13.3.6 Fibular Head Avulsions

An avulsion fracture of the fibular head has been referred to as the 'arcuate sign' and represents a sleeve of bone pulled away from the proximal fibula [27, 28] with the corresponding soft tissue attachments (Fig. 13.6). The size and location of the avulsed fragment is helpful to

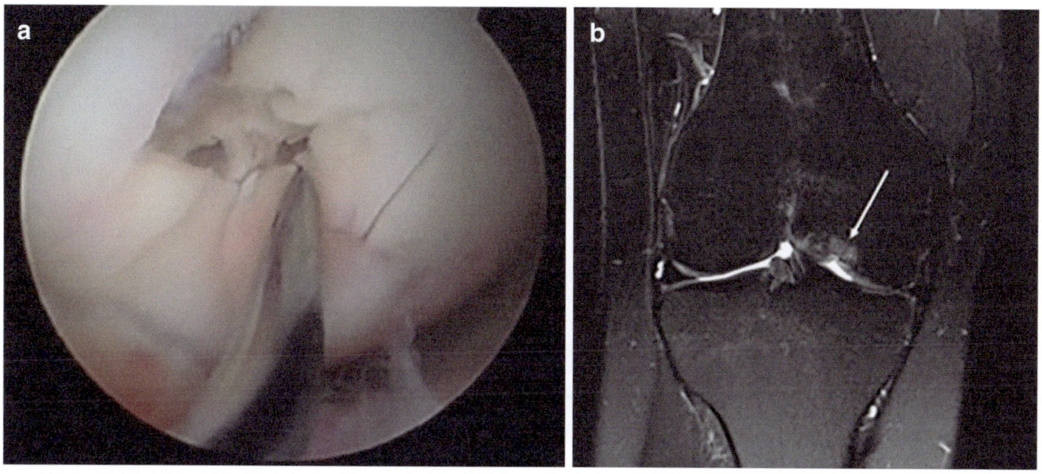

Fig. 13.5 (**a**) An arthroscopic view of the medial femoral condyle with an extensive impaction fracture of the chondral surface, which is highlighted by the arthroscopic probe; (**b**) A coronal T2 magnetic resonance image of the same knee depicting a depressed impaction fracture of the medial femoral condyle

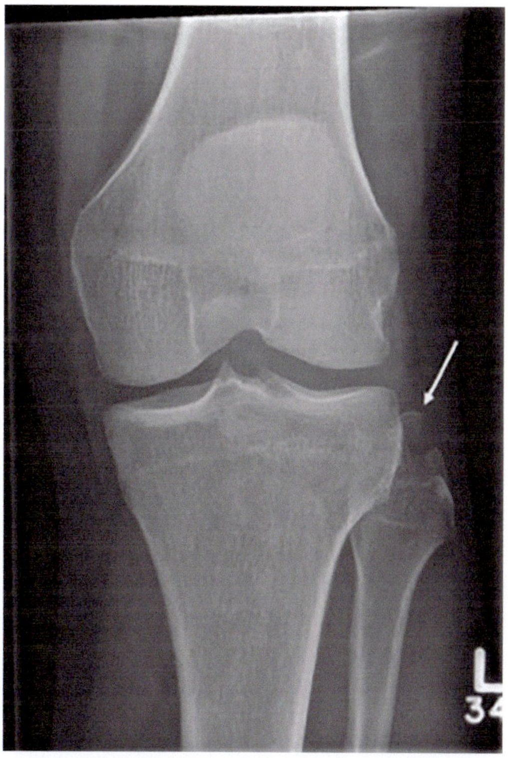

Fig. 13.6 Anteroposterior radiograph depicting an avulsion fracture of the fibular head (white arrow). This is also called an 'arcuate sign.' This fracture typically represents injury to the structures of the posterolateral corner. (Image courtesy of Dr. Ryan Martin, Calgary, Canada)

identify which of the PLC structures have been injured. The LCL, popliteofibular ligament, biceps femoris, fabellofibular, and arcuate ligaments all insert on the fibular head at different locations. Larger avulsions or a comminuted fibular head fracture may indicate a more extensive injury, whereas smaller avulsion may suggest that a solitary structure has been avulsed [29]. These fractures make reconstruction considerably more challenging. The fixation method depends on the size and extent of comminution of the fragment. Where possible, direct screw fixation of the fracture is best; however, a variety of techniques may need to be employed including Krakow sutures with bone anchors and tension band wiring.

13.3.7 Fractures Associated with Patella Dislocation

Patella dislocation may occur in conjunction with tibiofemoral dislocation or, more commonly, in isolation. Fracture associated with patella dislocation can range from osteochondral injury to avulsion fractures of the medial patellofemoral ligament [30] (MPFL) (Fig. 13.7). Osteochondral

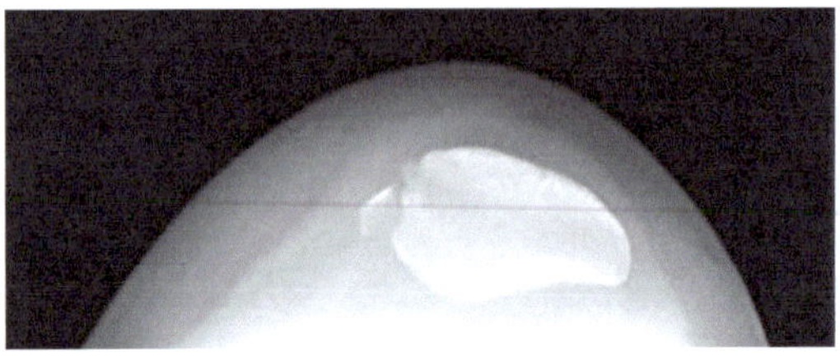

Fig. 13.7 Avulsion fracture of the medial patello femoral ligament

injury is said to be very common during patella dislocation, occurring in up to 95% of acute patella dislocations [30], and can range in severity from chondral impaction to displaced osteochondral fragments. They may be difficult to appreciate on plain radiography, requiring MRI for diagnosis. In general, impaction injuries are treated nonoperatively, and displaced osteochondral fragments should be considered for removal if small, or repair if large.

During acute patella dislocation, the MPFL is frequently injured and can range from intrasubstance ligament injury to avulsion of the attachment on the patella or femur. Avulsions may involve a large segment of patella chondral surface, which may benefit from fixation. However, the results of fixation of avulsions without chondral involvement may not indicate any benefit over nonsurgical management [31].

13.3.8 Osteochondral Fractures

Traumatic osteochondral fractures of the knee commonly occur in conjunction with soft tissue injuries such as ACL rupture or patella dislocation [32] (Fig. 13.8). The most common sites of injury are the patella or femoral condyles, and despite it being a common concurrent injury, there is little consensus as to an appropriate treatment algorithm [33]. There is much heterogeneity regarding different treatment options and indications, and therefore it is difficult to recommend one treatment over another. Options include excision or fixation with k-wires, bioabsorbable pins, and fibrin glue and range from arthroscopic to open surgery [33].

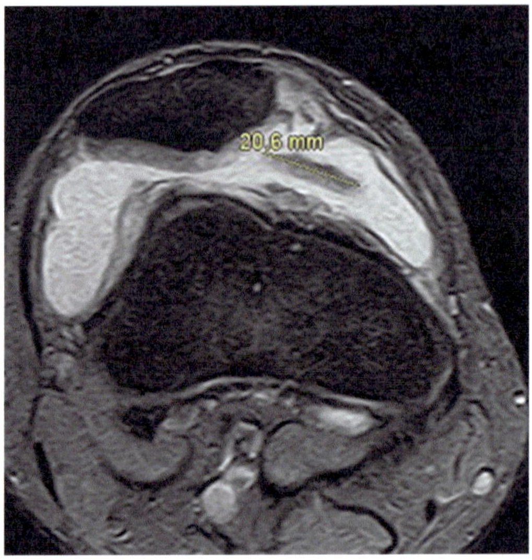

Fig. 13.8 An axial MRI which demonstrates a displaced osteochondral fragment (yellow line) from the medial patellar facet

13.4 Fractures and Associated Soft Tissue Injury

Severe fractures of the distal femur or proximal tibia represent a distinctly different problem compared to avulsion and marginal impaction fractures. The energy involved in these injuries is very high, and management of the fracture is normally independent of procedures required to confer ligamentous joint stability. The functional outcome of these injuries is worse than isolated ligamentous injuries, despite appropriate management of both the fracture and the soft tissue component.

13.4.1 Femoral Fractures

Periarticular and articular fractures of the femur include supracondylar fractures and femoral condyle fractures. Siliski et al. [34] reported supracondylar fractures with associated ligamentous injury; ACL injuries were found to be commonly associated with this fracture configuration. Interestingly, there were no reports of complete knee dislocation or multiple ligament injuries with supracondylar fractures.

Femoral condyle fractures have been associated with knee dislocation. In general the ligaments are preserved and attached to the fragment. However, despite fixation, these patients have only fair to good results with limited range of motion following fixation [35]. The 'Hoffa' fracture (Fig. 13.9) has been associated with disruption to the extensor mechanism, which typically occurs as a result of a shearing force when a load is transmitted to a flexed knee. Most references to these injuries in the literature are case reports; the consensus on treatment is that stiffness is a greater problem than instability. The recommendation is appropriate treatment of the fracture, typically via open reduction and internal fixation with compression screws and buttress plating, followed by nonoperative management of any ligamentous injury or delayed reconstruction once the fracture has healed, and range of motion has been re-established [35, 36].

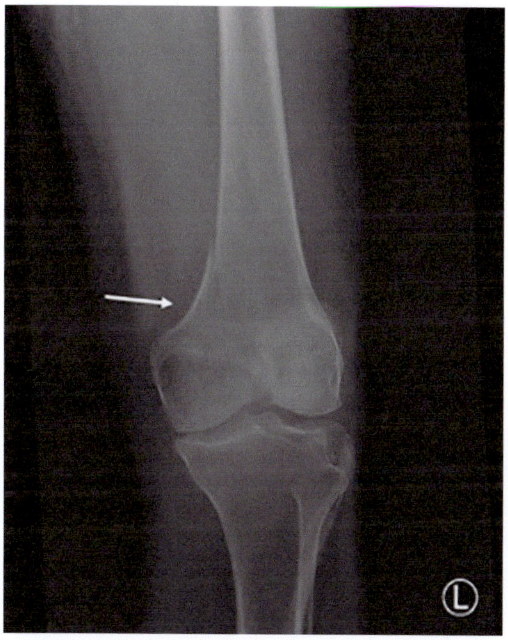

Fig. 13.9 An anteroposterior radiograph of the left knee showing an intra-articular fracture (white arrow) of the medial femoral condyle, the so-called 'Hoffa' fracture. Typically the ligamentous attachments of the knee are maintained and fixation of the fracture will restore stability

13.4.2 Tibial Fractures

The association of ligamentous injuries with tibial fractures is well recognized [5] (Fig. 13.10). Standard et al. [4] have found that up to 71% of patients tore at least one major ligament with a tibial plateau fracture. Using the Schatzker classification, the prevalence of the ligamentous injuries associated with the fracture type has been subcategorized: Type I, 46%; Type II, 45%; Type IV, 69%; Type V, 85%; and Type VI, 79%.

Standard's study revealed that a significant difference exists between groups regarding the incidence of ligament injuries and also regarding high-energy (types IV, V, VI) versus low-energy (types I, II, III) fracture patterns. Knee dislocations (dislocated on presentation, bicruciate

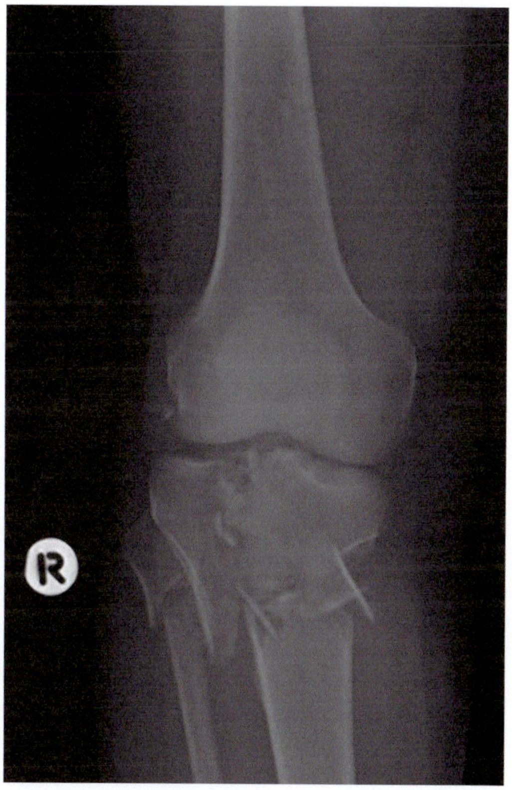

Fig. 13.10 An anteroposterior radiograph of the right knee demonstrating a highly comminuted tibial plateau fracture. These injuries are commonly associated with injury to the soft tissue structures of the knee

injury, or at least three ligament groups torn with a dislocatable knee) were most common in Schatzker type IV fractures (46%). The study concluded that high-energy fracture patterns (Schatzker types IV, V, VI) clearly have a significantly higher incidence of ligament injury and these patients should be carefully evaluated to rule out a spontaneously reduced knee dislocation. The authors recommend that MRI should be performed for all tibial plateau fractures caused by a high-energy mechanism, allowing identification and treatment of associated soft tissue injuries.

Typically, treatment involves appropriate nonoperative or operative fixation of the tibial fracture, with either delayed reconstruction or nonoperative ligamentous management.

13.4.3 Patellar Fractures

The extensor mechanism can be injured in the setting of knee injury by rupture of the patellar ligament or fracture of the patella (Fig. 13.11). In a series of 112 patellar fractures, Kosanovic et al. [37] reported 5% had ligamentous injuries of the knee and 4% had knee dislocations. The fractures were all comminuted and underwent osteosynthesis at the time of ligament reconstruction. Postoperative knee motion is critical to prevent stiffness. However, it is of course possible to sustain a soft tissue disruption of the extensor mechanism, where early range of motion is contraindicated following repair and, therefore, increases the risk of the development of arthrofibrosis [38].

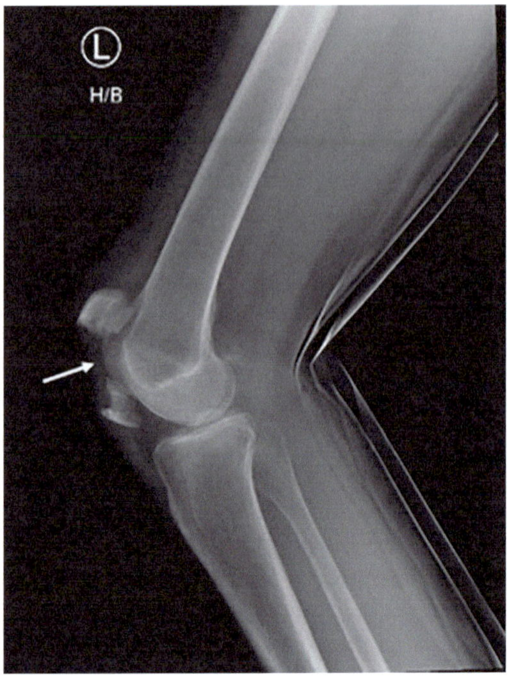

Fig. 13.11 A lateral radiograph of the left knee demonstrating a displaced transverse patellar fracture (white arrow)

13.4.4 Fractures Remote to the Knee

Bony injury may occur at an anatomical location separate to the concurrent knee injury and include fractures of the pelvis/acetabulum, hip, femoral and tibial shaft, distal tibia, plafond, foot, and upper extremity (Fig. 13.12). The very nature of multiple injuries indicates a high-energy injury with multisystem disruption. The presence of concomitant injury has a significant effect on clinical outcome and may affect surgical timing, rehabilitation, and the risk of the development of postoperative infection.

In general ipsilateral knee injuries are easier to rehabilitate, as the patient has a healthy contralateral limb. Surgery should proceed according to the standard principles for extremity injuries. Contralateral injuries present a bigger challenge. The surgeon must consider the benefits of early knee reconstruction against the risk of a bedridden patient. If reconstruction is to be performed, early range of motion should start as early as possible and weight bearing as best as possible.

Long bone injuries of the femur or tibia also pose a difficult problem. A number of studies have demonstrated the association with femoral and tibial shaft fractures and knee ligament injuries [5, 39]. The primary concern relates to the initial stabilization of the long bone injuries as part of the initial resuscitation effort and to establish limb alignment; this is often achieved with an intramedullary nail. It is very important that anatomic alignment and rotation are restored as this can compound an unstable knee leading to greater

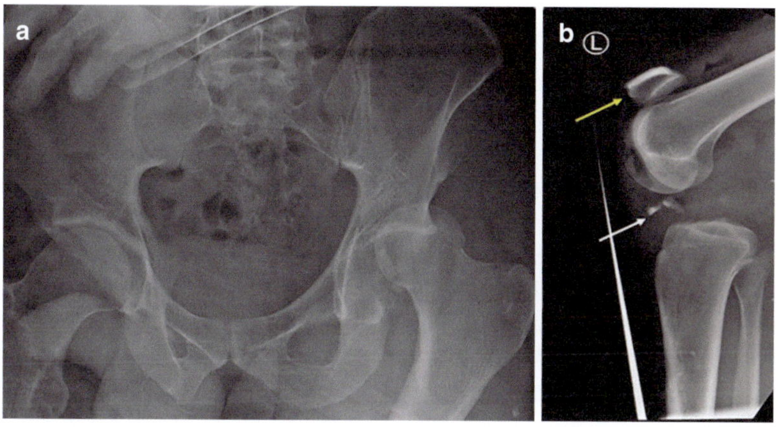

Fig. 13.12 (**a**) An anteroposterior pelvic radiograph taken in the trauma setting depicting a fracture-dislocation of the left hip that was sustained concurrently with a ipsilateral knee dislocation with disruption all major knee ligaments and the patella tendon (**b**). (**b**) A lateral radiograph of the left knee of the same patient depicted in (**a**) of the ipsilateral leg. The radiograph demonstrates a multiligamentous knee injury with avulsion of the patellar tendon (white arrow) and superior migration of the patella (yellow arrow). The tibia is also grossly subluxed

instability with an alteration in the mechanical axis. In addition, the surgeon should be cognizant of the need for further soft tissue reconstructive procedures in the future and leave sufficient room for tunnel placement in the proximal tibia and femur. Chahal et al. [40] have established an algorithm for the treatment of multiligamentous injuries in the setting of tibial fractures.

13.5 Surgical Timing, Rationale, and Order of Fixation

The timing and sequence of injury fixation in a multiple-injured patient can be difficult. The adage of life before limb is particularly appropriate in this setting, and the patient must be treated in concordance with advanced trauma principles. Equally, the fixation of life-threatening skeletal trauma must take precedence over knee bony and ligamentous injury. A clinical suspicion of associated knee ligamentous injury will allow the surgeon to make subtle adjustments in the fixation of long bones of the lower limb to accommodate delayed reconstructive procedures as necessary. Complex knee injuries may require temporary external fixation to stabilize the joint until it can be definitively treated or to allow urgent treatments such as wound management or vascular repair [41].

In general, in patients with bony avulsions [20, 21] or impaction fractures, the earlier the treatment is performed, the easier it is to achieve an anatomical repair or to correct the bony deformity. Ideally this should be performed in the first 2 weeks and incorporate reconstruction procedures, if necessary. This avoids the need for multiple procedures, allowing healing of the soft tissue injury, fracture, and reconstruction at the same time and reducing the potential rehabilitation time.

Soft tissue interventions can be considered after the patient has been stabilized, and life-threatening injuries are managed. Delaying these interventions also allows the use of arthroscopic techniques that may not be possible earlier due to capsular disruption and the risk of fluid extravasation. However, the surgeon must also consider the risk of waiting too long and encountering significant contracture and arthrofibrosis that will impair functional recovery.

Fractures involving the weight-bearing portion of the tibial plateau (Schatzker II–VI) should be fixed primarily with open reduction internal fixation, with reconstruction of the soft tissue being delayed. It may be possible to repair collateral ligament soft tissue avulsions at the initial surgery. It is important to achieve anatomical reduction as best as possible, to ensure future soft tissue reconstruction is not disadvantaged by subsequent angular deformity.

13.6 Conclusion

Fractures associated with knee injury are common. They may be broadly classified into soft tissue injuries with associated fractures, fractures with associated soft tissue injury, and fractures remote to knee injury. The treatment of each type of injury pattern must be considered in the broader context of the patient's overall condition, as many of these injuries are as a result of high-energy trauma.

References

1. Becker EH, Watson JD, Dreese JC. Investigation of multiligamentous knee injury patterns with associated injuries presenting at a level I trauma center. J Orthop Trauma. 2013;27(4):226–31.
2. Shepherd L, Abdollahi K, Lee J, Vangsness CT Jr. The prevalence of soft tissue injuries in nonoperative tibial plateau fractures as determined by magnetic resonance imaging. J Orthop Trauma. 2002;16(9):628–31.
3. Gardner MJ, et al. The incidence of soft tissue injury in operative tibial plateau fractures: a magnetic resonance imaging analysis of 103 patients. J Orthop Trauma. 2005;19(2):79–84.
4. Stannard JP, Lopez R, Volgas D. Soft tissue injury of the knee after tibial plateau fractur. J Knee Surg. 2010;23(4):187–92.
5. Moore TM, Patzakis MJ, Harvey JP Jr. Ipsilateral diaphyseal femur fractures and knee ligament injuries. Clin Orthop Relat Res. 1988;232(232):182–9.
6. Schenck RC Jr. The dislocated knee. Instr Course Lect. 1994;43:127–36.
7. Wascher DC, Dvirnak PC, DeCoster TA. Knee dislocation: initial assessment and implications for treatment. J Orthop Trauma. 1997;11(7):525–9.
8. Segond P. Reserches cliniques et experimentes sur les epanchements sanguins du genou par entorse. Prog Med. 1879. p. 297–419.
9. Albers M, et al. The iliotibial band and anterolateral capsule have a combined attachment to the Segond fracture. Knee Surg Sports Traumatol Arthrosc. 2018;26(5):1305–10.
10. Shaikh H, et al. The segond fracture is an avulsion of the anterolateral complex. Am J Sports Med. 2017;45(10):2247–52.
11. Goldman AB, Pavlov H, Rubenstein D. The Segond fracture of the proximal tibia: a small avulsion that reflects major ligamentous damage. 1988;151(6):1133–7.
12. Dietz GW, Wilcox DM, Montgomery JB. Segond tibial condyle fracture: lateral capsular ligament avulsion. Radiology. 1986;159(2):467–9.
13. Wharton R, Henckel J, Bhattee G, Ball S, Church S. Segond fracture in an adult is not pathognomonic for ACL injury. Knee Surg Sports Traumatol Arthrosc. 2014;23(7):1925–8.
14. Escobedo E, Mills WJ, Hunter JC. The 'reverse Segond' fracture: association with a tear of the posterior cruciate ligament and medial meniscus. AJR Am J Roentgenol. 2002;178(4):979–83.
15. Hall FM, Hochman MG. Medial Segond-type fracture: cortical avulsion off the medial tibial plateau associated with tears of the posterior cruciate ligament and medial meniscus. Skelet Radiol. 1997;26(9):553–5.
16. Merritt AL, Wahl C. Initial assessment of the acute and chronic multiple-ligament injured (dislocated) knee. Sports Med Arthrosc Rev. 2011;19(2):93–103. https://doi.org/10.1097/JSA.0b013e3182191a7e.
17. Sharma H, Singh GK, Gupta M, Moss M. Type IIIB tibial intercondylar eminence fracture associated with a complex knee dislocation in a grossly obese adult. Knee Surg Sports Traumatol Arthrosc. 2005;13(4):313–6.
18. Meyers MH, FM MK. Fracture of the intercondylar eminence of the tibia. J Bone Joint Surg Am. 1959;41-A(2):209–20. discussion 220-2
19. Anderson CN, Anderson AF. Tibial eminence fractures. Clin Sports Med. 2011;30(4):727–42.
20. Dhillon MS, Singh HP, Nagi ON. Posterior cruciate ligament avulsion from the tibia : fixation by a posteromedial approach. Acta Orthop Belg. 2003;69(2):162–7.
21. Horas UM, Meissner SA, Heiss C, Schnettler R. Arthroscopic fixation of posterior cruciate ligament avulsion fractures: a new minimally invasive technique. Knee Surg Sports Traumatol Arthrosc. 2015;18(6):781–3.
22. Archbold HA, Sloan S, Nicholas R. A tibial plateau fracture in a knee dislocation: a subtle sign of major ligamentous disruption. Injury. 2004;35(9):945–7.
23. Englesohn E, Umans H, Difelice GS. Maringal fractures of the medial tibial plateau: possible association with meniscal root tear. Skelet Radiol. 2007;36(1):73–6.
24. Cohen AP, King D, Gibbon AJ. Impingement fracture of the anteromedial tibial margin: a radiographic sign of combined posterolateral complex and posterior cruciate ligament disruption. Skelet Radiol. 2001;30(2):114–6.
25. Garth WP Jr, Wilson T. Open reduction of a lateral femoral notch associated with an acute anterior cruciate ligament tear. Arthroscopy. 2001;17(8):874–7.
26. Sadlo PA, Nebelung W. Arthroscopically assisted reduction of a lateral femoral noch in acute tear of the anterior cruciate ligament. Arthroscopy. 2006;22(5):574e1–3.
27. Huang GS, Yu JS, Munshi M, et al. Avulsion fracture of the head of the fibula(the "arcuate" sign): MR imaging findings predictive of injuries to the posterolateral ligaments and posterior cruciate ligament. AJR Am J Roentgenol. 2002;180(2):381–7.

28. Shindell R, Walsh WM, Connolly JF. Avulsion fracture of the fibula: the "arcuate sign" of posterolateral knee instability. Nebr Med J. 1984;69(11):369–71.
29. Nakhostine M, Perko M, Cross M. Isolated avulsion of the popliteus tendon. J Bone Joint Surg Br. 1995;77(2):242–4.
30. Nomura E, Inoue M, Kurimura M. Chondral and osteochondral injuries associated with acute patellar dislocation. Arthroscopy. 2003;19(7):717–21.
31. Sillanpaa PJ, Salonen E, Pihlajamaki H, Maenpaa HM. Medial patellofemoral ligament avulsion injury at the patella: classi cation and clinical outcome. Knee Surg Sports Traumatol Arthrosc. 2013;22:2414–8.
32. Brophy RH, et al. Anterior cruciate ligament reconstruction and concomitant articular cartilage injury: incidence and treatment. Arthroscopy. 2010;26(1):112–20.
33. Kuhle J, et al. Treatment of osteochondral fractures of the knee: a meta-analysis of available scientific evidence. Int Orthop. 2013;37(12):2385–94.
34. Siliski JM, Mahring M, Hofer HP. Supracondylar-intercondylar fractures of the femur. Treatment by internal fixation. J Bone Joint Surg Am. 1989;71(1):95–104.
35. Schenck RC Jr, McGanity PL, Heckman JD. Femoral-sided fracture-dislocation. J Orthop Trauma. 1997;11(6):416–21.
36. Shetty GM, et al. Incarcerated patellar tendon in Hoffa fracture: an unusual cause of irreducible knee dislocation. Knee Surg Sports Traumatol Arthrosc. 2008;16(4):378–81.
37. Kosanovic M, Komadina R, Batista M. Patella fractures associated with injuries of the knee ligament. Arch Orthop Trauma Surg. 1998;117(1-2):108–9.
38. Liow RY, et al. Ligament repair and reconstruction in traumatic dislocation of the knee. J Bone Joint Surg Br. 2003;85(6):845–51.
39. Szalay MJ, Hosking OR, Annear P. Injury of knee ligament associated with ipsilateral femoral shaft fractures and with ipsilateral femoral and tibial shaft fractures. Injury. 1990;21(6):398–400.
40. Chahal J, et al. PCL reconstruction with the tibial inlay technique following intra-medullary nail fixation of an ipsilateral tibial shaft fracture: a treatment algorithm. Knee Surg Sports Traumatol Arthrosc. 2010;18(6):777–80.
41. Boisrenoult P, et al. Vascular lesions associated with bicruciate and knee dislocation ligamentous injury. Orthop Traumatol Surg Res. 2009;95(8):621–6.

14 Osteotomy in Chronic Complex Ligament Injuries

Davide Edoardo Bonasia, Carola Pilone, and Annunziato Amendola

14.1 Introduction and Indications

High tibial osteotomy (HTO) and distal femoral osteotomy (DFO) are a valid treatment option for young (<60 years of age) and active patients with unicompartmental tibiofemoral osteoarthrosis (OA) and coronal malalignment [1].

Sometimes medial OA is combined with symptomatic anterior cruciate ligament (ACL) deficiency, and the surgeon has to address both problems. In addition, the natural history of chronic ACL tear is cartilage wear of the posteromedial tibial plateau with progression to varus deformity. In the later stages, a slackening of the lateral and posterolateral ligamentous structures results in a varus thrust (double varus) or varus recurvatum thrust (triple varus) [1].

The most common indications for valgus HTO and ACL reconstruction/revision include:

- Medial compartment OA (Ahlbäck 1–3) + varus malalignment + ACL tear (with symptomatic anteroposterior instability).
- Medial compartment OA (Ahlbäck 1–3) + varus malalignment + failed ACL reconstruction.
- Failed ACL reconstruction due to increased tibial slope.
- Double or triple varus and ACL tear (with symptomatic anteroposterior instability).
- Varus malalignment + ACL tear + chondral or meniscal injuries (requiring cartilage repair or meniscal transplant).

The most common indications for isolated valgus HTO (with possible delayed ACL reconstruction) include:

- Long-standing ACL deficiency + double or triple varus.
- Long-standing ACL deficiency + varus malalignment + symptomatic medial compartment OA.
- Long-standing ACL deficiency + double or triple varus + symptomatic medial compartment OA.

The results of conservative treatment of posterior cruciate ligament (PCL) tears (mostly grade I and II injuries) seem to produce favorable results also in the long term. However, in some patients, the natural history of chronic PCL tears, mostly when combined with posterolateral corner (PLC) injuries, entails a progressive degeneration of the medial and patellofemoral compartments with varus deformity (double or triple varus in the later

D. E. Bonasia (✉) · C. Pilone
Department of Orthopaedics and Traumatology, University of Torino, AO Ordine Mauriziano Hospital, Torino, Italy

A. Amendola
Department of Orthopaedics, Duke University, Durham, NC, USA
e-mail: ned.amendola@duke.edu

F. Margheritini et al. (eds.), *Complex Knee Ligament Injuries*,
https://doi.org/10.1007/978-3-662-58245-9_14

stages) [2]. The most common indications for isolated valgus HTO (with possible delayed PCL/PLC reconstruction) include:

- Long-standing PCL/PLC deficiency + double or triple varus.
- Long-standing PCL/PLC deficiency + varus malalignment + symptomatic medial compartment OA.
- Long-standing PCL/PLC deficiency + double or triple varus + symptomatic medial compartment OA.

Although the indications are more limited compared with valgus osteotomies, also varus-producing osteotomies (lateral opening wedge DFO, lateral opening wedge HTO, medial closing wedge HTO) can be indicated in the case of complex chronic knee ligament injuries [3]. The most common indications for isolated varus osteotomies, with concurrent or delayed medial collateral ligament (MCL) reconstruction, include:

- Valgus malalignment + chronic MCL or MCL/ACL injuries.
- Valgus malalignment + lateral compartment arthrosis + chronic MCL or MCL/ACL injuries.
- Valgus or valgus hyperextension thrust.

Although the choice between lateral opening wedge DFO, lateral opening wedge HTO, and medial closing wedge HTO is generally a matter of preference of the surgeon, some considerations can be made regarding the most appropriate indication. In the past, valgus deformity of the knee was generally attributed to femoral anatomical variants, i.e., lateral femoral epicondyle hypoplasia or decreased anatomic lateral distal femoral articular angle (aLDFA). For this reason, many authors adopted DFO as a preferred technique to correct these deformities: lateral opening wedge DFO for smaller corrections and medial closing wedge DFO for larger corrections and patients at high risk of nonunion (i.e., smokers). However, recent studies have shown that valgus malalignment was attributable to tibial deformity in the majority of patients and that a combined femoral- and tibial-based deformity was more common than an isolated femoral-based deformity [4, 5]. Therefore, in theory, varus osteotomies should be performed at the tibial site or as a double-level osteotomy in a relevant number of patients to avoid an oblique joint line [5]. In addition, DFO unloads the joint only in extension, and some authors proposed lateral opening wedge HTO with the goal of unloading the joint both in flexion and in extension. Another advantage of lateral opening wedge HTO is the possibility of changing the tibial slope, and this can be particularly useful in the case of valgus hyperextension thrust, in order to limit the recurvatum. Disadvantages of lateral opening wedge HTO include necessity of proximal tibiofibular joint disruption (or fibular osteotomy), possibility of correcting only small deformities, and the result of an oblique joint line, when preoperative aLDFA is markedly decreased (<81°) [3]. In the light of these considerations, classifying the valgus deformity based on the location of deformity is paramount, based on mechanical lateral distal femoral angle (mLDFA), mechanical medial proximal tibial angle (mMPTA), and joint-line convergence angle (JLCA) [5]:

1. Femoral-based valgus deformity (mLDFA > 90°).
2. Tibial-based valgus deformity (mMPTA < 85°).
3. Femoral- and tibial-based valgus deformity (mLDFA>90° and mMPTA<85°).
4. Intra-articular ligament-based valgus deformity (mLDFA and mMPTA normal, abnormal JLCA).

In the setting of HTO performed for complex knee instability, managing the tibial slope together with the coronal deformity is fundamental. It has been shown that increasing the tibial slope:

- Improves PCL deficiency.
- Reduces the recurvatum.

On the other hand, reducing the tibial slope:

- Improves ACL deficiency.
- Reduces the procurvatum.

Particularly difficult cases are ACL deficient (or failed ACL reconstruction) patients with recurvatum. In these cases, increasing the tibial slope improves the recurvatum but increases the stress on the neo-ligament (or worsens the anterior instability, if the ACL is not reconstructed). Understanding the main symptoms and identifying possible anatomical variants (i.e., markedly decreased tibial slope) are crucial in these patients.

14.2 Preoperative Planning

Long leg X-rays with anteroposterior and lateral views are required for the planning. In the case of medial OA, HTO is planned with a slight valgus overcorrection (3–5°, with the mechanical axis passing through a point located at 62.5% of the width of the tibial plateau from medial to lateral). In the case of HTO performed for knee instability or in varus-producing osteotomies (both HTO and DFO), a correction to a neutral alignment is preferable (50% of the tibial plateau). In addition, in the case of complex or chronic knee instability, part of the deformity is generally intra-articular (with abnormal JLCA). Once the knee is realigned, the JLCA is generally restored, adding some degrees of correction. This should be taken into account in the planning in order to avoid overcorrection.

The tibial slope is assessed on lateral views. The average normal tibial slope is 10.7° [6].

In the case of concomitant ligamentous reconstructions, these should be planned and allografts ordered, if necessary.

Even though bone block auto- or allograft (i.e., bone-patellar-tendon-bone) can be used for the ACL or PCL reconstruction/revision, the authors recommend soft tissue auto- (i.e., hamstring) or allograft (i.e., tibialis anterior) in order to overcome the possible complication of graft/tunnel mismatch and allow more flexibility in fixation methods around the osteotomy.

In the case of posteromedial (PMC) and posterolateral corner (PLC) reconstruction, soft tissue auto- or allografts are necessary. When still available, hamstrings are a good option for both procedures, particularly for PMC reconstruction, with the advantage of preserving the tibial insertion and avoiding tibial tunnels.

The planning for HTO and DFO is described in detail in Figs. 14.1, 14.2, 14.3, and 14.4.

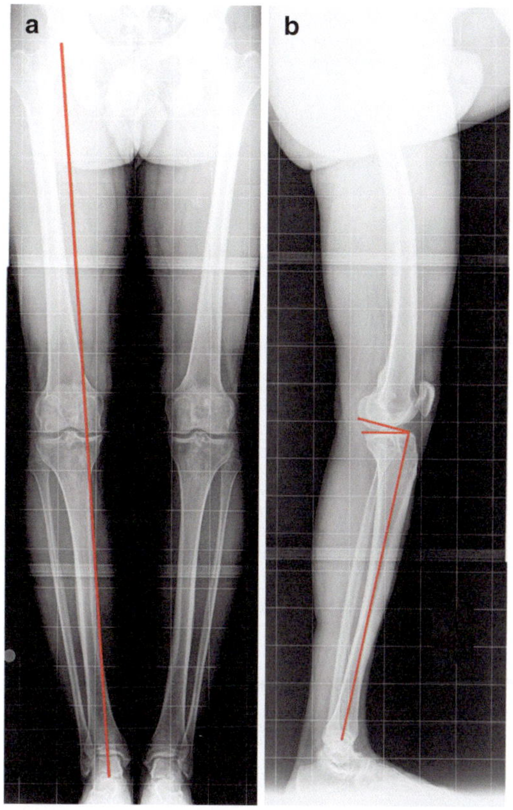

Fig. 14.1 (**a**) Long leg X-rays in AP view: evaluation of the mechanical axis (red line from the center of the femoral head to the center of the ankle joint) in a patient with failed ACL reconstruction, persistent instability, and medial arthritis. (**b**) Evaluation of the tibial slope on a long leg X-ray, lateral view

14.3 Surgical Techniques

14.3.1 Patient Positioning

Intravenous antibiotic prophylaxis is administered. The patient is positioned supine on a radiolucent table, in regional or general anesthesia, with a tourniquet at the proximal thigh. A lateral post at the level of the tourniquet is

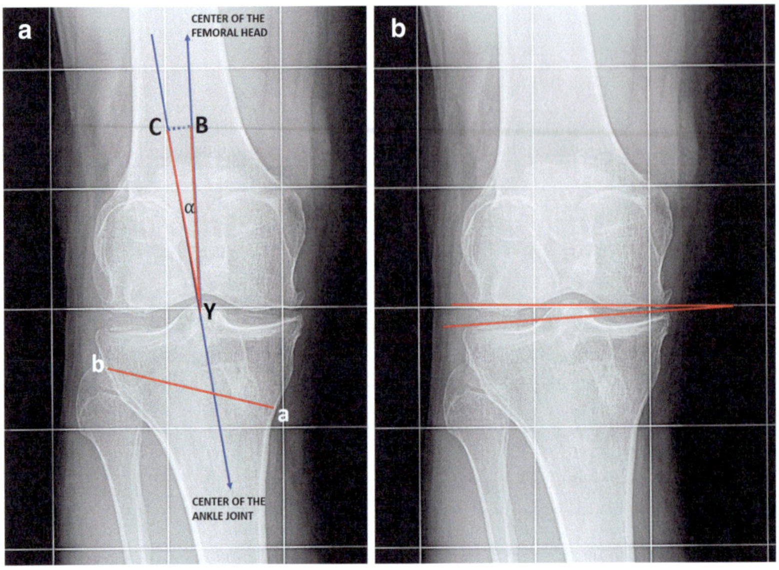

Fig. 14.2 Planning of opening wedge HTO. (**a**) Opening wedge HTO is planned with a line from Y (62.5% or 50%, like in this case, of the width of the tibial plateau) to the center of the femoral head and another line connecting Y with the center of the ankle joint. The angle between these two lines represents the angle of correction (α). The osteotomy line (ab) is defined from medial (around 4 cm below the joint line) to lateral (around 1 cm below the lateral joint line). This measurement is transferred to both rays (YB and YC) of the α angle from the vertex Y. The segment BC is equal to the opening of the osteotomy and the size of the tooth of the spacer plate. (**b**) Measurement of the joint-line convergence angle (JLCA)

placed. Positioning should allow for knee hyperflexion, if concurrent ACL reconstruction/revision is planned.

14.3.2 Arthroscopy and Knee Evaluation

Arthroscopy is performed through standard anteromedial (AM) and anterolateral (AL) portals. A complete knee evaluation is performed and concomitant meniscal and chondral injuries are treated. When concomitant ACL or PCL reconstruction is planned, preparation of tibial and femoral footprints is performed. If autologous graft harvesting is required, this is performed at this point of the procedure.

14.3.2.1 Medial Opening Wedge High Tibial Osteotomy

A 6 cm longitudinal incision is made on the anteromedial tibia (Fig. 14.5), starting 2 cm below the joint line and prolonged distally (midway between the tibial tubercle and the posteromedial tibial crest). The sartorial fascia is incised and the pes anserinus detached distally. The distal insertion of the superficial medial collateral ligament is partially detached. A Hohman retractor is positioned on the posteromedial tibia in order to improve visualization and protect the neurovascular structures (Fig. 14.5). The patellar tendon is identified and protected throughout the whole procedure.

A guide wire is positioned under fluoroscopic guidance from medial to lateral and from distal to proximal, starting around 4 cm below the medial joint line, aiming at the tip of the peroneal head (around 1 cm below the lateral joint line). The distal insertion of the superficial medial collateral ligament is partially detached (Fig. 14.5). The patellar tendon and the posterior neurovascular structures are protected with blunt retractors throughout the whole procedure. A 3-cm-wide, thin oscillating saw is used to cut the medial, anterior, and posteromedial cortices distal to the guide wire (Fig. 14.5). The

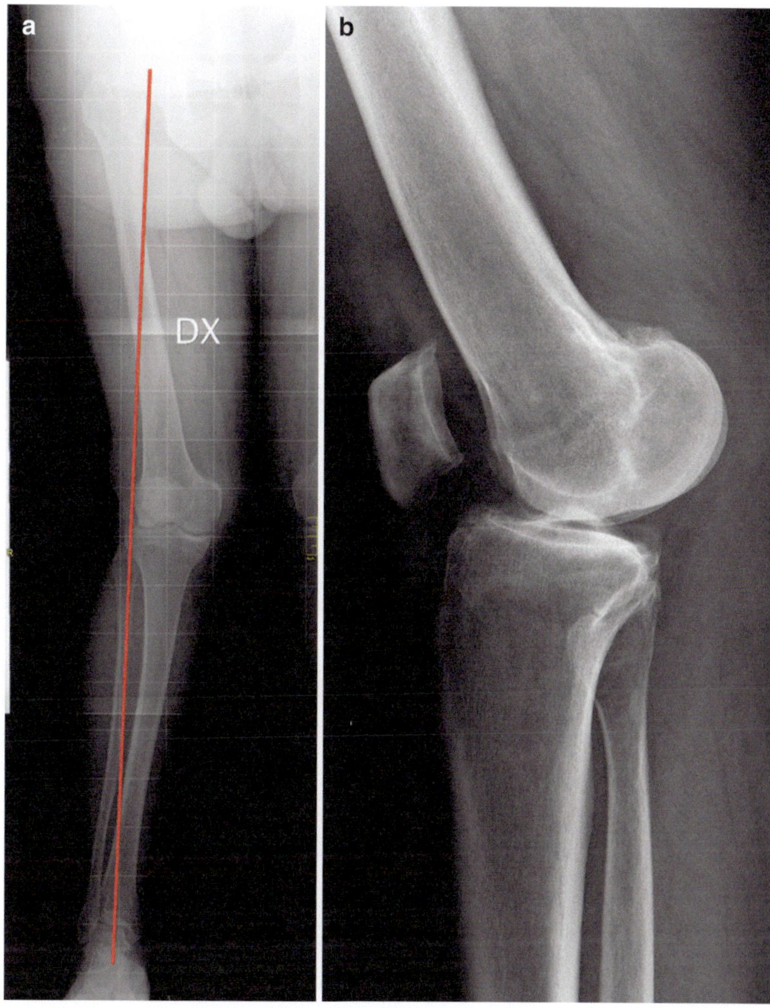

Fig. 14.3 (**a**) Preoperative long leg AP view of a patient with valgus recurvatum thrust. The mechanical axis (red line) shows the valgus alignment. (**b**) Preoperative lateral view of the same patients, showing the significant recurvatum deformity

osteotomy should be parallel to the tibial slope (with 10° of anteroposterior inclination). Wide thin osteotomes are used to complete the osteotomy, preserving a lateral cortical hinge (Fig. 14.5). With this goal, the blade of the osteotome should be advanced up to around 1 cm from the lateral tibial cortex; this distance should be less than the distance from the lateral joint line and the blade of the osteotome, in order to avoid intra-articular migration of the osteotomy. The mobility of the osteotomy is checked with a gentle valgus force or by pulling the handle of the last osteotome distally. If the osteotomy does not open, the surgeon should verify that the cut of the anterior and posterior cortices is complete. Graduated osteotomy wedges are then inserted up to the planned opening (Fig. 14.6). In this phase, the surgeon can vary the tibial slope by inserting the wedges in a more anterior position (increased tibial slope, for PCL deficient knees) or posterior position (decreased tibial slope, for ACL deficient knees) [7]. With fluoroscopy, a long alignment rod is placed from the center of the femoral head to the center of the ankle in order to check the mechanical axis at the level of the knee (Fig. 14.6). In the case of an increased JLCA, some authors suggested evaluating the alignment with a force under the foot (simulating a weight-bearing condition), in order to avoid overcorrection. When the desired alignment is achieved, fixation can be performed. The

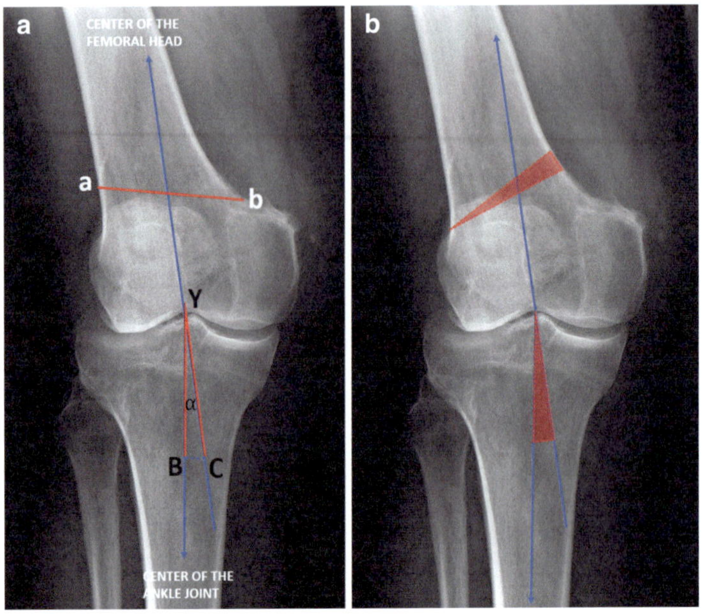

Fig. 14.4 (**a**) Planning of lateral opening wedge DFO (see legend of Fig. 14.2). In this type of surgery, no overcorrection should be achieved (50% of the tibial plateau width). (**b**) Planning of medial closing wedge DFO. The measurement of the angle of correction is as described before. The wedge to be removed medially should be an isosceles triangle with the base flush to the medial cortex. This avoids overlapping of the proximal and distal cortices after wedge removal

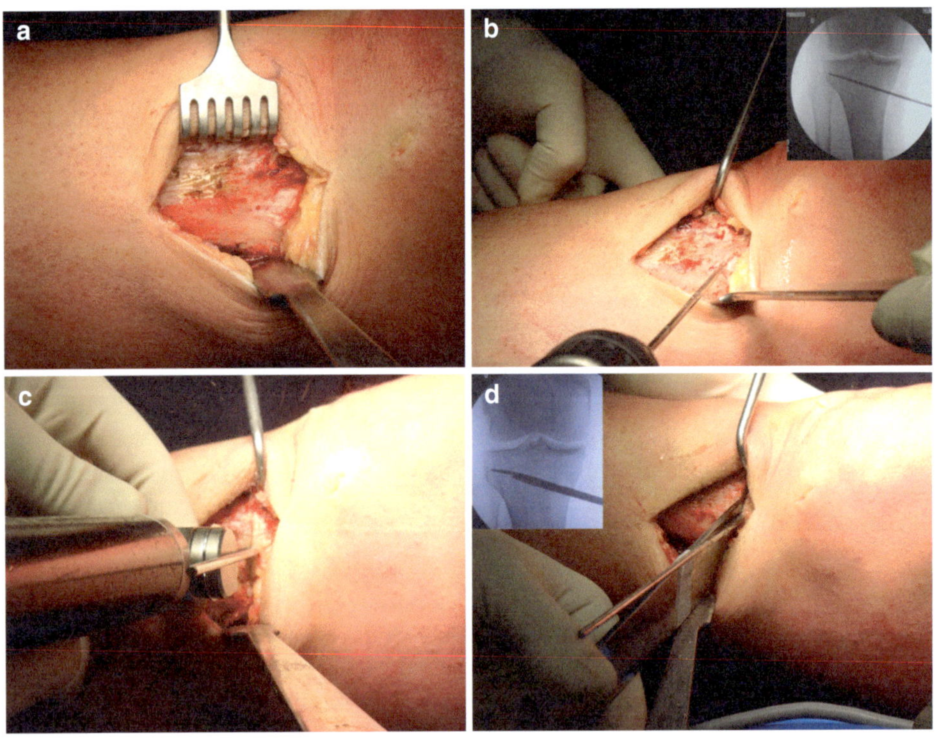

Fig. 14.5 Surgical technique for medial opening wedge HTO. (**a**) A 6 cm longitudinal incision is made on the anteromedial tibia, starting 2 cm below the joint line and prolonged distally. The pes anserinus is detached distally, and the distal insertion of the superficial medial collateral ligament is partially detached. A Hohman retractor is positioned on the posteromedial tibia. (**b**) The patellar tendon is identified and protected throughout the whole procedure. A guide wire is positioned under fluoroscopic guidance from medial to lateral and from distal to proximal, starting around 4 cm below the medial joint line, aiming at the tip of the peroneal head (around 1 cm below the lateral joint line). (**c**) A thin oscillating saw is used to cut the medial, anterior, and posteromedial cortices distal to the guide wire. The osteotomy should be parallel to the tibial slope (with 10° of anteroposterior inclination). (**d**) Wide thin osteotomes are used to complete the osteotomy, preserving a lateral cortical hinge, under fluoroscopic guidance (panel)

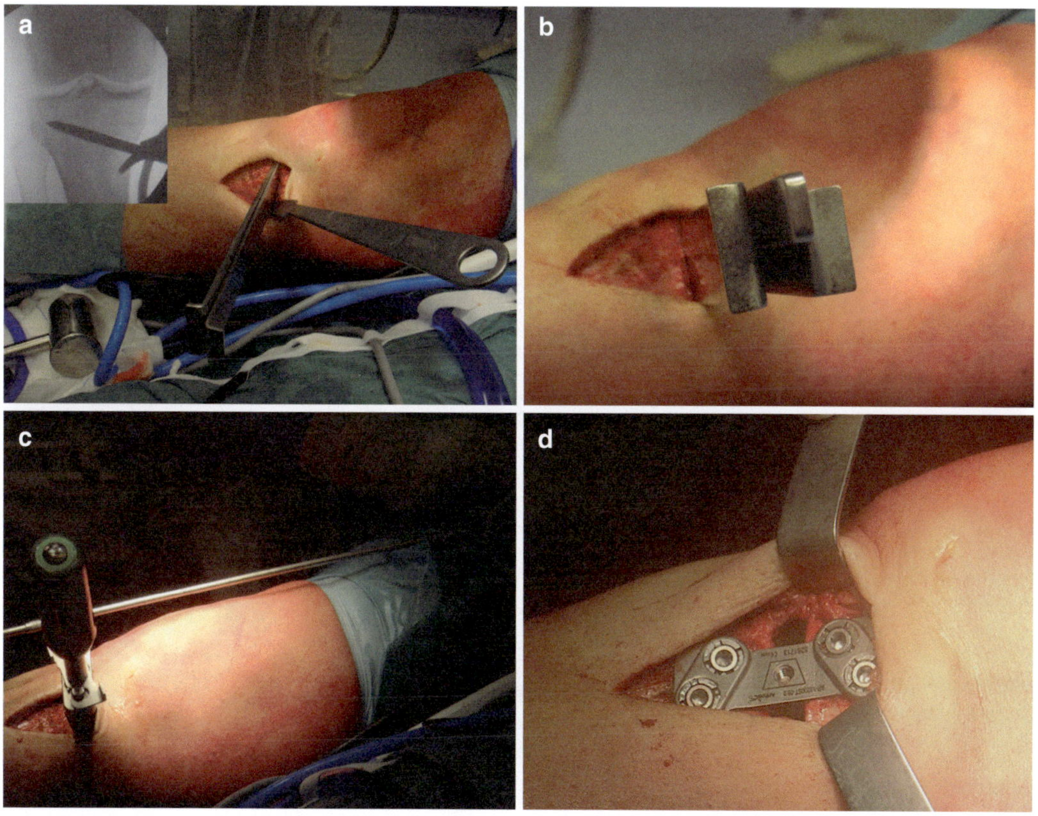

Fig. 14.6 (**a**) The completion and mobility of the osteotomy is checked with a gentle valgus force or by pulling the handle of the last osteotome distally. This is done under fluoroscopic guidance (panel). (**b**) Once the anterior and posterior cortices have been adequately cut, the opening of the osteotomy can be facilitated by piling three osteotomes. (**c**) Graduated osteotomy wedges are then inserted up to the planned opening. With fluoroscopy, a long alignment rod is placed from the center of the femoral head to the center of the ankle in order to check the mechanical axis at the level of the knee. (**d**) When the desired alignment is achieved, plating can be performed. In this case, a short locking spacer plate is used

authors' preferred fixation device is a short locking spacer plate (Figs. 14.6 and 14.7).

Also the position of the plate can determine the tibial slope correction. With a plate positioned posteriorly, the tibial slope is generally decreased, with the result of improved stability in ACL deficient knees or protection of the ACL graft from excessive tension. In the case of PCL deficient knees, the slope should be increased and the plate positioned anteriorly. When using short-tapered spacer plates in this scenario, these can be placed upside down (with the larger part of the taper anteriorly).

14.3.2.2 Lateral Closing Wedge High Tibial Osteotomy

An anterolateral inverted L-shaped incision is performed, with the vertical portion of the incision running along the lateral edge of the tibial tubercle and the horizontal portion running parallel to the lateral joint line (1 cm distal). The fascia of the anterior compartment is incised along the anterolateral crest of the tibia. A Cobb elevator is used to elevate the tibialis anterior muscle and the inferior portion of the iliotibial band from Gerdy's tubercle proximally. Dissection and protection of the common peroneal nerve throughout the procedure is not mandatory, since the osteotomy is proximal to it, but the nerve can be exposed based on the surgeon's preference. Many techniques have been described for addressing the proximal tibiofibular joint, including (1) joint excision or disruption, (2) fibular osteotomy (10 cm distal from the fibular head), and (3) excision of the fibular head. The lateral edge of the patellar tendon is identified and protected with a retractor.

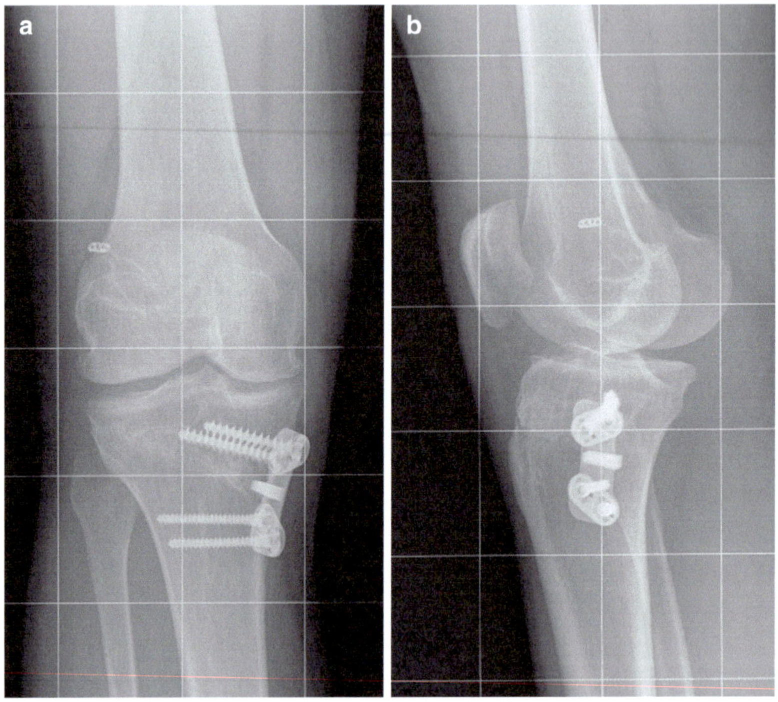

Fig. 14.7 (**a**) AP postoperative view after combined HTO and ACL reconstruction. (**b**) Lateral view of the same case

A second retractor is positioned on the posterolateral tibial edge to protect the neurovascular structures. A laterally based wedge is removed with an angular cutting guide. The base of the wedge should be 2–3 mm smaller than the planned osteotomy. During closure of the osteotomy, this will allow the distal cortex of the proximal fragment to overlap the proximal cortex of the distal fragment, without the risk of overcorrection.

To reduce the risk of intra-articular fracture, the outer cortex and a large portion of the wedge can be removed with saw cuts, using a combination of curettes, rongeurs, and osteotomes, to within 1 cm of the medial cortex. The completeness of wedge removal is assessed fluoroscopically. The osteotomy is closed, and alignment is checked under fluoroscopy. Fixation can be achieved with step staples driven from lateral to medial just anterior to the fibula. More rigid fixation can be achieved with laterally applied contoured T-plates or locking plates.

With a lateral closing wedge HTO, controlling the tibial slope is more difficult than with opening wedge HTO. Closing wedge HTOs generally result in a decreased tibial slope and therefore, in our point of view, should be contraindicated in PCL deficient knees [8].

14.3.2.3 Lateral Opening Wedge Distal Femoral Osteotomy

A 10–15 cm longitudinal lateral distal femoral incision is started 2 cm distal to the lateral femoral epicondyle and prolonged proximally (Fig. 14.8). The iliotibial band is split and the vastus lateralis is retracted anteriorly from the intermuscular septum using a curve blunt retractor. The bone is better exposed with a slight knee flexion (Fig. 14.8). Under fluoroscopic control, a guide wire is inserted in the middle of the lateral femur, with a cranio-caudal inclination of 20°, from lateral (6–7 cm above the joint line) to medial (4–5 cm above the joint line). The exposed cortex is cut with a small oscillating saw above the guide wire (Fig. 14.8). Sharp and thin osteotomes are then used to complete the osteotomy to within 1 cm from the medial cortex, under fluoroscopic guidance (Fig. 14.9). The site of osteotomy at this point is opened

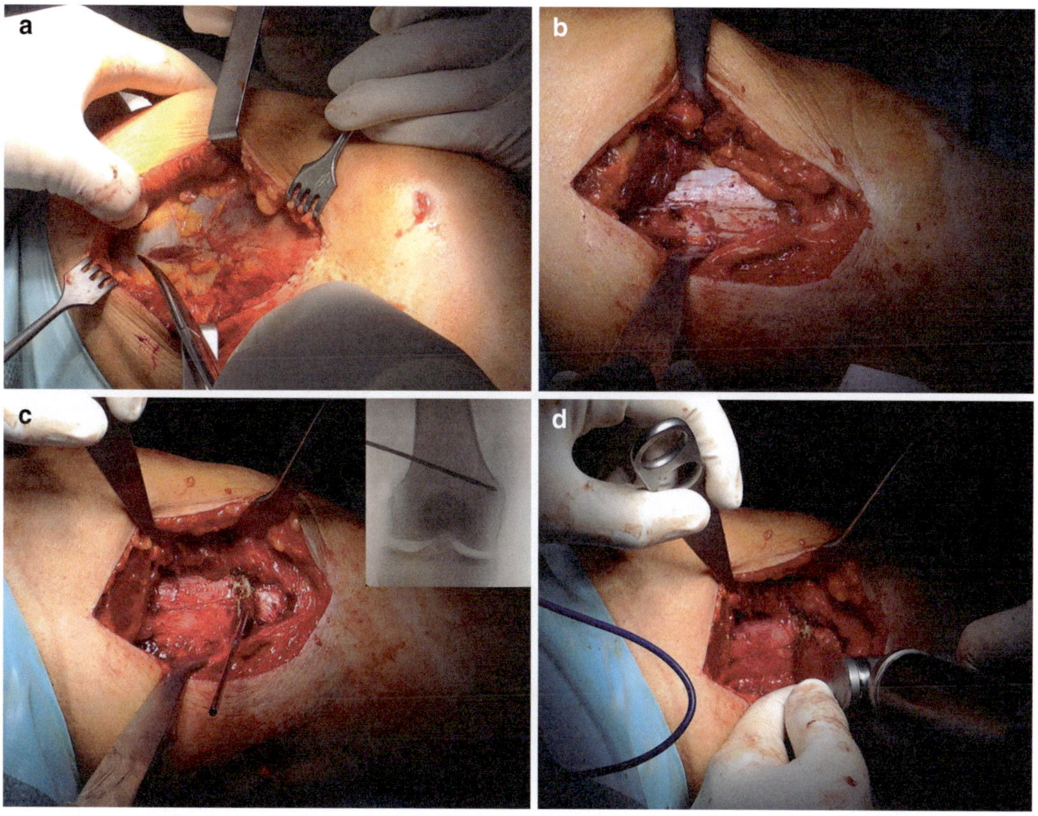

Fig. 14.8 Surgical technique for lateral opening wedge DFO. (**a**) A 10–15 cm longitudinal lateral distal femoral incision is started 2 cm distal to the lateral femoral epicondyle and prolonged proximally. (**b**) The iliotibial band is split, and the vastus lateralis is retracted anteriorly from the intermuscular septum using a curve blunt retractor. (**c**) Under fluoroscopic guidance (panel), a guide wire is inserted in the middle of the lateral femur, with a cranio-caudal inclination of 20°, from lateral (6–7 cm above the joint line) to medial (4–5 cm above the joint line). (**d**) The exposed cortex is cut with a small oscillating saw above the guide wire

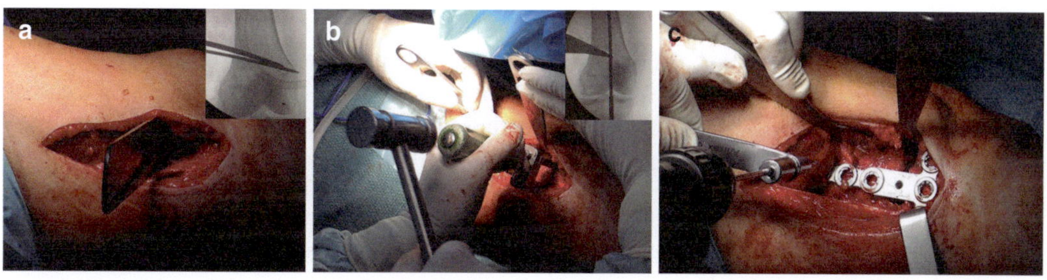

Fig. 14.9 (**a**) Sharp, thin osteotomes are then used to complete the osteotomy to within 1 cm from the medial cortex, under fluoroscopic guidance (panel). (**b**) The site of osteotomy at this point is opened with a wedge opener to the desired correction. Fluoroscopy and alignment rod are used to assess the limb correction (panel). (**c**) Plating can then be performed. In this case a distal femoral spacer plate (locked) was used

with a wedge opener to the desired correction. Fluoroscopy and alignment rod are used to assess the limb correction, as previously described (Fig. 14.9). A distal femoral spacer plate (regular or locked) is then used for fixation under image intensifier (Fig. 14.9). Bone grafting or bone substitutes are used to fill the gap [8] (Fig. 14.10).

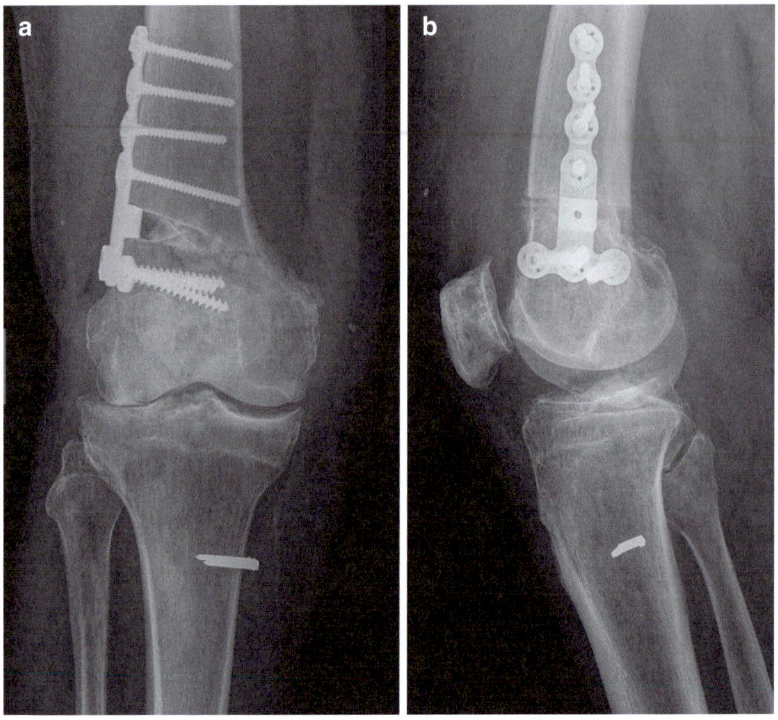

Fig. 14.10 (**a**) Postoperative X-ray AP view of the same patient described in Fig. 14.3, after lateral opening wedge DFO and medial collateral ligament reconstruction with autologous hamstrings. (**b**) Lateral view of the same case

14.3.2.4 Lateral Opening Wedge Proximal Tibial Osteotomy

A 6–8 cm anterolateral longitudinal incision is made lateral to the tibial tuberosity, extending distally from Gerdy's tubercle. Full-thickness skin flaps are created, and the fascia is then incised in line with the skin incision and the anterior compartment muscles elevated off the tibia and retracted posteriorly. The capsule of the proximal tibiofibular joint is incised anteriorly. No further disruption of this joint is usually required, as the desired osteotomy can usually be achieved after the capsulotomy. The patellar tendon is elevated, and in some cases, the release of the most proximal fibers at the insertion facilitates its mobilization. Posteriorly, the soft tissues are elevated carefully away from the tibia with a Cobb elevator. Retractors are passed along the posterior tibial cortex and beneath the patellar tendon to protect the posterior neurovascular structures and the patellar tendon, respectively.

The osteotomy is then performed in accordance with the surgical technique described for each implant. In all cases, a guide pin is inserted under fluoroscopic guidance along the line of the proposed osteotomy. The tip of this guide pin is positioned 1.5–2.0 cm below the level of the tibial articular surface and 1–1.5 cm from the medial tibial cortex. With fluoroscopy, the osteotomy is started with a micro-sagittal saw below the guide pin and completed with flexible and then solid osteotomes. The osteotomes are introduced parallel to the tibial slope. A spreading osteotome followed by a triangular wedge is introduced into the osteotomy site and distraction performed to the templated distance. The chosen plate is then applied and fixed according to the manufacturers' guidelines. The cancellous allograft bone is packed into the osteotomy site at the discretion of the surgeon. Fluoroscopy confirmed both the position of the plate and the osteotomy correction [3].

14.3.2.5 Medial Closing Wedge Distal Femoral Osteotomy

A longitudinal 10–15 cm anteromedial incision is performed on the distal femur. The fascia over the vastus medialis muscle is incised, and the muscle is separated from the intermuscular septum and retracted anteriorly.

When using a 90° blade plate, a guide wire is inserted parallel to the joint line. A slot for a blade plate is then prepared parallel to the guide wire, and an osteotomy is made about 2–3 cm proximal to the slot. The medial cortex and large portion of the wedge can be removed with saw cuts, along with the medial half using a combination of curettes, rongeurs, and osteotomes, to within 1 cm of the lateral cortex. The 90° angle blade plate is inserted in the prepared slot. Manual varus reduction is performed, allowing the medial spike of the proximal part to dig into the distal cancellous bone. The rigid fixation is achieved with the anatomic knee axis of 0°, after fluoroscopic assessment of the correction [8].

Since blade plates are currently hard to find in some countries' markets, locking plates can be used alternatively. In this case, the osteotomy wedge to be removed should be as much as possible an isosceles triangle. After osteotomy closure, this avoids significant overlapping of the cortices (proximal and distal to the osteotomy) and results in a better fit of the plate on the medial bone.

14.3.3 Postoperative Regimen

Immediate full range of motion exercises are allowed. The patient is kept partially weight bearing in a hinged knee brace for 6 weeks. At 6 weeks, after radiographic confirmation of bone healing, weight bearing is allowed, the brace is discontinued, and the rehabilitation protocol proceeds as in standard ligament reconstruction (if performed concurrently). The postoperative regimen may vary according to the fixation device used, the amount of opening required, and possible concomitant procedures on the cartilage, ligaments, and menisci.

14.4 Discussion

Osteotomies around the knee are rarely indicated to treat knee instability in the acute setting, unless significant deformities are present at the moment of ligament reconstruction. Both coronal and sagittal planes should be evaluated to rule out possible preexisting malalignment.

On the other hand, in the chronic setting, osteotomies are essential in treating knee instability, as an isolated procedure or combined with ligamentous reconstruction. Chronic instabilities treated with ligament reconstruction in a malaligned knee are likely to fail if realignment is not performed in advance or concurrently.

Compared to osteotomies performed for unicompartmental arthritis, when performing HTO and DFO for instability, the surgeon should take into account many more aspects:

- Tibial slope: The role of the tibial slope in anterior and posterior knee stability has been shown to be essential. In addition, abnormal tibial slope has shown to be correlated with a higher risk of re-rupture after ACL or PCL reconstruction. Finally, modifying the tibial slope is sometimes the only mean to correct excessive procurvatum or recurvatum deformities around the knee.
- Location of the deformity (femoral-based, tibial-based, combined, or intra-articular) can determine the choice between a procedure and another.
- JLCA: An abnormal JLCA contributes to the final amount of deformity. After realignment, this angle generally goes back almost to normal. When preoperative planning and intraoperative fluoroscopic evaluations are made without taking into account an abnormal JLCA, overcorrecting the knee becomes a risk.
- Unless a significant unicompartmental arthritis is present, generally correction to neutral alignment (no overcorrection) is indicated in osteotomies for knee instability.

References

1. Bonasia DE, Dettoni F, Palazzolo A, Rossi R. Opening wedge high tibial osteotomy and anterior cruciate ligament reconstruction or revision. Arthrosc Tech. 2017;6(5):e1735–41.

2. Naudie DD, Amendola A, Fowler PJ. Opening wedge high tibial osteotomy for symptomatic hyperextension-varus thrust. Am J Sports Med. 2004;32(1):60–70.
3. Collins B, Getgood A, Alomar AZ, Giffin JR, Willits K, Fowler PJ, Birmingham TB, Litchfield RB. A case series of lateral opening wedge high tibial osteotomy for valgus malalignment. Knee Surg Sports Traumatol Arthrosc. 2013;21(1):152–60.
4. Thienpont E, Schwab PE, Cornu O, Bellemans J, Victor J. Bone morphotypes of the varus and valgus knee. Arch Orthop Trauma Surg. 2017;137(3):393–400.
5. Eberbach H, Mehl J, Feucht MJ, Bode G, Südkamp NP, Niemeyer P. Geometry of the valgus knee: contradicting the dogma of a femoral-based deformity. Am J Sports Med. 2017;45(4):909–14.
6. Matsuda S, Miura H, Nagamine R, Urabe K, Ikenoue T, Okazaki K, Iwamoto Y. Posterior tibial slope in the normal and varus knee. Am J Knee Surg. 1999;12(3):165–8.
7. Ogawa H, Matsumoto K, Ogawa T, Takeuchi K, Akiyama H. Effect of wedge insertion angle on posterior tibial slope in medial opening wedge high tibial osteotomy. Orthop J Sports Med. 2016;4(2):2325967116630748.
8. Amendola A, Bonasia DE. Proximal tibial/distal femoral osteotomy for management of unicompartmental arthritis. In: Johnson DL, editor. Master techniques in orthopaedic surgery: reconstructive knee surgery. Alphen aan den Rijn: Wolters Kluwer Health; 2017.

15 Complex Knee Injuries in Young Patients

Pablo Rainaudi, Jorge Batista, and Rodrigo Maestu

Knee dislocation is an infrequent pathology, but its prevalence is believed to be underestimated owing to the absence of a diagnosis and also to the fact that in many cases they reduce spontaneously [1]. This prevalence has been increasing in later years due to a better understanding of the lesion and the advance in imaging diagnostic techniques [2]. Most of them are high-energy lesions which occur most frequently in traffic accidents and sports trauma. They might cause important articular damage with sequelae such as stiffness and multidirectional instability, but the associated neurovascular lesions are the most serious ones as they can end up in limb amputation.

In the case of dislocations that get to the shock room with no reduction, the diagnosis is evident. But in those cases in which there is a spontaneous reduction, there should be a high level of suspicion so as not to misdiagnose it.

The delay in the recognition of this lesion brings about a delay in diagnosing the most serious complication, which happens to be an arterial lesion with devastating consequences.

15.1 Conduct

These patients generally present a polytraumatic picture. Once the dislocation is reduced, a thorough neurovascular examination should be carried out. In those patients with no signs of vascular involvement, it is important to perform an evolution control with a regulated neurovascular examination, since very subtle damages to the popliteal artery may occur at later stages. In these cases the ankle/arm index might be very useful to control vascular status. If the patient requires CT studies, an angio CT of the popliteal artery can be performed. If there should be absence of pulse or if the latter diminishes along the studies, we indicate an arteriography.

When there is an imminent arterial lesion, a prompt surgical exploration is indicated with a multidisciplinary team [3].

Other possible lesions associated to knee dislocation are neurological lesions. It has been estimated that they are found in 10 and in 40% of cases, and the common peroneal nerve and popliteal sciatic nerve are the most commonly affected [4].

The neurological damage may be of variable seriousness, with partial or total functional recovery with rehabilitation, or it might be a complete

P. Rainaudi · R. Maestu (✉)
Arthroscopy and Knee Department, CETEA (Center for the Study and Treatment of Joint Diseases), Ciudad Autónoma de Buenos Aires, Buenos Aires, Argentina
e-mail: rmaestu@intramed.net

J. Batista
Arthroscopy Department, CABJ (Jorge Batista Arthroscopy Center), Ciudad Autónoma de Buenos Aires, Buenos Aires, Argentina

F. Margheritini et al. (eds.), *Complex Knee Ligament Injuries*,
https://doi.org/10.1007/978-3-662-58245-9_15

lesion which will require the transfer of the posterior tibial tendon to improve ankle functionality and hence walking ability.

Once the most serious complications are ruled out, and the patient is clinically stabilized, we focus on the knee. We carry out a thorough soft tissue, morbidity range, varus-valgus deformities and articular stability physical examination. Certainly, by this moment, we already have X-rays taken that rule out bone lesions and possibly CTs as well. Indicating an MRI is fundamental so as to allow us to see important details of the meniscal, ligament and capsular lesions.

15.2 Classification

To approach the treatment of knee dislocation, we base ourselves on the anatomic classification described by Robert Schenck [5].

	Lesion
KD I	Knee dislocation with ACL or intact PCL and variable involvement of collateral ligaments
KD II	Both cruciate ligaments injured, with intact collaterals
KD III	Both cruciate ligaments injured + one of the collaterals as well. M or L
KD IV	Both cruciate ligaments and both collaterals injured
KD V	Knee dislocation + peri articular fracture

There are specific indications for urgent surgery in the following cases [6]:

1. Irreducible dislocation.
2. Compartment syndrome.
3. Popliteal artery lesion.
4. Exposed dislocations.

Once the urgency has been treated, there are different treatments to apply according to the time elapsed since the injury occurred: during the acute period (before the 3 weeks), during the chronic stage or to plan a treatment in steps.

There are controversies concerning the optimal moment for surgery. Some authors conclude that treatment in the acute stage is the one that gets better results [7]. Other authors indicate that there is no difference, in long-term results, in patients treated in the acute or chronic stage [8].

And lastly, some authors propose that the best results are achieved approaching treatment for knee dislocation in stages [9].

We do believe that it is very important to evaluate each particular patient and to make individual decisions according to several factors. The presence of a vascular lesion, of associated lesions that require a priority approach; the status of soft tissues; the inflammatory process; and articular mobility are parameters that we really have to keep in mind at the moment of deciding the time for surgery as well as the techniques to be applied. We do obtain the best results performing surgical treatment as soon as possible. When we are able to perform the surgery in the acute period, we opt for performing a repair plus reconstruction with an allo- or autograft of the ligament structures involved.

We rarely do just repair since, coinciding with most published papers, the rate of residual laxity is high. That is the reason why we always associate it to the reconstruction.

When we approach treatment in the chronic stage, healing of the tissues makes it difficult to identify anatomical structures.

15.2.1 KD I

This type of dislocations is normally produced due to low-energy mechanisms, and they can very well be sports trauma. In such cases, there is a lesion of one of either cruciate ligaments and a variable involvement of one of the collateral ligaments. These patients usually present unidirectional instability which can be anterior or posterior. There might be a generally partial affectation of the medial collateral ligament. Depending on the medial collateral ligament involvement, we can indicate immobilization for 4 or 6 weeks to favour its healing process, to avoid residual laxity and to improve the inflammatory process of the joint. If one of the collateral ligaments is to be reconstructed, the surgery is carried out at the same time of the cruciate ligament reconstruction. The surgical techniques will be described ahead in this chapter.

Then we proceed to the ACL or PCL reconstruction according to the case. For this reconstruction, we can use bone–tendon-bone autograft (BTB) or semitendinosus gracilis autograft (hamstring tendon (HT)) or allograft (anterior tibial or Achilles).

We use anatomic reconstruction techniques either for ACL or PCL, respecting as much as possible anatomic ligament insertion footprints (Fig. 15.1 (a–d)).

In the post-op period, we do not use immobilizers for ACL reconstruction, but in PCL we do immobilize the knee for 6 weeks with posterior enhancement at the height of the calf to protect reconstruction, and then we indicate a knee brace for 3 months. For ACL, regarding partial weight bearing on crutches, the patient uses it according to their tolerance. And for PCL, they use them for 6 weeks. For collateral reconstruction we immobilize the knee and indicate weight bearing on crutches for 6 weeks. The patient starts with assisted passive mobility and physical and kinetic therapy from the second post-op day.

15.2.2 KD II

In this type of lesions, both cruciate ligaments are injured, and there is indemnity of both collateral ligaments. It is a rare lesion which usually occurs due to a hyperextension mechanism of the knee. Once mobility range of the knee is

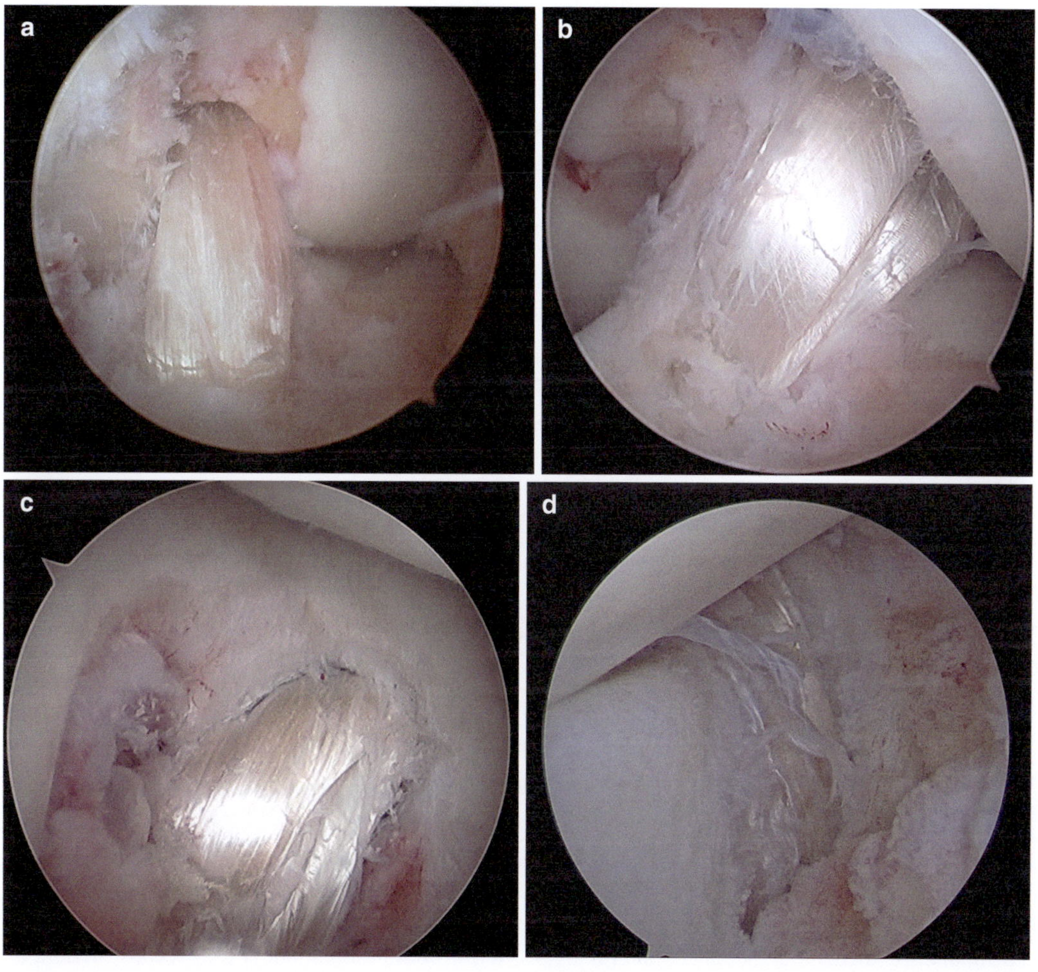

Fig. 15.1 (**a**) ACL reconstruction femoral view. (**b**) ACL reconstruction tibial view. (**c**) PCL reconstruction femoral view. (**d**) PCL reconstruction tibial view

recovered and joint swelling improved during the first days, we indicate reconstruction of both cruciate ligaments in one time. If we have the possibility to use allograft, we would rather use it since it diminishes knee morbidity and allows a faster rehabilitation and mobility range recovery. In these cases, we use anterior tibial or Achilles to reconstruct PCL and anterior tibial or BTB to reconstruct ACL.

In those cases in which it is not possible to use allograft, we resort to HT for PCL reconstruction and BTB for ACL reconstruction. We obtain both of them through the same medial anterior incision over the patellar tendon, slightly extended to distal, so as to be able to have access to the goose-leg insertion.

We start reconstruction from posterior to anterior: first, PCL femoral tunnel and ACL femoral tunnel then PCL tibial tunnel and then the ACL tibial one. Concerning graft passing, first we place the PCL graft and fix it proximal, and second we place ACL graft and fix it proximal too. The next step is to fix PCL, in 70–90°, distally. Finally we fix ACL, 0–10°, distally. The post-op is similar to PCL post-op.

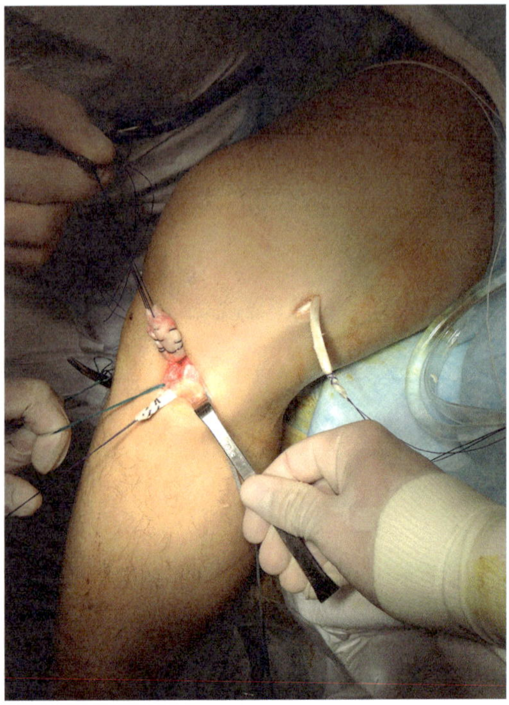

Fig. 15.2 Superficial band MCL reconstruction

15.2.3 KD III

In this type of dislocation, there is a lesion in both cruciate ligaments and in one of the collateral ligaments. Therefore, there are two subtypes: lesion of both cruciate ligaments + lesion of the MCL (KD III M) and lesion of both cruciate ligaments + lesion of the LCL (KDM III L). It is one of the most frequent types of knee dislocations.

These are patients that present an important anterior and posterior instability plus medial or lateral instability depending upon the affected collateral ligament.

15.2.4 KD III (M)

In this subtype, besides the lesion of both cruciate ligaments, there is a medial collateral ligament lesion as well. There is an anterior, posterior, medial or posteromedial instability. Our approach consists in the reconstruction of the three ligaments in only one time. We would rather use allograft not to add morbidity to the knee. We use anterior tibial tendon or semitendinosus for the reconstruction of MCL, anterior tibial tendon or Achilles' tendon for PCL reconstruction and anterior tibial or bone-patellar tendon-bone for ACL reconstruction. We always use anatomic reconstruction techniques; we do prefer the technique described by R. LaPrade for the case of medial collateral ligament lesion [10].

When instability is only medial, we reconstruct the superficial band of the MCL. We make tunnels on the anatomic bone footprints, and for fixation we use interferential screws. We perform this fixation in neutral rotation and in 30° of knee flexion (Fig. 15.2).

When there is a posteromedial corner (PMC) lesion, or on physical exam, we detect a medial instability in full extension; we carry out the posterior oblique ligament (POL) reconstruction, as LaPrade describes. This reconstruction is fixed in full knee extension (Fig. 15.3).

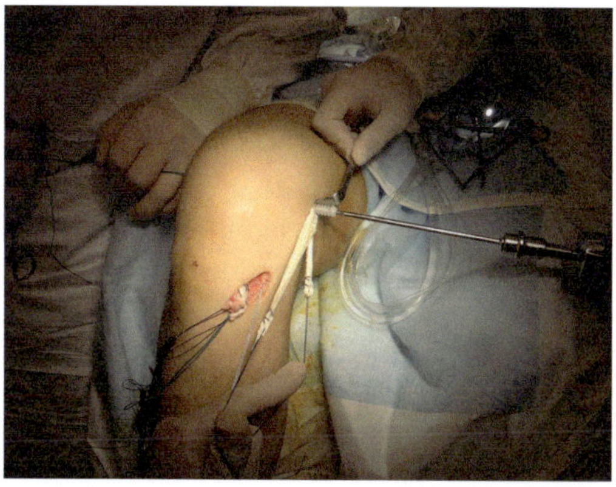

Fig. 15.3 Superficial band MCL and POL reconstruction

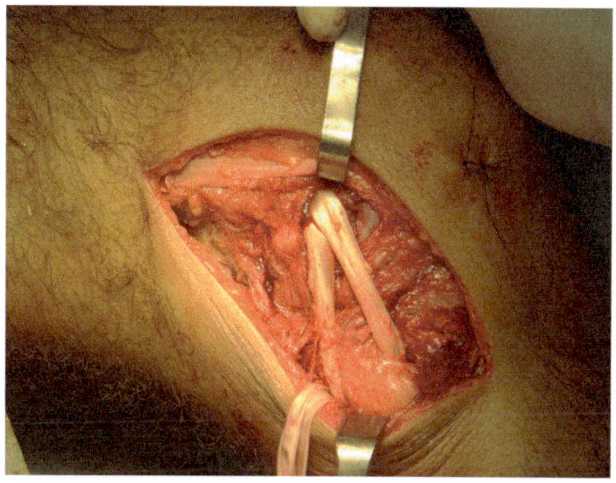

Fig. 15.4 Lateral knee Larson reconstruction

15.2.5 KD III (L)

In these cases, there is a lesion in both cruciate ligaments plus in the lateral side of the knee. The instability found is anterior, posterior and lateral or posterolateral. Like with the anterior type, we would rather perform the approach of all lesions in one time.

When, besides the lesion in both cruciate ligaments, we are faced with lateral instability, we use the technique described by Larson or Arciero to reconstruct the lateral collateral ligament [11, 12] (Fig. 15.4).

In those cases when instability is posterolateral, we prefer the anatomic reconstruction technique described by LaPrade (Fig. 15.5), even though there are papers that indicate the same rate of good results comparing it to Larson or Arciero's techniques [13].

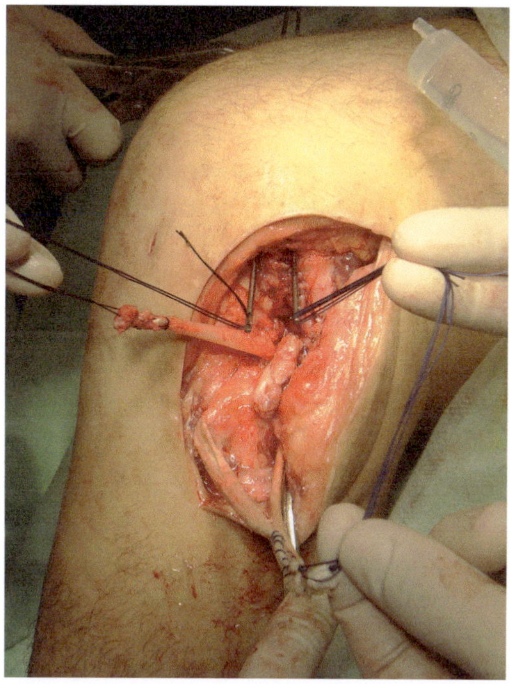

Fig. 15.5 Posterolateral knee LaPrade reconstruction

15.2.6 KD IV

In these cases, there is a complete disruption of the four main ligament structures of the knee. Both cruciate ligaments and both collateral ligaments are injured. In most cases, these lesions are caused by high-energy traffic accidents. We have to take into account several aspects when planning the surgical strategy in these patients. The general condition of patients and their associated lesions are factors that are going to condition us for the surgery. These patients usually present skull, chest or abdomen trauma of variable seriousness, and they demand priority. Likewise, vascular knee lesions due to the dislocation itself may delay the moment for surgery. The status of soft tissues and the inflammatory process are also conditioning factors to keep in mind.

Once the above-mentioned factors are solved, we have to plan the procedure to be performed.

The surgeons' experience is highly important. This can determine whether the procedure will be performed in one time or in stages to minimize the risks of ischemia of the thigh tourniquet. The availability of an allograft is crucial to minimize surgery morbidity. In case there is not one available, what can be considered is the use of an autograft from the contralateral knee.

Our conduct, whenever possible, is to plan just one surgical moment for the reconstruction of all lesioned structures. If we can use an allograft, our tendency is to apply one from the anterior tibial tendon or from Achilles tendon for PCL reconstruction, from anterior tibial or BTB for ACL reconstruction, anterior tibial or semitendinosus for medial structures and anterior tibial or Achilles for lateral structures.

Another option we draw upon is to handle both types of graft: allograft and autograft. In these cases, we employ allograft to reconstruct extra-articular structures (MCL; LCL) and autograft for the intra-articular ones (ACL; PCL). The techniques we use are the same ones which were previously described.

We indicate immobilization for 6 weeks, with crutches and partial weight bearing, and then knee brace for 3 months. The patient begins with active and passive mobility as from the second day post-op.

15.2.7 KD V

In these dislocations, a periarticular fracture is associated. The philosophy for their ligament approach does not vary from the anterior types, and the same premises are to be followed to plan the treatment strategy. But in these cases, the reduction and fixation of the associated fracture are added to allow for a rapid mobilization and rehabilitation of the articulation. Should it be impossible to resolve all lesions in only one surgical act, we have to take into account the possibility of proposing a treatment in stages, and it is in the first stage when the fracture must be resolved.

15.3 Conclusion

Knee dislocations in young patients are quite infrequent, and if they are not treated in time and correctly, they can have devastating consequences.

An accurate initial diagnosis is highly important. To achieve this, we must have an important rate of suspicion, bearing in mind that there are high number of cases that present already are spontaneously reduced.

We must always suspect a knee dislocation in those multiligament lesions or with important multidirectional instability.

The initial physical examination must be thorough so as not to misdiagnose a neurovascular lesion of extremely serious consequences. Currently, it has been demonstrated that surgical resolution of these lesions within the first 3 weeks leads to better results. It has also been demonstrated that the anatomic reconstruction of the injured structures versus their repair gets better results as well.

The availability of an allograft is relevant since it lowers morbidity and surgical time. Also, the surgeon's experience in the treatment of this type of lesions is crucial in the final results.

References

1. Hegyes MS, Richardson MW, Miller MD. Knee dislocation: complications of non-operative and operative management. Clin Sports Med. 2000;19(3):519–43.
2. Keating JF. Acute knee ligament injuries and knee dislocation. Eur Surg Orthop Traumatol. 2014:2949–71.
3. Schenck RC Jr, Richter DL, Wascher DC. Knee dislocations lessons learned from 20-Year follow-up. 2014. Investigation performed at the University of New Mexico School of Medicine, Albuquerque, New Mexico, USA.
4. Bonnevialle P, Dubrana F, Galau B, et al. Common peroneal nerve palsy complicating knee dislocation and bicruciate ligaments tears. Orthop Traumatol Surg Res. 2010;96:64–9.
5. Schenck RC Jr, Hunter RE, Ostrum RF, Perry CR. Knee dislocations. Instr Course Lect. 1999;48:515–22.
6. Rihn JA, Cha PS, Yram JG, Harner CD. The acutely dislocated knee: evaluation and management. J Am Acad Orthop Surg. 2004;12(5):334–46.
7. Hohmann E, Glatt V, Tetsworth K. Early or delayed reconstruction in multi-ligament knee injuries: a sys-

tematic review and meta-analysis THEKNE-02490; No of Pages 8.

8. Jiang W, Yao J, He Y, Sun W, Huang Y, Kong D. The timing of surgical treatment of knee dislocations: a systematic review. Knee Surg Sports Traumatol Arthrosc. 2014;
9. Ohkoshi Y, Nagasaki S, Shibata N, Yamamoto K, Hashimoto T, Yamane S. Two-stage reconstruction with autografts for knee dislocations. Clin Orthop Relat Res. 2002;398:169–75.
10. LaPrade RF, Engebretsen AH, Ly TV, Johansen S, Wentorf FA, Engebretsen L. The anatomy of the medial part of the knee. J Bone Joint Surg Am. 2010;. Current concepts review injuries to the MCL and associated medial structures of the Knee Wijdicks, Griffith, Johansen, Engebretsen and LaPrade J Bone Joint Surg Am. 2010
11. Fanelli y Larson. Practical management of posterolateral instability of the knee. Arthroscopy. 2002;18(2):1.
12. Arciero RA. Anatomic posterolateral corner knee reconstruction. Arthroscopy. 2005;
13. Treme G, Ortiz G, Gill GK, Menzer HM, Johnson PJ, Salas C, Qeadan F, Schenck RC, Richter DL, Wascher DC. A biomechanical comparison of knee stability after posterolateral corner reconstruction: Arciero vs. Laprade. 2017. Presented at: AOSSM Annual Meeting 2017; July 20–23; Toronto, Canada, Abstract.

Knee Dislocation in Athletes

16

Paul Herickhoff and Marc Safran

16.1 Introduction

Tibiofemoral dislocation is an uncommon but devastating injury to athletes. Less than 0.02% of all musculoskeletal injuries are knee dislocations [1]. In high school athletes, the knee represents 16% of all dislocated joints [2]. Three of the four major ligaments of the knee are typically injured, and there is often concomitant vascular or nerve injury or fracture [3]. Due to the potentially limb-threatening nature of this injury, knee dislocation represents a true orthopedic emergency, requiring expeditious evaluation and treatment [4].

Historically, treatment was primarily limited to closed reduction and casting or cast-brace immobilization. However, with the advent of better instrumentation, an improved understanding of the anatomy of the knee, and new reconstruction techniques, combined anterior and posterior cruciate ligament(ACL/PCL) tears with medial and/or lateral collateral ligament(MCL/LCL) disruption in the athlete is almost always managed surgically [5]. Due to the relative infrequency of these injuries, and the heterogeneity of injury patterns, there is little conclusive, high-level, scientific evidence to guide management. The purpose of this chapter is to review relevant knee anatomy, classification systems, mechanisms of injury, evaluation, treatment, rehabilitation, and outcomes of knee dislocations in athletes.

P. Herickhoff
Department of Orthopaedic Surgery, Pennsylvania State University, State College, PA, USA
e-mail: pherickhoff@pennstatehealth.psu.edu

M. Safran (✉)
Department of Orthopaedic Surgery, Stanford University, Redwood City, CA, USA
e-mail: Msafran@Stanford.edu

16.1.1 Anatomy

The anterior and posterior cruciate ligaments (ACL and PCL) and medial and lateral collateral ligaments (MCL and LCL) are the primary ligamentous stabilizers of the knee. The ACL is composed of two functional bundles, named anteromedial (AM) and posterolateral (PL), for their tibial attachment sites. For single-bundle ACL reconstruction (the recommended treatment for of ACL tears resulting from knee dislocation), the centerpoint of the ACL tibial footprint is located 15 mm anterior to the PCL and two-fifths of the medial-lateral interspinous distance [6]. The centerpoint of ACL femoral footprint is 24.8% of the proximal to distal distance measured from the proximal femoral cortex and 28.5% of the anterior to posterior distance, measured from the top of the notch [7].

The PCL is comprised of the anterolateral (AL) and posteromedial (PM) bundles, also named for their tibial attachments. For non-repairable PCL tears resulting from knee

F. Margheritini et al. (eds.), *Complex Knee Ligament Injuries*,
https://doi.org/10.1007/978-3-662-58245-9_16

dislocation, single-bundle reconstruction is also the recommended treatment. The centerpoint of the PCL tibial footprint is 7.4 mm anterior to the posterior tibial cortex or "champagne drop off" point and one-third of the medial to lateral distance between the medial groove and lateral cartilage point of the lateral tibial plateau. The centerpoint of the AL bundle is typically the chosen site for the femoral tunnel in single-bundle PCL reconstruction since its cross-sectional area is twice that of the PM bundle. The center of the AL bundle on the femur is 7.9 mm proximal to the distal articular cartilage and 7.4 mm posterior from the trochlear point, where the cartilage turns medially at the roof of the intercondylar notch [8].

The MCL of the knee has superficial and deep components. The superficial MCL femoral attachment is found in a depression 3.2 mm proximal and 4.8 mm posterior to the medial epicondyle. The superficial MCL has two distinct tibial attachments. The proximal attachment is to the semimembranosus anterior arm, while the distal attachment is broad-based, lies anterior to the posteromedial crest of the tibia, and forms the floor of the pes anserine bursa, approximately 6 cm distal to the joint line. The deep MCL is a thickening of the medial joint capsule parallel to the anterior border of the superficial MCL. The deep MCL consists of distinct meniscofemoral and meniscotibial attachments. The posterior oblique ligament is the main structure of the posteromedial corner of the knee. The central arm of the posterior oblique ligament originates from the distal aspect of the main semimembranosus and attaches to the femur 1.4 mm distal and 2.9 mm anterior to the gastrocnemius tubercle [9].

The LCL attaches to the femur 1.4 mm proximal and 3.1 mm posterior to the lateral femoral epicondyle. The fibular attachment of the LCL lies 8.2 mm posterior to the anterior border of the fibular head and 28.4 mm distal to the tip of the fibular styloid process. The LCL is one of several structures comprising the posterolateral corner of the knee, which includes important secondary stabilizers of the knee, namely, the popliteus and popliteofibular ligament. The popliteus tendon inserts into the femur 18.5 mm distal and anterior to the LCL femoral attachment. The popliteofibular ligament is composed of two bundles which attach 1.6 and 2.8 mm from the tip of the fibular styloid process, respectively [10]. Finally, the medial and lateral menisci, anterolateral capsule/ligament, and posterior capsule of the knee all provide secondary stabilization of the knee [11].

The popliteal artery is an "end artery" to the leg, with minimal collateral circulation through the superior and inferior genicular branches. It travels through the popliteal fossa, just posterior to the PCL and posterior horn of the lateral meniscus, and is the closest neurovascular structure to the knee. The distance between the popliteal artery and PCL increases from 5.4 mm with the knee in full extension to 9.3 mm with the knee at 100° of flexion [12]. The popliteal artery and vein are tethered proximally at the adductor hiatus, or Hunter's canal, and distally at the soleus arch, which increases their risk of injury with knee dislocation.

The sciatic nerve branches into the tibial and peroneal nerves in the popliteal fossa. The peroneal nerve travels laterally around the neck of the fibula and has less excursion than the tibial nerve, placing it at increased risk of injury with knee dislocation, particularly varus injury patterns [13]. Kadiyala and colleagues also demonstrated the precarious blood supply of the common peroneal nerve caused by its lack of intraneural vessels in the region of the fibular neck [14].

16.1.2 Classification

Historically, Kennedy classified knee dislocations into five types (anterior, posterior, medial, lateral, and rotatory) based on the direction of dislocation of the tibia relative to the femur [15]. Although this information is useful when the knee remains dislocated, knee dislocations often spontaneously reduce, which is typically the case in athletes, so the true direction of dislocation may be unknown. The major limitation of the Kennedy classification, however, is the variability in injured ligaments when only accounting for the direction of dislocation.

Table 16.1 Schenck classification of knee dislocation. "C" is added for concomitant arterial injuries, while "N" is added for nerve injury

Grade	Injured structure	Intact structure
I	1 cruciate + 1 collateral	1 cruciate + 1 collateral
II	Both cruciates	Both collaterals
IIIM	Both cruciates + MCL	LCL/PLC
IIIL	Both cruciates + LCL/PLC	MCL
IV	Both cruciates, both collaterals	–
V	Fracture dislocation	

Shelbourne and colleagues classified knee dislocations as low energy or high energy based upon the mechanism of injury [16]. Knee dislocations from sporting activities, with the exception of water-skiing, were classified as low energy, while motor vehicle collisions (MVC), crush injuries, and fall from high distances were classified as high-energy dislocations. Shelbourne reported only a 4.8% rate of vascular injury in low-energy dislocations. In contrast, McCoy and colleagues reported four cases of low-energy knee dislocation, three of which sustained vascular injuries requiring surgical repair [17]. Therefore, the physician must maintain a high index of suspicion for vascular injury in knee dislocation regardless of the mechanism of injury.

The most widely used and accepted classification of knee dislocations was developed by Schenck and is based on which anatomical structures are injured [18]. The Schenck classification accounts for injured ligaments, nerve and arterial injuries, and fractures. A summary of the Schenck classification is shown in Table 16.1.

16.1.3 Mechanism of Injury

Hyperextension of the knee, from either contact or noncontact injury, classically causes anterior dislocation of the knee and rupture of both cruciate ligaments and is a high-risk pattern for neurovascular injury due to stretch on the posterior structures of the knee [13]. In a cadaver study, Kennedy demonstrated that hyperextension of the knee past 30° resulted in tearing of the posterior capsule, while hyperextension to 50° ruptured the PCL and popliteal artery in all specimens [15].

A violent blow to the anterior proximal tibia of the flexed knee and falling directly onto a flexed knee are the typical patterns for posterior dislocations of the knee. Medial and lateral dislocations result from a varus or valgus force, often seen in contact sports such as rugby or American football, while rotatory dislocations result from twisting in combination with a varus/valgus stress or hyperextension, as may occur in skiing, wrestling, basketball, handball, or soccer [13]. In contact sports such as American football where multiple athletes are simultaneously competing with one another, the team physicians and athletic trainers may not witness the injury in real time. Therefore, asking the player "what happened to your knee" and reviewing instant replay video footage may be extremely helpful for making the diagnosis of knee dislocation.

16.1.4 Evaluation

16.1.4.1 General Considerations

The importance of immediate recognition of knee dislocation lies not with the treatment of instability but the recognition of potential vascular injury or vascular compromise [13]. Green and Allen reported an amputation rate of 86% when vascular repair associated with knee dislocations is delayed more than 8 hours after injury. Conversely, 89% of limbs remained viable when vascular repairs were performed less than 8 hours after injury [19].

On the field, a brief history is obtained from the patient, focusing on the mechanism of injury, location(s) of pain, and if there is any subjective numbness in the extremity. Socks and shoes are removed and athletic shorts pulled proximally to expose both lower extremities from the mid-thigh to the toes so that an adequate physical examination may be performed.

16.1.4.2 Physical Examination

Although the diagnosis may be obvious in cases where the knee is dislocated, signs and symptoms may be subtle in the spontaneously reduced knee. Capsular disruption may prevent the formation of a hemarthrosis, presenting instead as soft tissue swelling or bruising [20]. As soon as the diagnosis of knee dislocation is made or suspected, emergency medical services should be alerted to coordinate transportation to the hospital for further workup.

16.1.4.3 Closed Reduction

In cases where the knee dislocation has not spontaneously reduced, the physician should expeditiously palpate the patient's dorsalis pedis and posterior tibial pulses and check tibial and peroneal nerve motor and sensory function before proceeding with a closed reduction. Gentle inline traction with non-forceful manipulation is successful in reducing the majority of tibiofemoral knee dislocations on the field. Once the knee is reduced, a detailed physical examination is performed (below), including repeating the neurovascular exam. The extremity is then placed into a knee immobilizer or long leg splint, and the patient is transported to the hospital.

Occasionally, the knee will not completely reduce or not reduce at all. Clarke first described what is now known as the dimple sign in 1942 [20]. When the knee is gently brought into extension, a worsening skin dimple between the medial femoral condyle and the medial tibial plateau indicates that the medial femoral condyle has buttonholed through the medial joint capsule and the MCL has become entrapped within the joint. Emergent open reduction in the operating room is the appropriate treatment for irreducible knee dislocations [21].

16.1.4.4 Vascular Examination

The reported incidence of popliteal artery injury varies widely in the literature, from 3.3% to 65% [16, 19, 20, 22–25]. Anterior and posterior dislocations, higher-energy injuries, and dislocations where all four major ligaments are ruptured (Schenk classification KD IV) have been shown to be at higher risk of popliteal artery injury [13, 24].

The dorsalis pedis and posterior tibial pulses are palpated on both feet simultaneously. Asymmetry between the injured and uninjured legs and absent or weak pulses are indicative of arterial injury. In the training room, ankle-brachial index (ABI) should be obtained for both lower extremities. In an ABI examination, the patient is placed supine, and a blood pressure cuff is placed proximal to the ankle of the injured limb. Systolic pressure is determined with a Doppler probe at either the posterior tibial artery or the dorsalis pedis artery. The same measurement is made on the ipsilateral uninjured upper extremity limb. The ABI is calculated as the systolic pressure of the injured limb divided by the systolic pressure of the uninjured limb. Although the ABI measurement may be inaccurate in patients with peripheral arterial disease or vessel calcification, these conditions are rarely seen in the athlete. ABI less than 0.9 is strongly suggestive of vascular injury [5].

Controversy exists regarding the need for advanced imaging with an arteriogram, magnetic resonance arteriography, or computed tomographic angiography versus observation with serial physical examination to detect arterial injury. Part of the reasoning for this controversy is that popliteal artery intimal injuries may occur with knee dislocation and occlude many hours after the injury, resulting in a normal examination initially, only later to have occluded, resulting in vascular compromise. Some authors advocate for selective advanced imaging only in patients with abnormal physical exam or ABI [24–27], while others recommend arteriograms be obtained in every patient regardless of physical exam findings [19, 28]. It has been our practice to obtain computed tomography (CT) angiography in all athletes with knee dislocation, regardless of the physical examination or ABI, since, in our opinion, the potential benefits far outweigh the risks.

16.1.4.5 Neurologic Examination

The reported incidence of nerve injury associated with knee dislocation varies widely in the literature from 5% to 40.0% [15, 23, 29–32]. Most commonly, the common peroneal is the injured nerve, though isolated tibial nerve palsy has been reported [33]. The reported rate of peroneal nerve recovery after knee dislocation also varies; however, a general rule is that approximately one-third of injuries regain complete function, one-third regain partial function, and one-third do not regain any function [34, 35]. Multiple authors have demonstrated improved outcomes in patients with partial versus complete nerve injuries [36, 37]. A detailed neurologic examination includes sensation in the tibial, deep peroneal, and superficial peroneal distributions to light touch, pinprick, and temperature if available. Motor examination tests the flexor and extensor hallucis longus, tibialis anterior, and gastrocnemius to document baseline function [20].

16.1.4.6 Ligament Examination

Ligament testing in the acute multiple ligament-injured knee is often limited due to pain, and one must avoid inadvertent redislocation (e.g., by hyperextending the knee). ACL tears are diagnosed using Lachman's maneuver with the knee at 20° of flexion, while the PCL is evaluated with a posterior drawer test with the knee bent to 90°. Gentle testing of the collateral ligaments should be performed at 0 and 30° of flexion. Performing a dial test with external rotation of the feet at 30 and 90° of flexion is often difficult because of pain but is the best way to clinically evaluate the posterolateral corner [4].

16.1.4.7 Imaging

AP and lateral radiographs of the knee should be obtained to evaluate for fracture and to assess the joint reduction. Widening of the medial or lateral joint space in the AP view may be seen in cases of collateral ligament injury. PCL ruptured knees often demonstrate posterior sagging of the proximal tibia on the lateral view, which may be corrected by placing a soft, rolled blanket under the calf (with the splint or knee immobilizer in place). This maneuver helps remove tension off the posterior neurovascular structures. However, great care must be taken to ensure the rolled blanket does not migrate proximally up to the popliteal fossa, as this could cause obstruction of the popliteal artery and vein.

Magnetic resonance imaging is performed in all athletes with knee dislocation. MRI should be scrutinized not only for damage to the four major ligaments (ACL, PCL, MCL, LCL) but also for posterior capsular tears; avulsion injuries of the iliotibial band, biceps femoris, popliteus, and posterolateral corner; and extensor mechanism injuries.

16.1.5 Treatment

16.1.5.1 Arterial Injuries

Vascular surgery is consulted for emergent evaluation and treatment of all popliteal artery injuries. A dialogue between the orthopedic and vascular surgeon is necessary so that incisions made by the vascular surgeon will be appropriately placed for later ligament reconstruction [4]. The vascular surgeon may also request knee-spanning external fixation be placed to protect the arterial repair. After the leg is prepped and draped, two self-drilling, self-tapping, 5.0-mm-diameter pins are placed bicortically into the femur through stab incisions on the anterolateral aspect of the thigh. The pins should be spaced as far apart as possible to increase the stability of the construct; however, the pin closest to the knee must be at least 7.5 cm above the superior pole of the patella to avoid the suprapatellar pouch, in addition to avoiding future skin incisions [38]. Next, two self-drilling, self-tapping, 5.0-mm-diameter pins are placed bicortically into the tibia through small stab incisions over the anteromedial tibia. Similar to the femur, the pins are maximally spaced, with the most proximal pin at least 10 cm below the knee joint line to avoid future skin incisions. Standard radiolucent bars and pin-to-bar and bar-to-bar connectors are utilized to fashion the spanning external fixation construct. Finally, a large C-arm fluoroscope is brought in to verify proper pin depth and reduction of the knee.

16.1.6 Ligament Injuries

16.1.6.1 General Considerations

Goals of treatment include restoration of knee stability, full range of motion, and return of the athlete to their pre-injury level of play. Surgical treatment is recommended for all athletes, as several studies have demonstrated superiority over nonsurgical treatment of knee dislocations [39–41]. Optimal timing of surgery is 10–14 days after injury, when the soft tissues are amenable to repair and capsular tears have sufficiently healed to prevent fluid extravasation from the knee. It is not uncommon, however, for knee dislocations to initially be unrecognized or misdiagnosed and present several weeks out from injury, especially high school and recreational athletes without a team physician trained in musculoskeletal medicine. This becomes important in planning surgical treatment, as ligament contracture and scarring of the tissue planes prohibits repair of MCL/posteromedial corner and LCL/posterolateral corner when surgery is delayed more than 3 weeks from injury, and it becomes necessary to reconstruct these structures. The PCL and ACL are typically reconstructed regardless of time from injury to surgery, although repair of the PCL may be possible when avulsed from the femoral side or bony avulsion from the tibial side, and acute tibial eminence avulsion fractures of the ACL may also be amenable to repair. For all ligament reconstructions, allograft tissue is favored over autograft since multiple ligaments require reconstruction, autograft sources are limited, and donor site morbidity may be avoided, to minimize the duration of surgery and avoid additional trauma to the knee.

If the athlete is a high-level athlete, and good postoperative rehabilitation is available, then the senior author prefers to repair the collateral ligament(s)/corners, along with cruciate ligament reconstruction at 10–14 days post injury. There is some controversy about the outcomes of primary repair versus reconstruction acutely, as outcomes seem better for reconstruction of the collateral ligaments/corner than repair [42–44]. The senior author prefers repair and will augment the repair with allograft tissue for collateral ligament injury/corner injury, as the anatomy is more complex than just what is reconstructed with a graft. If the knee dislocation is not in an athlete, and/or rehabilitation by an experienced therapist is not available, it is the senior author's preference to reconstruct the PCL and fix/reconstruct the collateral ligament(s)/corner(s) first. Later, after the collateral ligament and corner are healed and the patient recovered from the PCL reconstruction, the ACL can be reconstructed if the patient has instability from insufficiency of the ACL. This approach is preferred, since rehabilitation is less complicated when compared to rehabilitation after reconstructing both cruciates. The PCL is reconstructed first, with the collateral ligament and corner, to reduce the knee in its anatomic tibiofemoral relationship, taking stress off the collateral ligament and corner. Reconstructing the ACL with the PCL torn may result in problems with appropriate ACL tensioning and/or tibiofemoral relationship, and the posterior sag will result in stretching out of the repaired/reconstructed collateral ligament(s)/corner(s).

Informed consent for surgery is obtained from the patient and/or family member and includes a review of the potential risks of surgery with the patient and family members, including neurovascular injury with subsequent risk of bleeding and possible need for transfusion, infection, stiffness, recurrent instability, arthritis, and need for further surgery. Multiligament knee surgeries are scheduled as "first-start" cases, allograft tissue is ordered, and vascular surgery is contacted to ensure their availability should any question of limb perfusion arises during the case.

16.1.7 Surgical Technique

16.1.7.1 Anesthesia and Room Setup

General anesthesia is preferred in all cases, and preoperative femoral and sciatic nerve blocks are often administered to aid postoperative pain control. Surgical instrument tables are situated on the side of the operative leg, while suction, the arthroscopy fluid tower, and C-arm fluoroscopy are positioned on the opposite side of the room. Exam under anesthesia is performed to confirm the ligament injuries suspected on preoperative exam and MRI and includes palpation of the posterior tibial and dorsalis pedis pulses. Doppler ultrasound should be available and utilized when pulses are not easily palpable.

A non-sterile tourniquet is placed as high as possible on the thigh, but is not typically used during the procedure. Care is taken to not create a venous tourniquet that may occur by wrapping the tourniquet tightly. The non-operative leg placed in an Allen stirrup with no varus or valgus stress on the knee, padding of the lateral leg to protect the peroneal nerve, and knee and hip flexion of 30–45°, each. The operative leg is placed in a circumferential thigh holder at the level of the upper to mid-thigh. Using sterile technique, the operative knee is insufflated with 60 cc of normal saline via a lateral mid-patellar approach. The foot of the bed is then lowered all the way and the table padding removed, which allows flexion of the knee to 120°.

The leg is prepped and draped using a sterile technique. Bony anatomy and skin incisions are identified with a skin marker. The anterolateral portal is just above the joint line, 5 mm lateral to the patellar tendon, while the anteromedial portal is at the same level, 1 cm medial to the patellar tendon. The tibial tubercle is identified, and the incision for ACL and PCL reconstructions is marked starting 2 cm medial to the tibial tubercle and extending distally 4 cm. This incision can be used in conjunction with a 2 cm incision centered over the medial epicondyle for MCL reconstruction or can be extended to the distal aspect of the medial epicondyle if a single incision is desired. For LCL repair or reconstruction, a hockey stick incision approximately 12 cm in length is marked out along the mid-IT band, curving distally at the lateral epicondyle and ending midway between Gerdy's tubercle and the fibular head.

16.1.7.2 Diagnostic Arthroscopy

Diagnostic arthroscopy is performed expeditiously, with gravity inflow instead of a pump to minimize the risk of fluid extravasation and compartment syndrome. Care should be taken throughout the case to ensure the calf muscle is supple; should firmness of the lower leg develop at any point during the case, fluid inflow is turned off, and dry arthroscopy is used for the remainder of the case.

A superolateral outflow cannula is placed, and the anterolateral and anteromedial portal incisions are made. Some prefer superomedial outflow cannula, particularly if a lateral collateral/posterolateral corner reconstruction is to be performed. A 30-degree arthroscope with gravity inflow attached is inserted in the anterolateral portal, and an arthroscopic probe is placed in the medial portal. Pictures are taken of the patellofemoral joint, gutters, and medial and lateral compartments, to document all ligament, cartilage, and meniscus injuries. Chondral lesions are debrided to a stable base. Meniscal tears with the capacity to heal are fixed using all-inside or inside-out sutures depending on the length and pattern of the tear.

16.1.7.3 Ligament Repair or Reconstruction

We recommend addressing the PCL and ACL first by drilling the tunnels, passing the grafts, and fixing them on the femoral side before proceeding with open repair or reconstruction of the MCL/posteromedial corner and LCL/posterolateral corner. Bone patellar tendon bone allografts are preferred for ACL and PCL reconstructions, while Achilles tendon allografts are preferred for MCL and LCL reconstructions. It is important to have a trained surgical assistant begin preparing the allografts as soon as the patient enters the operating room to avoid delays in the surgical procedure.

16.1.8 Posterior Cruciate Ligament

16.1.8.1 Repair

Arthroscopic repair of femoral avulsions of the PCL is our preferred treatment strategy, since it is faster and safer than PCL reconstruction, and can better replicate the anatomy (and potentially function) as compared with PCL reconstruction, while outcomes are comparable to, or better than, PCL reconstruction [45, 46].

After debridement of the ACL stump, the femoral insertion of the PCL is debrided to bleeding bone using an arthroscopic shaver. An arthroscopic suture passing device is used to pass a high strength, nonabsorbable suture through the PCL, typically grasping the tissue just above the medial tibial spine. The suture is reloaded and passed a second time through the PCL for a locking Bunnell suture configuration. The suture is shuttled out the anterolateral portal, and then another different-colored high-strength nonabsorbable suture is passed in similar fashion, just proximal to the first suture. A 2 cm incision is made along the posterior border of the vastus medialis, 3 cm proximal to the joint line. A PCL guide is placed through this incision and the anteromedial portal, and two bone tunnels, approximately 8–10 mm apart, are drilled retrograde using a 2.4 mm pin into the PCL femoral insertion. A Hewson suture passer is then used to shuttle each set of sutures out their respective bone tunnels, where they will eventually be tied over a button.

16.1.8.2 Reconstruction

Reconstruction of the PCL is our preferred treatment strategy for midsubstance ruptures and non-bony tibial PCL avulsions. An 11-mm-diameter bone-patellar tendon-bone allograft is fashioned on the back table with the femoral bone plug 20 mm in length and the tibial bone plug 25–30 mm in length. It is critical that the femoral bone plug be no more than 20 mm in length in order to facilitate passing the graft into the knee around the "killer turn." After debridement of the ACL remnant and anterior fibers of the PCL, a posteromedial portal is created under direct visualization using a spinal needle for localization, and a 5.5 mm cannula is inserted. A full-radius shaver is used through the posteromedial portal to resect the PCL to its tibial insertion. Switching to a 70-degree lens helps to visualize the tibial insertion with the arthroscope in the anterolateral portal.

The previously marked 4 cm incision is made on the anteromedial proximal tibia. The PCL tibial guide is placed through the anteromedial portal with the tip toward the lateral aspect of the PCL tibial insertion 7.4 mm anterior to the posterior tibial cortex and one-third of the medial to lateral distance between the medial groove and lateral cartilage point. The angle of the PCL guide is maximally opened (usually around 65°) so that the bullet of the guide is 6–7 cm below the joint line. Opening the guide to at least 65° will ensure adequate spacing between the PCL and ACL tibial tunnels and minimizes the angle of the so-called killer turn at the tibial tunnel aperture into the joint. A guidewire is then carefully drilled into the joint under direct visualization, choking up on the wire with the wire driver and gently drilling through the far cortex to prevent plunging into the joint and nearby neurovascular structures. Some PCL tibial guides have a flat surface to catch the guidewire, to reduce neurovascular injury by the guidewire. Fluoroscopy is brought in to check the position of the wire. After the proper position of the wire is confirmed, an 11 mm cannulated fully fluted reamer is then used to drill the tibial tunnel under arthroscopic visualization while covering the tip of the guidewire with a curette or a PCL tibial guidewire protector. Once the reamer contacts the far cortex, remove the guidewire before reaming into the joint.

The femoral PCL guide enters the joint through the anteromedial portal with the tip placed 7.9 mm proximal to the distal articular cartilage and 7.4 mm posterior from the trochlear point. A 2 cm incision is made along the posterior border of the vastus medialis, about 3 cm above the joint line, and the bullet of the guide is placed on the femur. A Beath needle is drilled into the joint outside-in, followed by retrograde drilling of the femoral tunnel with a cannulated 11 mm fully fluted reamer. To ensure that the graft will pass smoothly into the joint and femoral tunnels, the periosteum at all four apertures of the tunnels is liberally cleared with electrocautery. An 18-gauge metal wire is used to shuttle the sutures for the graft through the tunnels by bending the wire in half and pulling it retrograde through the femoral and tibial tunnels so that the looped end of the wire rests at the proximal tibia. The BPTB shuttling sutures and graft are then pulled up the tibial tunnel and through the joint until the femoral bone plug sits flush in the femoral tunnel. An 7 x 20-mm-diameter metal femoral interference screw is placed in the femoral tunnel from outside-in to fix the graft in the femur. When performing collateral ligament repair/reconstruction, PCL reconstruction is halted at this point to address these other structures. Once the ACL is fixed on the femoral side, and the collateral ligaments/corners are prepared for fixation, attention is returned to the PCL. While performing an anterior drawer maneuver with the knee at 90° of flexion such that the proximal medial tibia is 1 cm anterior to the medial femoral condyle, a 9 × 20 mm metal interference screw is placed into the tibial tunnel under direct visualization to secure the PCL graft in place.

16.1.8.3 Anterior Cruciate Ligament Reconstruction

A 10-mm bone-patellar tendon-bone allograft is fashioned on the back table with a 20-mm femoral bone plug and 25-mm tibial bone plug. To prevent graft-tunnel mismatch, the tendinous length of the allograft should be matched to the patient's height following the algorithm of Brown et al. [47]. A notchplasty is performed to create an upside-down "U"-shaped notch and allow clear visualization of the back wall. The tibial drill guide is inserted through the anteromedial portal with the tip two-fifths of the medial-lateral interspinous distance, centered in the remaining ACL footprint. The ACL drill guide is placed on the tibia so that after reaming the tibial tunnel, there will be at least a 1 cm bone bridge between the ACL and PCL tunnels (typically 45–50°). A Beath needle is then drilled into the joint. Once the proper location of the wire is confirmed, a cannulated, fully fluted, constant diameter 10 mm reamer is used to create the tibial tunnel.

A spinal needle is placed through the anteromedial portal to visualize the trajectory toward the femoral insertion of the ACL. Frequently, it is necessary to create an accessory anteromedial portal which is more medial and distal than the original AM portal to improve the angle of drilling the femoral tunnel and prevent blowing out the back wall. A 7 mm offset drill guide is then placed through the accessory AM portal and hooked on the back wall. The knee is flexed to 120°, and a Beath pin is drilled through the femoral insertion of the ACL, 24.8% of the proximal to distal distance measured from the proximal femoral cortex, and 28.5% of the anterior to posterior distance, measured from the top of the notch. The femoral tunnel is then drilled over the Beath pin using a cannulated hemispherical reamer to a depth of 23 mm. A passing suture is placed through the Beath pin, which is pulled out the lateral femoral cortex. The periosteum and soft tissue at the apertures of the tibial tunnel are removed with electrocautery, and then the passing suture is pulled from the joint down and out the tibial tunnel. The BPTB graft is shuttled up into the knee and then into the femoral tunnel with the cancellous surface of the graft oriented anteriorly. A nitinol wire is placed colinearly between the cancellous surface of the graft and the anterior wall of the femoral tunnel, and a 7 mm diameter metal screw with a rounded head is inserted to fix the graft on the femoral side. After the PCL and collateral ligaments have been secured, the tibial bone plug of the ACL is secured with a 9 × 20 mm metal interference screw.

16.1.8.4 Lateral Collateral Ligament/Posterolateral Corner

Repair of the lateral collateral ligament and posterolateral corner is our preferred treatment when surgery is performed less than 3 weeks out from injury, in cases of tendon avulsions from the bone, and when the tissue quality affords a robust repair. Injury patterns may vary substantially; therefore, thoughtful review of the preoperative MRI is essential for surgical planning. Care is taken to repair all damaged structures back to their anatomic insertions using double-loaded suture anchors with heavy nonabsorbable suture. Locking, Krackow suture configuration is utilized when suturing all damaged structures.

Reconstruction of the posterolateral corner is planned for all delayed surgical procedures but is also performed in acute cases (less than 3 weeks) when the tissue quality is poor, and it is not possible to obtain a robust repair. Because the final decision on repair or reconstruction will be made intraoperatively, Achilles tendon allograft must be made available for all knee dislocation surgeries regardless of the time from injury.

Our surgical technique for reconstruction of the posterolateral corner essentially mirrors the technique described by LaPrade et al., particularly for high-grade posterolateral injuries. For low-grade posterolateral corner injuries, that is, grade 3 injuries with lower degrees of laxity, Arciero's modification of Larson's lateral reconstruction through the fibular head is utilized to minimize the extra dissection of tissues to access the posterolateral aspect of the tibia [48]. The reader is directed to the original article referenced at the end of this chapter for a detailed description of the procedure [49]; however, an abbreviated summary of the procedure is discussed in the following paragraphs.

An Achilles tendon allograft is split into two grafts, each with a 9 mm × 18 mm bone block, and the tendinous portion trimmed to fit through a 7 mm graft sizer and tubularized with #2 nonabsorbable suture. The previously marked skin incision is made, and full-thickness skin flaps are developed above the fascia. The common peroneal nerve is identified through a fascial split posterior to the biceps femoris and approximately 2 cm below the fibular head. A neurolysis is performed so that the nerve is freely mobile and the nerve is protected throughout the remainder of the case.

The interval between the lateral head of the gastrocnemius and soleus is developed bluntly to identify the posterior fibular head and posterolateral surface of the tibia. Two incisions are made in line with the fibers of the iliotibial band, the first centered at the lateral epicondyle and the second centered 1 cm proximal to the tip of the fibula. The femoral insertion of the LCL is identified through the anterior fascial incision, 1.4 mm proximal and 3.1 mm posterior to the lateral femoral epicondyle, and a Beath pin is drilled transversely across the femur and through the skin on the medial side of the knee. The femoral insertion of the popliteus tendon is then identified 18.5 mm distal and posterior to the LCL, and a Beath pin is placed across the femur parallel to the LCL pin. Twenty millimeter length blind tunnels are then drilled over the top of each wire with a 9-mm-diameter cannulated reamer. A K-wire is then drilled from the fibular insertion of the LCL, 8.2 mm posterior to the anterior border of the fibular head and 28.4 mm distal to the tip of the fibular styloid process, aiming toward the tip of the surgeon's finger which is placed on the posteromedial downslope of the fibular styloid, at the attachment of the popliteofibular ligament. A 7 mm cannulated reamer is drilled over the K-wire through the fibular head, while a posteriorly placed retractor protects the peroneal nerve. Next, an ACL guide is placed on the bone of the proximal tibia, anterior to the popliteus, with the tip approximately 1 cm medial and 1 cm proximal to the posterior aperture of the fibular tunnel, and the bullet of the guide just distal and medial to Gerdy's tubercle. The guidewire is drilled and checked with fluoroscopy, and then a 10 mm fully fluted reamer is used to drill the tibial tunnel.

After all four tunnels have been drilled, the two Achilles allograft bone plugs are secured in the femur with 7 × 20 mm metal interference screws. The tendinous portion of both grafts are shuttled under the iliotibial band. A mosquito clamp to puncture the posterolateral capsule just above the lateral meniscus and pull the popliteus graft to the posterior aspect of the knee. The popliteus graft is then shuttled through the tibial tunnel from posterior to anterior using a Hewson suture passer to shuttle the sutures. The graft from the LCL insertion is passed superficial to the popliteus allograft tendon, passed from anterior to posterior through the fibula, and then shuttled from posterior to anterior through the tibial tunnel. After the PCL graft has been fixed to the tibia, a valgus force is applied to the knee in 20° of flexion, and the LCL graft is fixed to the fibula with a 7 × 20 mm metal interference screw. Finally, with the knee placed in 60° of flexion and neutral rotation, the tendinous ends of both grafts are fixed in the tibial tunnel with a 9 × 30 mm interference screw.

16.1.8.5 Medial Collateral Ligament/Posteromedial Corner

Similar to the lateral side of the knee, repair of the medial collateral ligament and posteromedial corner with suture anchors is our preferred technique when the MCL is avulsed from its femoral origin, the surgery is performed within 3 weeks of injury, and the tissue is of good quality for a robust repair. In all other cases, reconstruction of the MCL with an Achilles allograft as described by Marx et al. is our preferred technique [50]. The reader is referred to Marx's original article for a detailed description of the procedure; however, key points of the operation are summarized below.

An Achilles allograft is fashioned with a 9 × 18 mm bone block on the back Table. A 3 cm longitudinal incision is made centered over the medial epicondyle. The fascia is cut in line with the skin incision, and a subfascial tunnel is created distally toward the proximal tibial incision, under the sartorius and hamstring tendons. The origin of the superficial MCL is identified 3.2 mm proximal and 4.8 mm posterior to the medial epicondyle, and a Beath pin is driven across the femur, aiming slightly anteriorly to avoid the intercondylar notch. A nonabsorbable suture is passed through the subfascial tunnel and wrapped around the Beath pin. The isometric point on the tibia is identified by cycling the knee, typically posterior to the pes anserine insertion and marked with electrocautery. A cannulated 9 mm reamer is used to create a 20 mm blind tunnel in the femur over the Beath pin. The periosteum overlying the aperture of the femoral tunnel is removed with electrocautery. The Achilles bone block is pulled into the femoral tunnel and fixed with a 7 × 20 mm metal interference screw. The tendinous portion of the allograft is passed through the subfascial tunnel. After the PCL and LCL have been secured, the knee is flexed to 20°, a varus force is applied to the knee, and the graft is fixed at the previously marked isometric point with a 4.5 mm cortical screw and 17 mm spiked washer.

16.1.8.6 Postoperative Rehabilitation

At the conclusion of the surgical procedure, the patient is placed in a hinged knee brace locked in full extension after surgery and made non-weight-bearing with crutches for 6 weeks. If a standard brace is used, a couple of towels are placed between the upper calf and brace to provide an anterior directed force, to reduce the sag on the PCL. Alternatively, a brace with an anterior directed, spring-loaded force may be applied to reduce gravity forces that may result in stretching out of the PCL. Two weeks after surgery, the patient can unlock the brace to work on range of motion from 0 to 60°. At 4 weeks postoperatively, range of motion is increased to 0–90°. After 6 weeks, the brace is unlocked to allow full range of motion, and gradual progression of weight-bearing is allowed. The brace may be discontinued after 8 weeks when the patient has demonstrated functional quadriceps control. Running is delayed until at least 6 months after surgery. Patients typically return to sports 9–12 months after surgery.

16.1.8.7 Outcomes

Knee dislocation in athletes is an uncommon injury. Most of the available literature consists of level 4 evidence from retrospective case series with small numbers of patients and a variety of injury patterns and mechanisms, including high-energy motor vehicle collisions, low-energy sports injuries, and ultralow-energy dislocations in morbidly obese patients, limiting the applicability of some of the study findings to athletes. The prognosis for knee dislocations from sports injuries may be better than high-energy and ultralow-energy mechanisms; however, the prognosis for return to sports is fair to guard at best.

Richter and colleagues retrospectively reviewed 89 knee dislocations from all mechanisms of injury managed either conservatively or with surgery, 17 (19%) of whom dislocated their knee playing sports. Lysholm and IKDC scores were noted to be higher in the sports injury patients; however, the rate of return to sports among all patients was only 45%. Of these patients, 57% returned to the same level of play, 40% to a lower level of play, and 3% to a higher level of play [39]. Engebretsen and colleagues prospectively followed 85 patients for 2–9 years after surgical treatment of knee dislocation, of which 40 were low-energy sports-related injuries. Patients with knee dislocation performed significantly better in the triple hop test but showed similar Tegner, Lysholm, and IKDC scores and no significant difference in the one-leg hop test, crossover hop test, and 6 m timed hop test. The mean age of the sports injury patients, however, was significantly greater than the high-energy knee dislocations (47 vs. 38 years old), limiting the applicability of these findings to younger athletes [36].

Two retrospective case series have specifically been limited to knee dislocations in athletes. Shelbourne et al. reported 21 knee dislocations sustained in a variety of sports, including American football, wrestling, rugby, softball, running, and hurdling. Five patients were managed conservatively, while the other 16 underwent either repair or reconstruction of the torn ligaments. Seventy-seven percent of their patients were able to return to sports, but only 19% at the same level. Improved ROM was noted in patients treated with an accelerated rehabilitation protocol. Hirschmann and colleagues retrospectively reviewed their experience surgically treating knee dislocations in 26 elite athletes, of which 13 injured their knee playing sports. Medial and lateral ligament injuries were repaired in all patients, and the ACL and PCL were reconstructed with autograft BPTB and quadriceps tendon, respectively. Twenty-four patients were available for follow-up an average of 8 years after surgery. Seventy-nine percent of patients returned to sports, and 42% of these returned to their pre-injury level of play. Patients who underwent surgery greater than 40 days after injury had worse outcome scores and lower rates of return to sports than those who underwent early surgery.

Improved surgical outcomes with early surgery for knee dislocation has been demonstrated in several other studies. A systematic review by Levy et al. found five studies comparing early surgery (less than 3 weeks) with late surgery. Early treatment resulted in higher mean Lysholm scores (90 vs. 82) and a higher percentage of excellent/good IKDC scores (47% vs. 31%), as well as higher sports activity scores (89 vs. 69) on the Knee Outcome Survey [3].

16.2 Conclusion

Knee dislocation is a rare, potentially limb-threating injury in the athlete. The physician must have a high index of suspicion to avoid missing the diagnosis in spontaneously reduced knees. On-the-field management includes gentle closed reduction of dislocated knees, with splinting and transfer to the hospital. Magnetic resonance imaging and angiography are recommended for all athletes to evaluate for vascular injury and assist in preoperative planning. Optimal surgical timing is 10–14 days after injury, with repair or reconstruction of all damaged structures. ACL reconstruction with allograft is recommended for all athletes. The PCL may be repaired when avulsed from the femur or bony avulsion from the tibia but is reconstructed for other tear patterns. The LCL/posterolateral corner and MCL/posteromedial corners are repaired when surgery is performed within 3 weeks of injury, the tissue quality is good, and the ligaments have avulsed from both; in all other cases, reconstruction with allograft is recommended. Nine to twelve months of rehabilitation is typically required before returning to sports. Published rates of return to play range between 50 and 80%.

References

1. Peskun CJ, et al. Diagnosis and management of knee dislocations. Phys Sportsmed. 2010;38(4):101–11. http://www.ncbi.nlm.nih.gov/pubmed/21150149
2. Kerr ZY, et al. Dislocation/separation injuries among US high school athletes in 9 selected sports: 2005-2009. Clin J Sport Med. 2011;21(2):101–8.
3. Levy BA, Stannard JP, et al. Decision making in the multiligament-injured knee: an evidence-based systematic review. Arthroscopy. 2009b;25(4):430–8. https://doi.org/10.1016/j.arthro.2009.01.008.
4. Cole B, Harner C. The multiple ligament injured knee. Clin Sports Med. 1999;18(1):241–62.
5. Levy BA, Fanelli GC, et al. Controversies in the treatment of knee dislocations and multiligament reconstruction. J Am Acad Orthop Surg. 2009a;17(4):197–206.
6. Hwang MD, Piefer JW, Lubowitz JH. Anterior cruciate ligament tibial footprint anatomy: systematic review of the 21st century literature. Arthroscopy. 2012;28(5):728–34. https://doi.org/10.1016/j.arthro.2011.11.025.
7. Bernard M, et al. Femoral insertion of the ACL. Radiographic quadrant method. Am J Knee Surg. 1997;10:14–22.
8. Anderson CJ, et al. Arthroscopically pertinent anatomy of the anterolateral and posteromedial bundles of the posterior cruciate ligament. J Bone Joint Surg Am. 2012;94(21):1936–45. http://www.ncbi.nlm.nih.gov/pubmed/23138236%5Cn http://ovidsp.tx.ovid.com/ovftpdfs/FPDDNCGCHFIAGI00/fs046/ovft/live/gv023/00004623/00004623-201211070-00003.pdf
9. LaPrade RF, et al. The anatomy of the medial part of the knee. J Bone Joint Surg Am. 2007;89(9):2000–10. http://jbjs.org/article.aspx?doi=10.2106/JBJS.F.01176%5Cnpapers2://publication/doi/10.2106/JBJS.F.01176

10. LaPrade RF, et al. The posterolateral attachments of the knee: a qualitative and quantitative morphologic analysis of the fibular collateral ligament, popliteus tendon, popliteofibular ligament, and lateral gastrocnemius tendon. Am J Sports Med. 2003;31(6):854–60. http://www.ncbi.nlm.nih.gov/pubmed/14623649
11. Musahl V, et al. The influence of meniscal and anterolateral capsular injury on knee laxity in patients with anterior cruciate ligament injuries. Am J Sports Med. 2016;20(10):1–6.
12. Matava MJ, Sethi NS, Totty WG. Proximity of the posterior cruciate ligament insertion to the popliteal artery as a function of the knee flexion angle: implications for posterior cruciate ligament reconstruction. Arthroscopy. 2000;16(8):796–804. http://www.ncbi.nlm.nih.gov/pubmed/11078535
13. Fanelli GC, Orcutt DR, Edson CJ. Current concepts. The multiple-ligament injured knee: evaluation, treatment, and results. Arthroscopy. 2005;21(4):471–86.
14. Kadiyala RK, et al. The blood supply of the common peroneal nerve in the popliteal fossa. J Bone Joint Surg [Br]. 2005;87_B(3):337–42.
15. Kennedy JC. Complete dislocation of the knee joint. J Bone Joint Surg Am. 1963;45–A(5):889–904.
16. Shelbourne K, et al. Low-velocity knee dislocation. Orthop Rev. 1991;20(11):995–1004.
17. McCoy G, et al. Vascular injury associated with low-velocity dislocations of the knee. J Bone Joint Surg Am. 1987;69(2):285–7.
18. Schenck R. Classification of knee dislocations. Oper Tech Sports Med. 2003;11(3):193–8.
19. Green NE, Allen BL. Vascular injuries associated with dislocation of the knee. J Bone Joint Surg Am. 1977;59–A(2):236–9.
20. Lachman JR, Rehman S, Do PSP. Traumatic Knee dislocations treatment. Orthop Clin North Am. 2017;2015 https://doi.org/10.1016/j.ocl.2015.06.004.
21. Wand JS. A physical sign denoting irreducibility of a dislocated knee. J Bone Joint Surg. 1989;71(5):862. http://www.ncbi.nlm.nih.gov/pubmed/2584265
22. Natsuhara KM, et al. What is the frequency of vascular injury after knee dislocation ? Clin Orthop Relat Res. 2014;472:2615–20.
23. Sisto DJ, Warren RF. Complete knee dislocation. A follow-up study of operative treatment. Clin Orthop Relat Res. 1985;(198):94–101. http://www.ncbi.nlm.nih.gov/pubmed/4028570
24. Stannard JP, et al. Vascular injuries in knee dislocations: the role of physical examination in determining the need for arteriography. J Bone Joint Surg Am. 2004;86–A(5):910–5.
25. Treiman GS, et al. Examination of the patient with a knee dislocation. The case for selective arteriography. Arch Surg. 1992;127(9):1056–62. 3. http://www.ncbi.nlm.nih.gov/pubmed/1514907
26. Hollis JD, Daley BJ. 10-year review of knee dislocations : is arteriography. J Trauma. 2005;59(3):672–6.
27. Klineberg EO, et al. The role of arteriography in assessing popliteal artery injury in knee dislocations. J Trauma. 2004;56(4):786–90.
28. McCutchan JDS, Gillham NR. Injury to the popliteal artery associated with dislocation of the knee: palpable distal pulses do not negate the requirement for arteriography. Injury. 1989;20(5):307–10.
29. Liow RYL, et al. Ligament repair and reconstruction in traumatic dislocation of the knee. J Bone Joint Surg [Br]. 2001;85–B(6):845–51.
30. Meyers M, Harvey JP. Traumatic dislocation of the knee joint. A study of eighteen cases. J Bone Joint Surg Am. 1971;53–A(1):16–29.
31. Shields L, Mital M, Cave E. Complete dislocation of the knee: experience at the massachusetts general hospital. J Trauma. 1969;9(3):192–215.
32. Twaddle BC, Bidwell TA, Chapman JR. Knee dislocations : where are the lesions ? A prospective evaluation of surgical findings in 63 cases. J Orthop Trauma. 2003;17(3):198–202.
33. Frassica FJ, et al. Dislocation of the knee. Clin Orthop Relat Res. 1991;(263):200–5.
34. Niall DM, Nutton RW, Keating JF. Palsy of the common peroneal nerve after traumatic dislocation of the knee. J Bone Joint Surg [Br]. 2005;87–B(5):664–7.
35. Peskun CJ, Whelan DB. Outcomes of operative and nonoperative treatment of multiligament knee injuries: an evidence-based review. Sports Med Arthrosc Rev. 2011;19(2):167–73.
36. Engebretsen L, et al. Outcome after knee dislocations: a 2–9 years follow-up of 85 consecutive patients. Knee Surg Sports Traumatol Arthrosc. 2009;17:1013–26.
37. Krych AJ, et al. Is peroneal nerve injury associated with worse function after knee dislocation ? Clin Orthop Relat Res. 2014;472(9):2630–6.
38. Beltran MJ, et al. The safe zone for external fixator pins in the femur. J Orthop Trauma. 2012;26(11):643–7. http://content.wkhealth.com/linkback/openurl?sid=WKPTLP:landingpage&an=00005131-201211000-00007%5Cnpapers2://publication/doi/10.1097/BOT.0b013e31824aed95
39. Richter M, et al. Comparison of surgical repair or reconstruction of the cruciate ligaments versus nonsurgical treatment in patients with traumatic knee dislocations. Am J Sports Med. 2002;30(5):718–27.
40. Ríos A, et al. Results after treatment of traumatic knee dislocations: a report of 26 cases. J Trauma. 2003;55(3):489–94.
41. Wong CH, et al. Knee dislocations - a retrospective study comparing operative versus closed immobilization treatment outcomes. Knee Surg Sports Traumatol Arthrosc. 2004;12(6):540–4.
42. Levy BA, et al. Repair versus reconstruction of the fibular collateral ligament and posterolateral corner in the multiligament-injured knee. Am J Sports Med. 2010;38(4):804–9.
43. Stannard JP, et al. 2012. Posteromedial corner injury in knee dislocations posteromedial corner injury in knee dislocations. (November).

44. Stannard JP, et al. 2000. The posterolateral corner of the knee repair versus reconstruction. 3–8.
45. DiFelice GS, Lissy M, Haynes P. When to arthroscopically repair the torn posterior cruciate ligament. Clin Orthop Relat Res. 2012;470(3):861–8.
46. Wheatley WB, et al. Arthroscopic posterior cruciate ligament repair. Arthroscopy. 2002;18(7):695–702.
47. Brown JA, et al. Avoiding allograft length mismatch during anterior cruciate ligament reconstruction: patient height as an indicator of appropriate graft length. Am J Sports Med. 2007;35(6):986–9. http://www.ncbi.nlm.nih.gov/pubmed/17337725
48. Rios CG, et al. Posterolateral corner reconstruction of the knee evaluation of a technique with clinical outcomes and stress radiography. Am J Sports Med. 2010;38(8):1564–74.
49. Laprade RF, Johansen S, Engebretsen L. Outcomes of an anatomic posterolateral knee reconstruction surgical technique. J Bone Joint Surg AmJ. 2011;93(92):16–22.
50. Marx RG, Hetsroni I. Surgical technique: medial collateral ligament reconstruction using achilles allograft for combined knee ligament injury. Clin Orthop Relat Res. 2012;470(3):798–805.

Complications in Complex Knee Ligament Injuries

17

Sung-Jae Kim and Min Jung

17.1 Introduction

Complications in complex knee ligament injuries consist of a wide variety of conditions. Complex knee ligament injuries are usually the result of knee dislocations following high energy injury, and complications are frequent. Diagnosis of these injuries often can be difficult, because some of dislocated knees are reduced spontaneously and could appear to be benign on plain radiographs. Accordingly, in situations where complex knee ligament injuries are suspected based on mechanism of injury, condition of soft tissue injury, and severity of the ligament instability, early recognition and thorough neurovascular assessments are necessary to prevent serious complications. In this chapter, relatively common complications associated with complex knee ligament injuries are described.

17.2 Persistent Instability

Persistent instability arises as one of the common complication in complex knee ligament injury. Instability is continued in almost all patients, who were treated with nonsurgical method and even with surgical treatment. Some of patients who were treated conservatively are capable of performing reasonable amount of various daily activities without much difficulty although they experience persistent instability. This capability in daily activities by some stability is thought to be the result of capsular adhesion or scarring rather than mechanical stabilization by ligament [1]. Also in surgically treated patients, persistent instability present in at least one plane has been discovered in 42% on average [2]. Plancher and Siliski reported that 76.9% of conservatively treated patients and 80% of patients with surgical treatment had returned to their previous occupations [3]. However, returning to sport activity showed substantially lower rate in the conservatively treated group (31%) than the surgically treated group (74%). Other studies also noted similar results of higher IKDC score and significantly more patients returning to sports in surgically treated patients [4].

In analysis of Becker et al. on 82 cases with complex knee ligament injury, they found that there were 90% of anterior cruciate ligament involvement, 79% of posterior cruciate ligament involvement, 78% of posterolateral corner involvement, and 28% having accompanying medial collateral ligament injury [5]. Persistent instability occurring postoperatively could be caused by negligence of these concurrent injuries and malalignment arising from poor correction of combined extra-articular fracture. Woodmass et al. reported that about 47.8% and 17.4% of

S.-J. Kim · M. Jung (✉)
Department of Orthopedic Surgery, Yonsei University College of Medicine, Seoul, Republic of Korea
e-mail: sungjaekim@yuhs.ac; jmin1103@yuhs.ac

F. Margheritini et al. (eds.), *Complex Knee Ligament Injuries*,
https://doi.org/10.1007/978-3-662-58245-9_17

failed reconstructions of complex knee ligament injury are induced by unaddressed concurrent ligament injury and malalignment, respectively [6]. Thorough radiologic evaluation of all accompanying ligament injuries is necessary preoperatively to prevent failure after the surgery, and for any suspected injury, it needs to be reevaluated prior to surgery by performing stress tests after inducing anesthesia. In patients without correction of malalignment in the lower limb, persistent postoperative instability may be caused by sustained abnormal force applied to reconstructed tendons. Accordingly, it is necessary to maintain the normal alignment of lower limb to prevent persistent instability after complex knee ligament injuries.

Consequently, surgical treatment has significantly better outcome than conservative management in preventing persistent instability after complex knee ligament injuries. So thorough evaluation of combined ligament injury followed by appropriate surgical treatment for instability is necessary.

17.3 Arthrofibrosis

Arthrofibrosis is the most common long-term complication after complex knee ligament injury. Severe loss of knee motion following injury can be a more serious complication than persistent instability. This is also a substantial source of pain and disability. The prevalence has ranged from 5% to 71% in the published literature [7]. Recent studies have reported 9~11% of the rates of manipulation or arthrolysis after surgical treatment [8].

Several risk factors of arthrofibrosis have been discussed in various studies [1], including severity of injury, excessive scarring due to immobilization, complex regional pain syndrome, infection, heterotopic ossification and surgical factors such as tunnel placement, excessive graft tension, and timing of surgery. Reconstruction of both the anterior cruciate ligament and posterior cruciate ligament was reported to be associated with higher risk of loss of motion (up to 45%). Reconstruction of medial collateral ligament also can cause higher rate of motion loss after surgery involving both flexion and extension. Meanwhile, repair of lateral collateral ligament has not been known to influence significantly on postoperative range of motion. Intercondylar notch scarring is one of the common causes of extension block after ligament reconstruction. Heterotopic ossification can occur following musculoskeletal trauma. The incidence of radiological heterotopic ossification has been reported as 26~44% [8]. About 10% of heterotopic ossification after complex knee ligament injury requires management for loss of motion with less than 70° of flexion. Timing and type of surgery had no significant effect on the degree of heterotopic ossification formation. The role of prophylactic anti-inflammatory drugs or low-dose radiation has not been clearly identified in the complex knee ligament injury. Timing of surgery is a considerable risk factor of arthrofibrosis. Harner et al. reported about 21% manipulation rate for patients who underwent surgery for complex knee ligament injury before 3 weeks from the time of injury, whereas no manipulation was performed for patients who underwent surgery after 3 weeks [4].

17.4 Vascular Injury

Vascular injury is a fatal and not uncommon complication of complex knee ligament injuries. Recent systematic review showed that the frequency of vascular injury is 18% in overall, of which high energy injury ranges from 7% to 43% and low energy knee injury ranges from 5% to 11% [9]. A thorough and complete vascular examination should be performed at initial evaluation of a knee with complex knee ligament injuries. Failure to recognize a vascular injury can cause serious consequences such as limb dysfunction and amputation. Vascular lesions include intimal injury, arterial occlusions, avulsion injuries, ruptures, or transections. Vascular assessment includes physical examination, the use of the ankle-brachial index, duplex ultrasound, conventional angiography, and CT angiography. When a patient presents with a cool and pulseless dysvascular limb, immediate vascular intervention is needed. However, when a patient has a palpable but asymmetric pulse, and asymmetric warmth and color of the limb, further assessment is needed. The ankle-brachial index lower than 0.9 is considered abnormal requiring angiography, and patients with ankle-brachial index of 0.9 or greater have low risk of major arterial injury. But because delayed thrombus is also a risk, serial vascular evaluation at least every 4–6 h for a minimum of 48 h is necessary [10]. Duplex ultrasonography is a highly sensitive and specific test for detecting arterial injury but is operator-dependent. CT angiography is a minimally invasive method with high sensitivity and specificity for evaluating arterial injuries with advantages over conventional angiography.

The popliteal artery is the most commonly injured because it is tethered by the tendinous hiatus of the adductor magnus muscle proximally and the tendinous arch of the soleus distally [5]. Other possible injured vessels included the medial genicular artery, anterior tibial artery, posterior tibial artery, superficial femoral artery, and common femoral artery. Restoration of blood flow is the mainstay goal of the treatment. Surgical options include primary end-to-end anastomosis, saphenous vein interposition graft, and vein patch angioplasty. Balloon angioplasty and endovascular stent placement are other treatment options for vascular injuries. Recent systematic review found that 80% of vascular injuries underwent surgical intervention, and of these patients, 12% of vascular injuries resulted in amputation [9]. Early recognition and rapid intervention are keys for treatment of vascular injuries. Delays exceeding 8 h in treatment of vascular injury resulted in an amputation rate of 86% [11]. In addition, care must be taken to avoid intraoperative iatrogenic vascular injury or damage to vascular reconstructions.

17.5 Neurological Injury

Neurological injury is another serious complication frequently encountered in complex knee ligament injuries as well as vascular injury. The incidence of neurological injuries following complex knee ligament injuries has been reported variously. A recent systemic review reported that the frequency of nerve injuries after knee dislocation was 25% [9]. Both the common peroneal nerve and the tibial nerve can be involved, but the common peroneal nerve injury was reported to be more frequently injured. Compared with the tibial nerve located within the popliteal fossa surrounded by popliteal muscle and fascia, the common peroneal nerve is more vulnerable to injury due to its anatomical characteristics, which is tethered around the proximal fibula. The common mechanism of injury of the peroneal nerve is usually a combination of varus, hyperextension, and tibia external rotation forces, which is usually observed in posterolateral corner injury of the knee. This subsequently causes the traction or stretching of the nerve.

Thorough neurological examination should be carried out in patients suspected of complex knee ligament injuries. All motor and sensory functions of the common peroneal nerve and the tibial nerves should be tested even in the case which is spontaneously reduced after knee dislocation. The clinical manifestations of the peroneal nerve injury appear as a dysfunction of the innervated anatomical structure, depending on whether superficial or deep division is injured. It usually results in foot drop and gait impairment, as well as sensory disturbances. In the same way, tibial nerve injury may result in the disturbance in the sense of where the nerve innervates and motor dysfunction including loss of ankle plantar flexion, loss of toe flexion, and weakened inversion. Furthermore, compartment syndrome should be differentiated from a neurological injury, since both motor and sensory disturbance can be caused by compartment syndrome. As assessment tool, electromyography and nerve conduction velocity studies are commonly used assessment tools to determine the severity and location of injury, as well as predicting prognosis. However, since pathologic findings secondary to nerve injury are not differentiated for approximately 3 weeks after injury, they have limited value in immediate post-injury period. These studies are useful in subsequently comparing the progress of recovery at 3 and

6 months and determining whether further treatment is needed. Magnetic resonance imaging (MRI) can help to detect the presence and location of a nerve injury, and ultrasonography helps to discriminate between complete and incomplete interruption of nerves.

Although various treatment modalities have been proposed, treatment of neurological injury in complex knee ligament injuries remains controversial. These include physical therapy, neurolysis, nerve repair, nerve grafting, and tendon transfer. Every patient with common peroneal nerve injury should begin to be treated with ankle-foot-orthosis to prevent equinovarus deformity. Exploration and neurolysis is indicated if early surgical treatment of concomitant ligament injuries is planned, evidence of complete nerve injury is identified, or spontaneous recovery is unlikely. In the case of incomplete nerve injury, serial clinical and electro-diagnostic test can be performed waiting to see nerve regeneration, but opinions on the observation period vary between studies [10]. Primary nerve repair is direct end-to-end reanastomosis procedure performed when the nerve is not in continuity and the extent of lesion is short. However, due to the mechanism of injury characterized by traction or stretching of the nerve, the damaged nerve can be too long to repair without tension. If it is not feasible to repair damaged nerve with tension-free fashion, nerve graft is recommended. Tendon transfer can be used to restore function when all of the above-mentioned treatments fail or are not applicable or in combination with other treatments. The posterior tibialis tendon is the most commonly used tendon. Despite these various treatment modalities, overall prognosis of neurological injury is not satisfactory. A systematic review reported that 87% of patients with an incomplete peroneal nerve injury regained full motor function, while 38% of patients with a complete peroneal nerve injury regained the ability to dorsiflex the ankle against gravity [12]. In contrast, tibial nerve injury is reported to have a relatively good prognosis. Kim et al. reported that most of their patients (95%, 36 of 38) with tibial nerve injuries at knee or leg level recovered motor grade 3 or better function after surgical treatment [13].

17.6 Compartment Syndrome

Compartment syndrome can occur at the time of injury or after revascularization procedure due to ischemia induced by vascular injury. Incidence of compartment syndrome at complex knee ligament injury is unclear, but one retrospective study reported that 16% of compartment syndrome occurred following multiligamentous knee injury [5]. When compartment syndrome is diagnosed, a fasciotomy should be done, and wounds are closed before any reconstruction of ligaments. Compartment syndrome can also occur after arthroscopic knee surgery, because capsular disruption or fascial defect can happen after complex knee ligament injury. Extravasation of arthroscopic fluid can be a potential cause of compartment syndrome in arthroscopic surgery. Delayed arthroscopic ligament reconstruction until capsular and fascial healing for 1–2 weeks may decrease the risk of compartment syndrome. Low flow pump or no pump, dry arthroscopy can be another strategy to reduce the risk.

17.7 Miscellaneous Complications

Complications such as wound problem, complex regional pain syndrome, deep vein thrombosis, and pulmonary embolism are not the only problems found in complex knee ligament injuries. However, these miscellaneous complications can give rise to significant morbidity and they should be kept in mind during the treatment process for complex knee ligament injuries.

Wound complication can be a fatal problem for patients with complex knee ligament injuries that require a variety of surgical treatments. If the immediate surgical intervention is not planned, the surgeon should consider the proper timing of surgery and the location of the incision depending on the condition of the skin. In situations where the skin is swollen, ecchymotic, or fragile, it is recommended to delay the surgery until the skin condition improves. In particular, special care must be taken in the case of open knee dislocation. King et al. reported that the average number of the irrigation and debridement procedure per patients was 6.6 and their patients needed to take delayed wound closure with various methods of skin graft and muscle flap in their retrospective review of seven patients with open knee dislocation [14].

Since complex regional pain syndrome can occur after various situations secondary to limb injury such as fracture, soft tissue injury, prolonged immobilization, or surgical procedure, the occurrence of complex regional pain syndrome in complex knee ligament injuries must also be considered. The incidence of complex regional pain syndrome in complex knee ligament injuries has not yet been known. However, complex regional pain syndrome should be taken care of during treatment process because it can decelerate recovery as it causes disproportionate pain, periarticular swelling of the knee, and soft tissue contracture.

Patients with complex knee ligament injuries are at increased risk of deep vein thrombosis or pulmonary embolism because of the complexity of the injury needing prolonged immobilization and surgical procedure. In analysis of Engebretsen et al., on 85 cases with knee dislocation, they reported that there were three patients diagnosed with deep vein thrombosis [15]. Also, Becker et al. reported that pulmonary embolism was found in 5% (5 of 102 patients) [5]. Hence, adequate evaluation of deep vein thrombosis should be performed before planned surgery, and appropriate anticoagulant treatment should be considered throughout the treatment process, especially in the setting of prolonged immobilization.

17.8 Summary

There have been several studies that have investigated surgical outcomes including complications after complex knee ligament injuries. However, these are mostly case series, and comparative study with high level of evidence has been scarce. This rarity is due to varied heterogenicity in injury mechanism of patients with complex knee ligament injuries and wide range of surgical methods to treat these patients. Also, because of significantly fewer incidences of the complex knee ligament injuries and difficulty of making a prospective study, there is still a limitation in reaching a concrete conclusion regarding management and complications in complex knee ligament injuries. Nevertheless, significant complications in practice are common after complex knee ligament injuries. It is important to accurately diagnose complex knee ligament injuries, prevent possible complications, and properly address complications.

Acknowledgment The authors would like to thank professor Tae-Hwan Yoon and clinical fellows (Kwangho Chung, Jinyoung Jang, Hyun-Soo Moon, Chan-Myoung Woo) for their support in writing this chapter.

References

1. Tay AK, MacDonald PB. Complications associated with treatment of multiple ligament injured (dislocated) knee. Sports Med Arthrosc Rev. 2011;19:153–61.
2. Fanelli GC, Stannard JP, Stuart MJ, et al. Management of complex knee ligament injuries. J Bone Joint Surg Am. 2010;92:2235–46.
3. Plancher KD, Siliski J. Long-term functional results and complications in patients with knee dislocations. J Knee Surg. 2008;21:261–8.
4. Harner CD, Waltrip RL, Bennett CH, Francis KA, Cole B, Irrgang JJ. Surgical management of knee dislocations. JBJS. 2004;86:262–73.
5. Becker EH, Watson JD, Dreese JC. Investigation of multiligamentous knee injury patterns with associated injuries presenting at a level I trauma center. J Orthop Trauma. 2013;27:226–31.
6. Woodmass JM, O'Malley MP, Krych AJ, et al. Revision multiligament knee reconstruction: clinical outcomes and proposed treatment algorithm. Arthroscopy. 2018;34:736–744.e733.
7. Stannard J, Schenck RC Jr, Fanelli G. Knee dislocations and fracture-dislocations. In: Bucholz RW, Heckman JD, Court-Brown CM, Tornetta P, editors. Rockwood and green's fractures in adults. 7th ed. Philadelphia: Lippincott Williams & Wilkins; 2009. p. 1832–66.
8. Levy BA, Krych AJ, Shah JP, Morgan JA, Stuart MJ. Staged protocol for initial management of the dislocated knee. Knee Surg Sports Traumatol Arthrosc. 2010;18:1630–7.
9. Medina O, Arom GA, Yeranosian MG, Petrigliano FA, McAllister DR. Vascular and nerve injury after knee dislocation: a systematic review. Clin Orthop Relat Res. 2014;472:2621–9.
10. Johnson ME, Foster L, DeLee JC. Neurologic and vascular injuries associated with knee ligament injuries. Am J Sports Med. 2008;36:2448–62.

11. Green NE, Allen BL. Vascular injuries associated with dislocation of the knee. J Bone Joint Surg Am. 1977;59:236–9.
12. Woodmass JM, Romatowski NP, Esposito JG, Mohtadi NG, Longino PD. A systematic review of peroneal nerve palsy and recovery following traumatic knee dislocation. Knee Surg Sports Traumatol Arthrosc. 2015;23:2992–3002.
13. Kim DH, Cho Y-J, Ryu S, Tiel RL, Kline DG. Surgical management and results of 135 tibial nerve lesions at the Louisiana State University Health Sciences Center. Neurosurgery. 2003;53:1114–25.
14. King JJ 3rd, Cerynik DL, Blair JA, Harding SP, Tom JA. Surgical outcomes after traumatic open knee dislocation. Knee Surg Sports Traumatol Arthrosc. 2009;17:1027–32.
15. Engebretsen L, Risberg MA, Robertson B, Ludvigsen TC, Johansen S. Outcome after knee dislocations: a 2-9 years follow-up of 85 consecutive patients. Knee Surg Sports Traumatol Arthrosc. 2009;17:1013–26.

Future Trends in Ligament Surgery: The Role of Biology

18

Graeme P. Whyte, Ignacio Dallo, Katarzyna Herman, and Alberto Gobbi

18.1 Introduction

There have been numerous treatments developed to address ligament injury, given the functional impact of such injury on lifestyle and participation in physical activities at all levels of recreational and competitive endeavors. With regard to commonly diagnosed knee injuries, anterior cruciate ligament (ACL) insufficiency is a frequently encountered pathology that often requires surgical treatment to restore the desired level of function. Considering that ligament injuries most commonly affect active individuals who tend to be younger, such injuries can lead to substantial alterations in lifestyle, and therapeutic treatments that restore near-anatomic function of damaged ligaments have the potential to overcome some of the shortcomings associated with current methods of reconstruction, particularly in the case of ACL insufficiency. The incidence of complete injury to the posterior cruciate ligament (PCL) is considerably lower than that of the ACL and is estimated to occur at a rate of 2 per 100,000; however, the prevalence of asymptomatic PCL injury is considered to be not ably higher [1]. Injury to collateral ligaments represents a significant proportion of knee injuries that present to emergency rooms, and high rates of medial and collateral ligament injuries are associated with collegiate sporting activities, with many of these cases involving noncontact competition [2].

Despite advances in sports medicine, there remains controversy in the treatment of ligament injury, particularly when there is functional insufficiency associated with partial ligament injury. For instance, reconstruction of the ACL is the current gold standard treatment for symptomatic ACL insufficiency, irrespective of injury pattern, and high rates of return to sport are expected [3, 4]. Disadvantages of ACL reconstruction include donor site morbidity, inability to restore normal joint kinematics, and an increased incidence of premature degenerative joint changes [5–8].

There are challenges associated with restoring anatomic function in cases of ligament injury, and biologic therapies have great potential to address some of these concerns. Therapeutic interventions that utilize bioactive growth factors and cellular elements may be used to augment ligament repair processes and can be used in

G. P. Whyte
Orthopaedic Arthroscopic Surgery International (OASI) Bioresearch Foundation, Milan, Italy

Weill Medical College, Cornell University, New York, NY, USA

New York Presbyterian Hospital/Queens, New York, NY, USA

I. Dallo
Unit of Regenerative Therapy and Arthroscopic Surgery, Sanatorio Garay, Santa Fe, Argentina

K. Herman · A. Gobbi (✉)
Orthopaedic Arthroscopic Surgery International (OASI) Bioresearch Foundation, Milan, Italy
e-mail: gobbi@cartilagedoctor.it

F. Margheritini et al. (eds.), *Complex Knee Ligament Injuries*,
https://doi.org/10.1007/978-3-662-58245-9_18

conjunction with surgical treatment modalities. These biologic treatments may be a prominent feature of treatment algorithms as these technologies develop and understanding of reparative processes at the cellular level advances.

18.2 Basic Science and Anatomic Considerations of Ligament Healing and Repair

The ACL and PCL receive vascular supply from the middle genicular artery, after branching from the popliteal artery. There are synovial sheath vessels that are associated with the cruciate ligaments, as well as capsular vessels that supply the distal fibers of the PCL, which branch from the popliteal and inferior genicular arteries [9]. While the ACL and PCL both share blood supply arising from the middle genicular artery, anatomic differences in the vascular supply may impact the improved healing capacity of the PCL. Anastomosing branches of the middle genicular artery and infrapatellar fat pad are an important vascular contributor to the ACL, whereas the PCL derives a more direct arterial supply. Moreover, there is greater synovial encapsulation of the PCL.

Collateral ligaments have a greater inherent healing potential, and there are anatomic factors related to vascular supply that should be considered. Differences in the healing capabilities of the ACL and MCL have been examined in animal models that have highlighted the positive impact of vascular supply on the healing potential of these ligaments [10]. There are multiple branching vessels about the medial collateral ligament (MCL), and several vessels directly supply the ligament tissue [11, 12], whereas the vascular supply of the ACL consists of one or two branches of the middle genicular artery that course beneath the synovial sheath [12, 13]. The body of the ACL has sparse or no direct vascular supply and is relatively hypovascular, and this may be a major contributor to the reduced healing capacity of the ACL as a result of the diminished physiologic and metabolic response to injury.

There are anatomic and physiologic factors related to the intra- or extra-articular location of ligaments that impact the healing potential. Processes of cell signaling, migration, proliferation, and differentiation, as well as the proficiency of collagen production, affect the inherent capacity for ligamentous repair and regeneration. Fibrin clot formation at the site of ligament injury sequesters reparative cells and provides a microenvironment that favors healing and repair. Due to the intra-articular position of the ACL, the process of fibrin clot formation is deficient, and tissue repair processes are impaired. Moreover, circulating plasmin within the intra-articular space can inhibit fibrin clot formation, and synovial fluid may inhibit fibroblast proliferation and migration [14, 15].

18.3 Growth Factors and Platelet-Rich Plasma (PRP) in Ligament Repair

Numerous bioactive substances coordinate the complex processes of cellular regenerative activation and response after tendon injury [16]. Certain growth factors are capable of directing cellular proliferation, migration, and differentiation while also enhancing collagen production. Bioactive growth factors are upregulated in response to ligament and tendon injury and act at several phases of the regenerative cascade, of which transforming growth factor beta (TGF-β), insulin-like growth factor-1 (IGF-1), basic fibroblast growth factor (bFGF), bone morphogenetic protein (BMP), and vascular endothelial growth factor (VEGF) have been shown to have particularly considerable contributions to processes critical to ligament healing [17–20]. PDGF could also play a significant role in the early stages of healing as the application of PDGF-BB has been shown to improve the structural composition of rabbit and rat ligaments [21, 22].

Platelet-rich plasma is generally defined as an isolate of plasma that has a concentration of platelets above the baseline concentration in whole blood. Autologous PRP can be prepared after venous blood extraction using a variety of commercially available preparation systems. Within platelets, there are important regulatory bioactive factors that coordinate processes of ligament repair, including cellular proliferation, chemotaxis, differentiation, and deposition of extracellular matrix. Applying PRP to a site of tissue injury is performed to provide a concentrated release of platelet-derived growth factors to stimulate and augment reparative processes. There is variability in the protocols used for PRP preparation, and there is debate as to the ideal constituency. Plasma isolates can generally be categorized as platelet-poor plasma (PPP) or platelet-rich plasma (PRP). PRP can then be further categorized as either leucocyte-poor platelet-rich plasma (LP-PRP) or leucocyte-rich platelet-rich plasma (L-PRP) [23]. When PRP is applied to injured tissue, thrombin or intra-articular collagen will activate the platelets, leading to sustained release of regenerative growth factors capable of augmenting repair processes. A variety of biologic growth factor preparations have been studied to treat ligament and tendon injury, and these treatments are being increasingly utilized in the clinical setting [24, 25].

The application of growth factors contained within platelets has been studied in several animal models. TGF-β1, bone morphogenetic protein 2 (BMP2), and growth differentiation factor 5 (GDF5) have shown increased collagen synthesis and healing in response to ligament injury [26, 27]. There continues to be contrasting findings in the literature related to the use of growth factors in ACL repair. The application of basic fibroblast growth factor (bFGF) has shown enhanced vascularity and ligament healing in cases of canine ACL injury [28], whereas other research examining the use of PRP for ACL injury in animal models has failed to demonstrate superior ligament repair. In examining the clinical use of growth factors to treat ligament injury in humans, preliminary research has demonstrated that the use of such therapy in partial ACL injury may enable high rates of return to pre-injury activity levels. There is, however, inconsistency in the literature, and there may be important differences in the expected outcome of biologic treatments depending on the concentration of bioactive factors, the type of ligament treated, and also the specific injury pattern. Recent work by LaPrade et al. [29] examined the use of PRP to treat complete MCL disruption in a rabbit model. While treatment with a PRP isolate of two times the baseline platelet concentration did not improve healing, it was actually found that treatment with a PRP isolate containing four times the baseline platelet concentration negatively impacted the quality of repair tissue compared to controls.

18.4 Cellular Therapy in Ligament Repair

Mesenchymal stem cells (MSCs) are multipotent cells that have an inherent self-renewal capability and contain a large assortment of growth factors that direct regenerative processes. These cells can be isolated from a number of readily accessible tissues that include the bone marrow and fat tissue [30] (Fig. 18.1). There has been increasing interest in the clinical use of such cells in recent

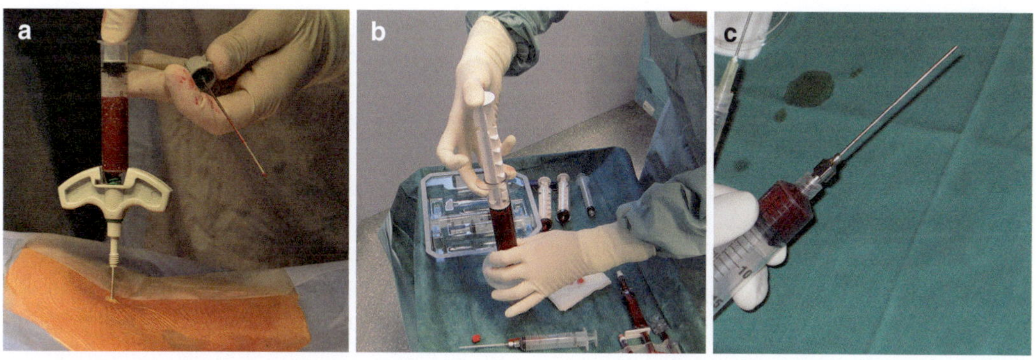

Fig. 18.1 Bone marrow aspiration from the iliac crest (**a**). Processing of bone marrow aspirate in a commercially available system to isolate bone marrow aspirate concentrate (**b**). Final preparation of bone marrow aspirate concentrate (BMAC) for clinical application (**c**)

years due to the wide range of potential therapeutic applications [31, 32]. These multipotent cellular isolates have been used successfully to restore healthy and functional tissues for a variety of pathologies, including challenging cases of high-grade articular cartilage injury [33–35]. Therapies that utilize MSCs have the capacity to coordinate regenerative processes at the molecular level, and there are similar cellular characteristics with ligament outgrowth cells that are important for ligament repair [6, 36]. Intra-articular injection therapy of multipotent cells sourced from bone marrow aspirate concentrate to treat ligament injury has demonstrated improvement in tissue integrity according to MRI examination [37].

18.5 Scaffolds and Cell-Scaffold Composites in Ligament Repair

Scaffolds may be used to provide structural biomechanical support to healing ligamentous tissue and to contain concentrations of endogenous cells, while extracellular matrix is deposited and remodeled, thereby contributing to stability of the repair and optimizing the local regenerative microenvironment. Scaffolds may be used to facilitate cellular proliferation and differentiation and can encourage growth factor attachment while promoting extracellular matrix production and remodeling into ligament repair tissue [38].

Combining cellular isolates with biologic scaffolding has demonstrated promising clinical utility in the treatment of chondral and osteochondral lesions [39–42], and there are great potential advantages for this treatment in cases of ligament injury. Biologics such as PRP and MSC preparations contain regenerative growth factors and cellular elements important for ligament repair, and combining these bioactive isolates with scaffolding can provide a supportive matrix to facilitate cellular processes while also providing biomechanical support to the destabilized injured tissue. Moreover, when undertaking primary repair of injured ligament tissue, such scaffolding can act to protect the repair site from the effects of plasmin, thereby stabilizing the microenvironment for tissue regeneration to proceed. Randomized controlled trials are needed to further study the extent of expected clinical benefits of such techniques, as there has been limited critical evaluation of outcomes in human trials.

18.6 Surgical Techniques of Ligament Repair

There continues to be debate among clinicians regarding treatment of ligament injuries, particularly in cases of partial tears that are associated with instability. Noyes et al. determined that conservative treatment of partial ACL injury would lead to complete ACL insufficiency in 50% of those treated where more than 50% of the ligament was injured [43].

Historical data indicates that surgical repair of the ACL leads to a failure rate that is excessively high for this method to be considered a preferential treatment [44, 45]. Short-term follow-up in a military cohort of patients by Feagin demonstrated good outcomes; however, 94% of these cases suffered from knee instability 5 years postoperatively [46]. There have been cohorts of patients treated with primary ACL repair that have had successful outcomes and maintained knee stability long-term [45], and so it is thought that a subset of injury types could benefit from a primary repair procedure, when properly indicated.

Reconstruction of the ACL is widely considered the gold standard surgical treatment to restore stability and enable return to physical activity in cases of complete or partial ligament instability that is associated with functional limitation [3, 4]. Reconstruction of the ACL is associated with a number of complications that include donor site morbidity, altered proprioception, bone tunnel widening, the inability to replicate anatomic joint kinematics, and degenerative changes to the articular cartilage [6–8]. With reconstructive methods, the incorporation of the graft is typically slow due to the hypovascular and hypocellular characteristics of the graft tissue [47].

18.6.1 Biologic Augmentation of Surgical Ligament Repair

Regeneration of the ACL and restored stability after primary repair procedures that have been augmented by biologic growth factors and cellular therapy has been demonstrated [48–52]. Augmenting the healing processes of ligament repair with multipotent cellular elements provides an array of regenerative growth factors to support healing processes. Early methods of providing such augmentation have been described by Steadman and involved releasing marrow elements from the bone marrow to assist with ligament repair [51, 53]. Phenotypically, these cells are capable of great plasticity, and several methods have been developed to strategically isolate and proliferate cell lines with these capabilities to treat a growing number of musculoskeletal disorders, including ligament injury. These regenerative cells can be readily isolated from tissues such as bone, synovium, fat, muscle, connective tissue, and skin.

Our center has used bone marrow stimulation to augment primary repair for certain injury patterns of the ACL and PCL for over a decade [54–56] and has demonstrated in clinical series that partial tears of the ACL can successfully be treated by primary repair with biologic augmentation, in lesions that are indicated appropriately [48, 57]. The most recent clinical outcomes after long-term follow-up of up to a 14-year duration in a series of patients who underwent treatment of symptomatic partial ACL injury with primary ligament repair with biologic augmentation demonstrated good to excellent outcomes and restored knee stability, and these benefits were maintained at a high rate over the course of follow-up.

18.6.2 Preferred Technique of Primary ACL or PCL Repair with Biologic Augmentation

Patient positioning and perioperative setup are performed according to surgeon preference for ligament reconstruction. In cases where bone marrow aspirate concentrate (BMAC) will be isolated to provide biologic augmentation, the ipsilateral iliac crest is included in the prepared surgical field. Examination under anesthesia of the operative knee and diagnostic arthroscopy are performed to determine the degree of ligamentous instability and to identify associated lesions that are treated concurrently. Partial ligament tears are visualized and probed while varying the degree of knee flexion and with the knee aligned in a figure-of-4 position. Jerk and Lachman tests are also performed during diagnostic arthroscopy to supplement the examination of ligament sufficiency. To repair the torn ligament fibers, PDS no. 1 suture is passed through fibers of the distal stump followed by fibers of the proximal stump using a standard clever hook or other suture passing devices. Two or three sutures are typically passed, and a Duncan loop is tied to reapproximate the injured ligament tissue, thereby restoring continuity and eliminating gapping between injured fibers (Fig. 18.2a).

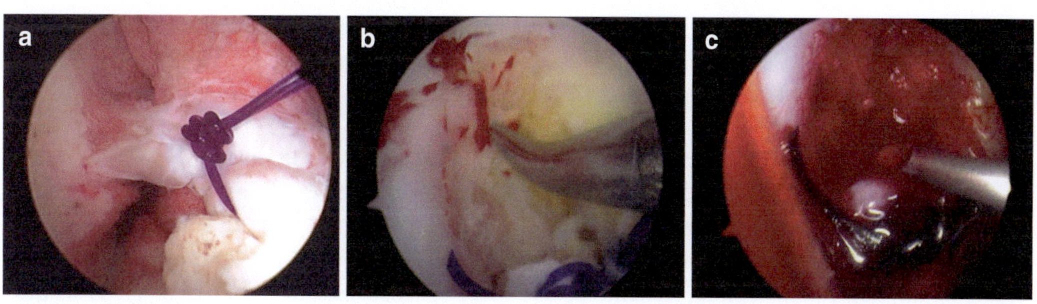

Fig. 18.2 Partial anterior cruciate ligament (ACL) arthroscopic suture repair of torn anteromedial bundle (**a**). Microfracture of intercondylar notch to release marrow elements about the repair site (**b**). Biologic augmentation of primary ACL repair with clot-activated bone marrow aspirate concentrate (**c**)

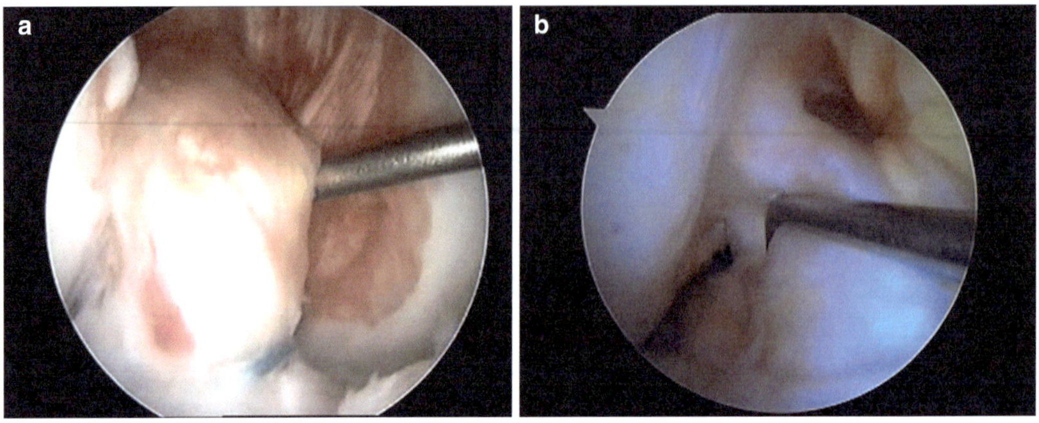

Fig. 18.3 Second-look arthroscopic examinations of healed anterior cruciate ligaments after treatment by primary repair and biologic augmentation depicted 4 months postoperatively (**a**) and 6 months postoperatively (**b**)

Bone marrow elements are then released by performing microfracture perforations within the intercondylar notch about the anatomic origin of the injured ligament (Fig. 18.2b). Careful examination of remaining tissue about the footprint ensures that residual ligament fibers are protected while performing marrow stimulation. The available reparative biologic factors are then supplemented with PRP or BMAC. The chosen biologic is isolated using a commercial system and is then activated with batroxobin enzyme or autologous thrombin to create an adhesive biologic gel. Intra-articular fluid is removed to provide a working space for dry arthroscopy. The biologic gel is then applied over and about the ligament, further enhancing the regenerative microenvironment and minimizing the effects of plasmin at the repair site (Fig. 18.2c). Second-look arthroscopic examination of primary ACL repair with biologic augmentation is depicted in Fig. 18.3.

18.6.3 Postoperative Rehabilitation

Mechanical stimulation is an important consideration during rehabilitation and physical therapy. Mechanotransduction provides stimuli to the cellular elements that act synergistically with this surgical repair technique. Bracing is used initially postoperatively, with continuous passive motion and weight bearing recommended early in the rehabilitation. Running activities are usually allowed 3 months postoperatively, with more intense activities and contact sports avoided until at least 4 to 5 months, depending on the extent of ligament repair and the rehabilitation progression.

18.7 Conclusion

The understanding of tissue healing processes is progressing at a rapid pace, and there has been increasing interest in treatments that are capable of retaining functional ligament tissue and optimizing the regenerative environment, particularly in cases of partial ligament injury. There are several important advantages of therapies that restore native ligament anatomy, with restoration of anatomic joint kinematics being of crucial importance. A number of biologic isolates have been developed for clinical application that have the potential to enhance ligament repair by providing growth factors and cellular elements, and there is also continued development of biologic scaffolding that can be used in conjunction with biologics to sequester a regenerative microenvironment. There has been an acceleration in the publication of literature that examines the clinical outcomes of ligament repair procedures over recent time. In the case of ACL insufficiency, initial findings have been most supportive of primary repair and biologic augmentation in the setting of acute, partial, and proximal ligament injury. This ongoing work will have great clinical importance in the identification and characterization of specific injury patterns that would benefit most from these regenerative treatments.

References

1. Sanders TL, Pareek A, Barrett IJ, Kremers HM, Bryan AJ, Stuart MJ, Levy BA, Krych AJ. Incidence and long-term follow-up of isolated posterior cruciate ligament tears. Knee Surg, Sport Traumatol Arthrosc. 2017;25:3017–23.
2. Yawn BP, Amadio P, Harmsen WS, Hill J, Ilstrup D, Gabriel S. Isolated acute knee injuries in the general population. J Trauma. 2000;48:716–23.
3. Gobbi A, Francisco R. Factors affecting return to sports after anterior cruciate ligament reconstruction with patellar tendon and hamstring graft: a prospective clinical investigation. Knee Surg Sports Traumatol Arthrosc. 2006;14:1021–8.
4. Gobbi A, Mahajan V, Karnatzikos G, Nakamura N. Single- versus double-bundle ACL reconstruction: is there any difference in stability and function at 3-year followup? Clin Orthop Relat Res. 2012;470:824–34.
5. Cohen M, Amaro JT, Ejnisman B, Carvalho RT, Nakano KK, Peccin MS, Teixeira R, Laurino CFS, Abdalla RJ. Anterior cruciate ligament reconstruction after 10 to 15 years: association between meniscectomy and osteoarthrosis. Arthroscopy. 2007;23:629–34.
6. Gobbi A, Domzalski M, Pascual J, Zanazzo M. Hamstring anterior cruciate ligament reconstruction: is it necessary to sacrifice the gracilis? Arthroscopy. 2005;21:275–80.
7. Kartus J, Movin T, Karlsson J. Donor-site morbidity and anterior knee problems after anterior cruciate ligament reconstruction using autografts. Arthroscopy. 2001;17:971–80.
8. Lohmander LS, Englund PM, Dahl LL, Roos EM. The long-term consequence of anterior cruciate ligament and meniscus injuries: osteoarthritis. Am J Sports Med. 2007;35:1756–69.
9. Vladimirov B. Arterial sources of blood supply of the knee-joint in man. Nauchni Tr Vissh Med Inst Sofiia. 1968;47:1–10.
10. Bray RC, Leonard CA, Salo PT. Vascular physiology and long-term healing of partial ligament tears. J Orthop Res. 2002;20:984–9.
11. Bray RC, Fisher AW, Frank CB. Fine vascular anatomy of adult rabbit knee ligaments. J Anat. 1990;172:69–79.
12. Wallace CD, Amiel D. Vascular assessment of the periarticular ligaments of the rabbit knee. J Orthop Res. 1991;9:787–91.
13. Arnoczky SP. Blood supply to the anterior cruciate ligament and supporting structures. Orthop Clin North Am. 1985;16:15–28.
14. Andrish J, Holmes R. Effects of synovial fluid on fibroblasts in tissue culture. Clin Orthop Relat Res. 1979:279–83.
15. Rość D, Powierza W, Zastawna E, Drewniak W, Michalski A, Kotschy M. Post-traumatic plasminogenesis in intraarticular exudate in the knee joint. Med Sci Monit. 2002;8:CR371–8.
16. Andia I, Sanchez M, Maffulli N. Tendon healing and platelet-rich plasma therapies. Expert Opin Biol Ther. 2010;10:1415–26.
17. Chen CH, Cao Y, Wu YF, Bais AJ, Gao JS, Tang JB. Tendon healing in vivo: gene expression and production of multiple growth factors in early tendon healing period. J Hand Surg Am. 2008;33:1834–42.
18. Kobayashi M, Itoi E, Minagawa H, Miyakoshi N, Takahashi S, Tuoheti Y, Okada K, Shimada Y. Expression of growth factors in the early phase of supraspinatus tendon healing in rabbits. J Shoulder Elb Surg. 2006;15:371–7.
19. Molloy T, Wang Y, Murrell G. The roles of growth factors in tendon and ligament healing. Sports Med. 2003;33:381–94.
20. Würgler-Hauri CC, Dourte LM, Baradet TC, Williams GR, Soslowsky LJ. Temporal expression of 8 growth factors in tendon-to-bone healing in a rat supraspinatus model. J Shoulder Elb Surg. 2007;16:S198–203.
21. Batten ML, Hansen JC, Dahners LE. Influence of dosage and timing of application of platelet-derived growth factor on early healing of the rat medial collateral ligament. J Orthop Res. 1996;14:736–41.
22. Lee J, Harwood FL, Akeson WH, Amiel D. Growth factor expression in healing rabbit medial collateral and anterior cruciate ligaments. Iowa Orthop J. 1998;18:19–25.
23. Dohan Ehrenfest DM, Rasmusson L, Albrektsson T. Classification of platelet concentrates: from pure platelet-rich plasma (P-PRP) to leucocyte- and platelet-rich fibrin (L-PRF). Trends Biotechnol. 2009;27:158–67.
24. Gobbi A, Whyte GP. Emerging orthobiologic approaches to ligament injury. In: Bio-orthopaedics. Berlin, Heidelberg: Springer; 2017. p. 313–24.
25. Whyte GP, Gobbi A, Lane JG (2018) The role of orthobiologics in return to play. Return to play in football Springer, Berlin, Heidelberg, pp 273–282.
26. Aspenberg P, Forslund C. Enhanced tendon healing with GDF 5 and 6. Acta Orthop Scand. 1999;70:51–4.
27. Marui T, Niyibizi C, Georgescu HI, Cao M, Kavalkovich KW, Levine RE, Woo SL. Effect of growth factors on matrix synthesis by ligament fibroblasts. J Orthop Res. 1997;15:18–23.
28. Kobayashi D, Kurosaka M, Yoshiya S, Mizuno K. Effect of basic fibroblast growth factor on the healing of defects in the canine anterior cruciate

ligament. Knee Surg Sports Traumatol Arthrosc. 1997;5:189–94.
29. LaPrade RF, Goodrich LR, Phillips J, Dornan GJ, Turnbull TL, Hawes ML, Dahl KD, Coggins AN, Kisiday J, Frisbie D, Chahla J. Use of platelet-rich plasma immediately after an injury did not improve ligament healing, and increasing platelet concentrations was detrimental in an in vivo animal model. Am J Sport Med. 2018;46:702–12.
30. Gobbi A, de Girolamo L, Whyte GP, Sciarretta FV. Clinical applications of adipose tissue-derived stem cells. In: Bio-orthopaedics. Berlin, Heidelberg: Springer; 2017. p. 553–9.
31. Gobbi A, Karnatzikos G, Scotti C, Mahajan V, Mazzucco L, Grigolo B. One-step cartilage repair with bone marrow aspirate concentrated cells and collagen matrix in full-thickness knee cartilage lesions: results at 2-year follow-up. Cartilage. 2011;2:286–99.
32. Gobbi A, Scotti C, Karnatzikos G, Mudhigere A, Castro M, Peretti GM. One-step surgery with multipotent stem cells and Hyaluronan-based scaffold for the treatment of full-thickness chondral defects of the knee in patients older than 45 years. Knee Surg Sports Traumatol Arthrosc. 2017;25:2494–501.
33. Gobbi A, Espregueira-Mendes J, Karahan M, Cohen M, Whyte GP. Osteochondritis dissecans of the knee in football players. In: Injuries and health problems in football. Berlin, Heidelberg: Springer; 2017. p. 189–200.
34. Gobbi A, Whyte GP. Osteochondritis dissecans: pathoanatomy, classification, and advances in biologic surgical treatment. In: Bio-orthopaedics. Berlin, Heidelberg: Springer; 2017. p. 489–501.
35. Whyte GP, Gobbi A. Biologic knee Arthroplasty for cartilage injury and early osteoarthritis. In: Bio-orthopaedics. Berlin, Heidelberg: Springer; 2017. p. 517–25.
36. Steinert AF, Kunz M, Prager P, Barthel T, Jakob F, Nöth U, Murray MM, Evans CH, Porter RM. Mesenchymal stem cell characteristics of human anterior cruciate ligament outgrowth cells. Tissue Eng Part A. 2011;17:1375–88.
37. Centeno CJ, Pitts J, Al-Sayegh H, Freeman MD. Anterior cruciate ligament tears treated with percutaneous injection of autologous bone marrow nucleated cells: a case series. J Pain Res. 2015;8:437–47.
38. Liu Y, Ramanath HS, Wang D-A. Tendon tissue engineering using scaffold enhancing strategies. Trends Biotechnol. 2008;26:201–9.
39. Gobbi A, Whyte GP. One-stage cartilage repair using a hyaluronic acid-based scaffold with activated bone marrow-derived mesenchymal stem cells compared with microfracture: five-year follow-up. Am J Sports Med. 2016;44:2846–54.
40. Sadlik B, Gobbi A, Puszkarz M, Klon W, Whyte GP. Biologic inlay osteochondral reconstruction: arthroscopic one-step osteochondral lesion repair in the knee using morselized bone grafting and hyaluronic acid-based scaffold embedded with bone marrow aspirate concentrate. Arthrosc Tech. 2017;6:e383–9.
41. Sadlik B, Kolodziej L, Puszkarz M, Laprus H, Mojzesz M, Whyte GP. Surgical repair of osteochondral lesions of the talus using biologic inlay osteochondral reconstruction: clinical outcomes after treatment using a medial malleolar osteotomy approach compared to an arthroscopically-assisted approach. Foot Ankle Surg. 2018;
42. Whyte GP, Gobbi A, Sadlik B. Dry arthroscopic single-stage cartilage repair of the knee using a hyaluronic acid-based scaffold with activated bone marrow-derived mesenchymal stem cells. Arthrosc Tech. 2016;5:e913–8.
43. Noyes FR, Mooar LA, Moorman CT, McGinniss GH. Partial tears of the anterior cruciate ligament. Progression to complete ligament deficiency. J Bone Joint Surg Br. 1989;71:825–33.
44. Strand T, Mølster A, Hordvik M, Krukhaug Y. Long-term follow-up after primary repair of the anterior cruciate ligament: clinical and radiological evaluation 15–23 years postoperatively. Arch Orthop Trauma Surg. 2005;125:217–21.
45. Taylor DC, Posner M, Curl WW, Feagin JA. Isolated tears of the anterior cruciate ligament: over 30-year follow-up of patients treated with arthrotomy and primary repair. Am J Sports Med. 2009;37:65–71.
46. Feagin JA, Curl WW. Isolated tear of the anterior cruciate ligament: five-year follow-up study. J Orthop Sport Phys Ther. 1990;12:232–6.
47. Liu C-F, Aschbacher-Smith L, Barthelery NJ, Dyment N, Butler D, Wylie C. What we should know before using tissue engineering techniques to repair injured tendons: a developmental biology perspective. Tissue Eng Part B Rev. 2011;17:165–76.
48. Gobbi A, Bathan L, Boldrini L. Primary repair combined with bone marrow stimulation in acute anterior cruciate ligament lesions: results in a group of athletes. Am J Sports Med. 2009;37:571–8.
49. Kaplan N, Wickiewicz TL, Warren RF. Primary surgical treatment of anterior cruciate ligament ruptures. A long-term follow-up study. Am J Sports Med. 1990;18:354–8.
50. Sherman MF, Lieber L, Bonamo JR, Podesta L, Reiter I. The long-term followup of primary anterior cruciate ligament repair. Defining a rationale for augmentation. Am J Sports Med. 1991;19:243–55.
51. Steadman JR, Cameron-Donaldson ML, Briggs KK, Rodkey WG. A minimally invasive technique ("healing response") to treat proximal ACL injuries in skeletally immature athletes. J Knee Surg. 2006;19:8–13.
52. Steadman JR, Rodkey WG. Role of primary anterior cruciate ligament repair with or without augmentation. Clin Sports Med. 1993;12:685–95.
53. Steadman JR, Matheny LM, Briggs KK, Rodkey WG, Carreira DS. Outcomes following healing

response in older, active patients: a primary anterior cruciate ligament repair technique. J Knee Surg. 2012;25:255–60.
54. Gobbi A, Whyte GP. Biological augmentation in acute ACL repair. In: Bio-orthopaedics. Berlin, Heidelberg: Springer; 2017. p. 325–35.
55. Gobbi A, Whyte GP, Karnatzikos G. Acute ACL rupture: a biological approach through primary ACL repair and augmentation with bone marrow stimulation and growth factor injection. In: Controversies in the technical aspects of ACL reconstruction. Berlin, Heidelberg: Springer; 2017. p. 135–44.
56. Whyte GP, Gobbi A, Szwedowski D. Partial anterior cruciate ligament lesions: a biological approach to repair. In: Bio-orthopaedics. Berlin, Heidelberg: Springer; 2017. p. 665–70.
57. Gobbi A, Karnatzikos G, Sankineani SR, Petrera M. Biological augmentation of ACL refixation in partial lesions in a group of athletes: results at the 5-year follow-up. Tech Orthop. 2013;28:180–4.

Correction to: Acute Knee Dislocations

Conor I. Murphy, Philip P. Roessler, Tracye J. Lawyer, and Volker Musahl

Correction to:
Chapter 11 in: F. Margheritini et al. (eds.), *Complex Knee Ligament Injuries*, https://doi.org/10.1007/978-3-662-58245-9_11

Dr. Philip P. Roessler's name had been missed out in chapter 11. The authors' name has now been updated.

The updated online version of this chapter can be found at
https://doi.org/10.1007/978-3-662-58245-9_11

C. I. Murphy · P. P. Roessler · T. J. Lawyer
V. Musahl (✉)
Department of Orthopaedic Surgery, University of Pittsburgh, Pittsburgh, PA, USA
e-mail: murphyci@upmc.edu; musahlv@upmc.edu

F. Margheritini et al. (eds.), *Complex Knee Ligament Injuries*,
https://doi.org/10.1007/978-3-662-58245-9_19

MIX
Papier aus verantwortungsvollen Quellen
Paper from responsible sources
FSC® C105338

If you have any concerns about our products,
you can contact us on
ProductSafety@springernature.com

In case Publisher is established outside the EU,
the EU authorized representative is:
Springer Nature Customer Service Center GmbH
Europaplatz 3, 69115 Heidelberg, Germany

Printed by Libri Plureos GmbH
in Hamburg, Germany